MCQs in
ENDOCRINOLOGY
for DM Entrance Examination

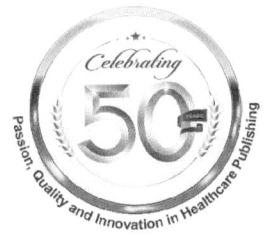

MCQs in
ENDOCRINOLOGY
for DM Entrance Examination

Amritava Ghosh
MBBS MD (General Medicine)
DM (Endocrinology)
Assistant Professor and Head
Department of Endocrinology and
Metabolism
All India Institute of Medical Sciences
Raipur, Chhattisgarh, India

Sowrabha Bhat
MBBS MD (Med)
Senior Resident
Department of Endocrinology
Institute of Postgraduate Medical
Education and Research
Kolkata, West Bengal, India

Sarita Bajaj
MD DM (Endocrinology, AIIMS) FRCP
(London, Glasgow, Edin)
Director-Professor and Head
Department of Medicine
MLN Medical College,
Allahabad, Uttar Pradesh, India

Sujoy Ghosh
DM FRCP FACE
Associate Professor
Department of Endocrinology
Institute of Postgraduate Medical
Education and Research
Kolkata, West Bengal, India

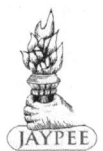

JAYPEE BROTHERS MEDICAL PUBLISHERS
The Health Sciences Publisher
New Delhi | London | Panama

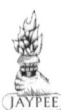 **Jaypee Brothers Medical Publishers (P) Ltd**

Headquarters
Jaypee Brothers Medical Publishers (P) Ltd
4838/24, Ansari Road, Daryaganj
New Delhi 110 002, India
Phone: +91-11-43574357
Fax: +91-11-43574314
E-mail: jaypee@jaypeebrothers.com

Overseas Offices

J P Medical Ltd
83 Victoria Street, London
SW1H 0HW (UK)
Phone: +44 20 3170 8910
Fax: +44 (0)20 3008 6180
E-mail: info@jpmedpub.com

Jaypee-Highlights Medical Publishers Inc
City of Knowledge, Bld. 235, 2nd Floor, Clayton
Panama City, Panama
Phone: +1 507-301-0496
Fax: +1 507-301-0499
E-mail: cservice@jphmedical.com

Jaypee Brothers Medical Publishers (P) Ltd
Bhotahity, Kathmandu, Nepal
Phone: +977-9741283608
E-mail: kathmandu@jaypeebrothers.com

Website: www.jaypeebrothers.com
Website: www.jaypeedigital.com

© 2019, Jaypee Brothers Medical Publishers

The views and opinions expressed in this book are solely those of the original contributor(s)/author(s) and do not necessarily represent those of editor(s) of the book.

All rights reserved. No part of this publication may be reproduced, stored or transmitted in any form or by any means, electronic, mechanical, photocopying, recording or otherwise, without the prior permission in writing of the publishers.

All brand names and product names used in this book are trade names, service marks, trademarks or registered trademarks of their respective owners. The publisher is not associated with any product or vendor mentioned in this book.

Medical knowledge and practice change constantly. This book is designed to provide accurate, authoritative information about the subject matter in question. However, readers are advised to check the most current information available on procedures included and check information from the manufacturer of each product to be administered, to verify the recommended dose, formula, method and duration of administration, adverse effects and contraindications. It is the responsibility of the practitioner to take all appropriate safety precautions. Neither the publisher nor the author(s)/editor(s) assume any liability for any injury and/or damage to persons or property arising from or related to use of material in this book.

This book is sold on the understanding that the publisher is not engaged in providing professional medical services. If such advice or services are required, the services of a competent medical professional should be sought.

Every effort has been made where necessary to contact holders of copyright to obtain permission to reproduce copyright material. If any have been inadvertently overlooked, the publisher will be pleased to make the necessary arrangements at the first opportunity. The **CD/DVD-ROM** (if any) provided in the sealed envelope with this book is complimentary and free of cost. **Not meant for sale.**

Inquiries for bulk sales may be solicited at: jaypee@jaypeebrothers.com

MCQs in Endocrinology for DM Entrance Examination

First Edition: **2019**
ISBN: 978-93-89188-25-7

Printed at Repro India Limited

Dedicated to

All future endocrinologists

Preface

The authors have attempted to produce *MCQs in Endocrinology for DM Entrance Examination*, which reflects the layout of NEET DM Endocrinology Examination MCQ paper. The book is divided into several chapters.

The questions and answers are both well laid out, clear and easy to read through. The answers are well written and concise. There are a number of useful diagrams or tables included with some of the answers to explain particular topics in further details. Each set of answers relative to a particular question stem includes a reference, if further reading is required. The various textbooks referred to are all widely available to trainees.

The standard and difficulty of the questions are a reasonable reflection of that found in an actual examination paper. Some emphasis is given to particular areas. The same emphasis is likely to be seen by a candidate in an actual MCQ paper.

A sound knowledge base is a prerequisite to crack the entrance examination.

Like most MCQ-based books, the book, *MCQs in Endocrinology for DM Entrance Examination*, is of a size that allows a trainee to carry it with him/her during a normal working day and easily make use of a spare half an hour. It will certainly go a long way in helping them with that necessary practice.

Amritava Ghosh
Sowrabha Bhat
Sarita Bajaj
Sujoy Ghosh

Acknowledgments

The authors are grateful to all those students who appeared in various DM Endocrinology Entrance Examinations, and did their best to try and recollect the questions and helped us to collate the same for this book. Special thanks to Dr Manoj Kataria and Dr Deep Dutta for their help. We wish to also thank Dr Arijit Singha (aspiring candidate for DM Entrance Examinations) for having reviewed the questions/proof. Finally, we wish to thank Mr Pradip Mondal who helped us to type out the first draft of the manuscript.

We greatly value and appreciate the cooperative work of the staff of M/s Jaypee Brothers Medical Publishers (P) Ltd, New Delhi, India, for their assistance, thoroughness, patience and professional work. We are thankful to Shri Jitendar P Vij (Group Chairman), Mr Ankit Vij (Managing Director), Ms Chetna Malhotra Vohra (Associate Director—Content Strategy), and Ms Prerna Bajaj (Development Editor) of M/s Jaypee Brothers Medical Publishers (P) Ltd, New Delhi, India, for giving a go-ahead at the very beginning and helping us in every way possible to bring out this book.

Contents

1. Principles of Hormone Action 1
2. Genetics of Endocrinology 17
3. Laboratory Techniques for Recognition of Endocrine Disorders 23
4. Neuroendocrinology 27
5. Pituitary Physiology and Diagnostic Evaluation 34
6. Pituitary Masses and Tumors 50
7. Posterior Pituitary 65
8. Thyroid 77
9. Adrenal Cortex 106
10. Endocrine Hypertension 125
11. Female Reproductive Axis 142
12. Testicular Disorders 164
13. Multiple Endocrine Neoplasia 177
14. Endocrine Changes in Pregnancy 180
15. Endocrinology of Fetal Development 185
16. Pediatric Disorders of Sexual Development 189
17. Normal and Aberrant Growth 202
18. Puberty 213
19. Mineral Metabolism 226

20. **Kidney Stones** 247

21. **Diabetes** 250

22. **Hypoglycemia** 274

23. **Obesity** 287

24. **Disorders of Lipid Metabolism** 293

25. **Statistics** 301

CHAPTER 1

Principles of Hormone Action

QUESTIONS

1. **Peptide hormones:**
   a. Oxytocin-Vasopressin-Somatostatin
   b. Oxytocin-Vasopressin-Epinephrine
   c. Oxytocin-Vasopressin-Thyroxine
   d. Testosterone-Vasopressin-Oxytocin

2. **All use second messengers except:**
   a. Calcitriol
   b. Catecholamines
   c. Glycoproteins
   d. Pituitary hormones

3. **Steroid receptors act through:**
   a. Ligand activated transcription factor
   b. Activation of the JAK-STAT pathway
   c. Heterotrimeric G proteins
   d. Stimulation of tyrosine kinases

4. **Which of the following is lipophilic?**
   a. Insulin
   b. Steroids
   c. Polypeptides
   d. Polysaccharide

5. **Glycoprotein hormones share structural homology due to:**
   a. α chain
   b. β chain
   c. γ chain
   d. δ chain

6. **Which of the following is a peptide?**
   a. Catecholamine
   b. Thyroxine
   c. TSH
   d. Estradiol

7. **RIA is used for measurement of:**
   a. Hormone
   b. Glucose
   c. Calcium
   d. Creatinine

8. Which of the following is not a polypeptide?
   a. Melatonin   b. Oxytocin
   c. Vasopressin   d. TRH

9. Orphan receptors include all except:
   a. SF-1   b. DAX-1
   c. HNF-4α   d. LXR

10. Dysfunction of GPCR is associated with all except:
    a. Severe neonatal hyperparathyroidism
    b. Precocious puberty
    c. Pseudohypoparathyroidism
    d. Nephrogenic DI

11. Nuclear receptor for all except:
    a. Inhibin   b. Aldosterone
    c. T4   d. Vit-D

12. Lipophilic hormone is:
    a. Calcitonin   b. Calcitriol
    c. hCG   d. CRH

13. Immunomodulators- all except:
    a. Prolactin   b. Steroid
    c. Vit-D   d. FSH

14. Orphan receptor:
    a. Exact site not yet located
    b. No definite binders
    c. Exact action not defined
    d. Structure not known

15. Not a second messenger:
    a. ATP   b. cAMP
    c. Tyrosine kinase d. Ca^{++}

16. Glucocorticoid acts on:
    a. Cell membrane   b. Nucleus
    c. Nuclear membrane d. Cytoplasm

17. Post-translational events in hormone secretion include all except:
    a. Phosphorylation   b. Polypeptide folding
    c. Prohormone → hormone d. mRNA

18. Which of the following is not an orphan receptor?
    a. HNF4α   b. SF1
    c. DAX1   d. Androgen receptor

19. GPCR all except:
    a. ACTH   b. TSH
    c. CaSR   d. Insulin

20. **GPCR all except:**
    a. ACTH
    b. PTH
    c. GH
    d. Glucagon

21. **Which of the following is least likely to have ectopic production?**
    a. Insulin
    b. Thyroid hormone
    c. GH
    d. Cortisol

22. **Prohormone converting enzyme:**
    a. Proinsulin to insulin
    b. T4 -> T3
    c. Androgen to estrogen
    d. Cortisol to cortisone

23. **GPCR:**
    a. LH
    b. Prolactin
    c. GH
    d. Insulin

24. **True about G protein is:**
    a. Binds to DNA
    b. Situated at membrane
    c. Intracellular
    d. Glucocorticoids act through them

25. **Not true about insulin:**
    a. Secreted as proinsulin
    b. It is a steroid
    c. Increases protein synthesis
    d. Metabolic function

26. **Nuclear receptor:**
    a. AVP
    b. PTH
    c. Ca
    d. VDR
    e. GnRH

27. **Action of thyroid hormone involves all except:**
    a. TR
    b. RXR
    c. CoA
    d. CoR
    e. HRE

28. **Each of the following hormones is an amino acid derivative except:**
    a. Epinephrine
    b. Melatonin
    c. Thyroxine (T4)
    d. Thyroid stimulating hormone (TSH)
    e. Norepinephrine

29. **When adenyl cyclase is activated?**
    a. cAMP is formed
    b. cAMP is broken
    c. G-proteins bind to cAMP
    d. Steroid hormones enter the cell

30. Which of the following hormones does not act by a second messenger system?
    a. Glucagon
    b. Epinephrine
    c. Growth hormone
    d. Testosterone
    e. ACTH

31. The action of glucocorticoids involves many functions, but only one of the following is a correct one:
    a. Increases inflammatory responses
    b. Decreases lipid hydrolysis (lipolysis)
    c. Increases glucose levels
    d. Retention of electrolytes by the kidneys
    e. Increases osteoclast activity

32. This hormone acts on the intestines and causes increased calcium absorption:
    a. Calcitonin
    b. Calcitriol
    c. Thyroxine
    d. Pancreatic polypeptide
    e. Corticotropin releasing factor (CRF)

33. Thyroid stimulating hormone (TSH) causes all of the following except:
    a. Activation of thyroid follicular cells
    b. Increased iodide trapping in thyroid follicles
    c. Increased thyroglobulin synthesis
    d. Increased release of T3/T4
    e. All of the above are correct

34. Which of the following characteristics is the same for the nervous and endocrine systems?
    a. Target cells affected
    b. Time to onset of actions
    c. Duration of actions
    d. Mechanism of signaling and communication
    e. None of the above

35. Which one of the following G-protein-coupled receptor does not match with the clinical conditions associated with their receptor mutations?
    a. Inactivating mutation of melanocortin-4 receptor leads to obesity in childhood
    b. Inactivating mutation of LH receptor in males lead to Leydig cell hypoplasia
    c. Activating mutation of calcium-sensing receptor associated with autosomal-dominant hypercalciuric hypocalcemia
    d. Inactivation mutation of GnRH receptor leads to isolated hypogonadotropic hypogonadism
    e. Activation mutation of TSH receptor associated with non-autoimmune hypothyroidism

36. **Prolactin acts by one of the following receptor:**
    a. G protein coupled receptor
    b. Intracellular receptor
    c. JAK-STAT receptor
    d. Ion channel

37. **All of the following are examples of nuclear receptor except:**
    a. Bile acid receptor
    b. Liver X receptor
    c. Progesterone receptor
    d. Adrenergic receptor

38. **In absence of their ligand, which of the following nuclear receptors normally resides in cytoplasm?**
    a. Glucocorticoid receptor
    b. Vitamin D receptor
    c. Thyroid hormone receptor
    d. Mineralocorticoid receptor

39. **Which of the following is not a GPCR?**
    a. LH receptor
    b. VIP receptor
    c. PPAR
    d. Calcium sensing receptor

ANSWERS

1. **Ans. (a) Oxytocin-Vasopressin-Somatostatin**
   [Williams 13th ed pg 18, 19, 20, 123, 129, 137, 145, 152, 183, 188, 199, 207, 301, 492, 494, 595, 606, 704, 1256, 1267, 1269, 1270, 1703-1714; Clinical Chemistry, Immunology and Laboratory Quality Control: A Comprehensive Review for Board Preparation, Certification and Clinical Practice, pg 149]

   Hormones vary widely in terms of their chemical composition. These include:
   - Peptides/Proteins
     - Thyrotropin-releasing hormone (TRH) (3 amino acids)
     - Corticotropin-releasing hormone (CRH) (41 amino acids)
     - Growth hormone–releasing hormone (GHRH) (2 forms-44 amino acids and 40 amino acids)
     - Somatostatin (2 forms-14 amino acids and 28 amino acids)
     - Gonadotropin-releasing hormone (GnRH) (10 amino acids)
     - Prolactin (199 amino acids)
     - Growth hormone (GH) (191 amino acids)
     - Adrenocorticotropic hormone or corticotrophin (ACTH) (39 amino acids)
     - LH, FSH, TSH, hCG (heterodimeric glycoproteins; common α subunit, and unique β subunit; α subunit- 92 amino acids; LHβ subunit- 121 amino acids; FSHβ- 117 amino acids; hCGβ subunit- 145 amino acids; TSHβ subunit- 112 amino acids
     - Vasopressin or antidiuretic hormone (ADH) (9 amino acids)
     - Oxytocin (9 amino acids)
     - Parathyroid hormone (PTH) (84 amino acids)
     - Calcitonin (32 amino acids)
     - Pancreatic and gut hormones (e.g. Insulin- 51 amino acids; Glucagon- 29 amino acids)
     - Inhibin
   - Amino acid derivatives
     - Thyroid hormones: Triiodothyronine (T3), Tetraiodothyronine or Thyroxine (T4)
     - Monoamines: Dopamine, norepinephrine or noradrenaline, epinephrine or adrenaline, serotonin, melatonin
   - Vitamin derivative
     - $1,25(OH)_2D_3$
   - Steroids
     - Adrenal steroids (Mineralocorticoids, e.g. Deoxycorticosterone, aldosterone; Glucocorticoids, e.g. Cortisol, corticosterone; Androgens, e.g. Dehydroepiandrosterone, androstenedione)
     - Gonadal steroids (Ovary, e.g. Progesterone, estradiol; Testes, e.g. Testosterone)
   - Eicosanoids
     - Prostaglandins (e.g. PGA1, PGA2, PGE2)

2. **Ans. (a) Calcitriol**
   [Williams 13th ed pg 18, 19, 37]
   Hormones can be divided into two groups
   1. Hormones that act through cell surface receptors, e.g. polypeptide hormones, monoamines, and prostaglandins. See discussion of Chapter 1, Question 1.
   2. Hormones that act through nuclear receptors, e.g. thyroid hormones, steroid hormones, $1,25(OH)_2D_3$.

   In case of hormones acting through cell surface receptors, second messengers, which are soluble, intracellular signaling molecules generated by hormone-receptor association, are responsible for translating the extracellular signal into an intracellular response.

3. **Ans. (a) Ligand activated transcription factor**
   [Harrison's Endocrinology 3rd ed pg 6, 7]

   Nuclear Receptors
   - Nuclear receptors may be located in
     - Cytoplasm (e.g. glucocorticoid receptor)—translocate to the nucleus after ligand binding.
     - Nucleus (e.g. thyroid hormone receptor).
   - Nuclear receptors ultimately act to increase or decrease gene transcription
   - Structures of nuclear receptors:
     - The DNA-binding domain, consisting of two zinc fingers, contacts specific DNA recognition sequences in target genes.
       Most nuclear receptors bind to DNA as dimers:
       - Homodimers—e.g. steroid receptors (glucocorticoid, estrogen, progesterone, and androgen receptors)
       - Heterodimers—in combination with retinoid X receptors (RXRs); e.g. thyroid, retinoid, peroxisome proliferator-activated, and vitamin D receptors
     - The carboxy-terminal hormone-binding domain mediates transcriptional control.
     - For type 2 receptors, e.g. TR and retinoic acid receptor (RAR), co-repressor proteins bind to the receptor in the absence of ligand and silence gene transcription. Hormone binding induces conformational changes, triggering the release of co-repressors and inducing the recruitment of coactivators that stimulate transcription.
     - Most type 1 steroid receptors interact weakly with co-repressors, but ligand binding induces interactions with coactivators.
   - The receptor-coactivator complex stimulates gene transcription by several pathways, including
     1. Recruitment of enzymes (histone acetyl transferases) that modify chromatin structure
     2. Interactions with additional transcription factors on the target gene, and

3. Direct interactions with components of the general transcription apparatus to enhance the rate of RNA polymerase II–mediated transcription.

4. **Ans. (b) Steroids**
   [Harrison's Endocrinology 3rd ed pg 2; Williams 13th ed pg 5]
   Steroids, thyroid hormones, vitamin D, and retinoids are lipid-soluble (interact with intracellular nuclear receptors). Such molecules are bound to 50- to 60-kDa carrier plasma glycoproteins such as thyroxine-binding globulin (TBG), sex hormone-binding globulin (SHBG), and corticosteroid binding globulin (CBG) as well as to albumin.
   Protein hormones and some small molecules, such as the catecholamines are water-soluble. They are readily transported via the circulatory system.
   See discussion of Chapter 1, Question 1.

5. **Ans. (a) α chain**
   [Williams 13th ed pg 204, 212]
   The four heterodimeric glycoprotein hormones—LH, FSH, TSH, and hCG—share structural homology. The α-subunit is common to TSH, LH, FSH, and hCG, whereas the β-subunit is unique and confers specificity of action.

6. **Ans. (c) TSH**
   [Williams 13th ed pg 18, 19, 20, 123, 129, 137, 145, 152, 183, 188, 199, 207, 301, 492, 494, 595, 606, 704, 1256, 1267, 1269, 1270, 1703-1714; Clinical Chemistry, Immunology and Laboratory Quality Control: A Comprehensive Review for Board Preparation, Certification and Clinical Practice, pg 149]
   See discussion of Chapter 1, Question 1.

7. **Ans. (a) Hormone**
   [Williams 13th ed pg 9]

8. **Ans. (a) Melatonin**
   [Williams 13th ed pg 18, 19, 20, 123, 129, 137, 145, 152, 183, 188, 199, 207, 301, 492, 494, 595, 606, 704, 1256, 1267, 1269, 1270, 1703-1714; Clinical Chemistry, Immunology and Laboratory Quality Control: A Comprehensive Review for Board Preparation, Certification and Clinical Practice, pg 149]
   See discussion of Chapter 1, Question 1.

9. **Ans. (d) LXR**
   [Williams 13th ed pg 4, 11, 38, 217, 867, 1391]
   Orphan receptors are receptors for which no clear ligand is known. Include:
   - Nuclear receptors—e.g. SF1, DAX1, HNF-4α
   - G-protein–coupled receptors—e.g. GPR161

Oxygenated derivatives of cholesterol are the ligands for liver X receptor (LXR), which regulates genes involved in cholesterol and fatty acid metabolism.

10. **Ans. (c) Pseudohypoparathyroidism**
    [Williams 12th ed pg 78; Williams 13th ed pg 10, 1297]
    See discussion of Chapter 2, Question 6.

11. **Ans. (a) Inhibin**
    [Williams 13th ed pg 18, 19, 37]
    See discussion of Chapter 1, Questions 1 and 2.

12. **Ans. (b) Calcitriol**
    [Harrison's Endocrinology 3rd ed pg 2; Williams 13th ed pg 5]
    See discussion of Chapter 1, Questions 1 and 4.

13. **Ans. (d) FSH**
    [Williams 13th ed pg 185, 505; De Groot 7th ed pg 1028]

14. **Ans. (b) No definite binders**
    [Williams 13th ed pg 11, 38, 217, 867, 1391]
    See discussion of Chapter 1, Question 9.

15. **Ans. (a) ATP**
    [Harrison's Endocrinology 3rd ed pg 2; De Groot 6th ed pg 85]

Membrane Receptor Families and Signaling Pathways

Receptors	Effectors	Signaling pathways
G Protein–Coupled Seven-Transmembrane (GPCR)		
β-Adrenergic, LH, FSH, TSH, Vasopressin V_2, Calcitonin, VIP	Gsα, adenylate cyclase	Stimulation of cyclic AMP production, protein kinase A
Glucagon, PTH, PTHrP, ACTH, MSH, GHRH, CRH	Ca^{2+} channels	Calmodulin, Ca^{2+}-dependent kinases
α-Adrenergic Somatostatin	Giα	Inhibition of cyclic AMP production; Activation of K^+, Ca^{2+} channels
TRH, GnRH, Vasopressin $V_{1a,1b}$, Calcium sensor (CaSR), Oxytocin	Gq, G11	Phospholipase C, diacylglycerol, IP3, protein kinase C, voltage-dependent Ca^{2+} channels
Receptor Tyrosine Kinase		
Insulin, IGF-I	Tyrosine kinases, IRS	MAP kinases, PI 3-kinase; AKT, also known as protein kinase B, PKB
EGF, NGF	Tyrosine kinases, ras	Raf, MAP kinases, RSK

Contd...

Contd...

Receptors	Effectors	Signaling pathways
Cytokine Receptor–Linked Kinase		
GH, PRL	JAK, tyrosine kinases	STAT, MAP kinase, PI 3-kinase, IRS-1
Serine Kinase		
Activin, TGF-β, MIS	Serine kinase	Smads

Note: IP3, inositol triphosphate; IRS, insulin receptor substrates; MAP, mitogen-activated protein; MSH, melanocyte-stimulating hormone; NGF, nerve growth factor; PI, phosphatylinositol; RSK, ribosomal S6 kinase; TGF-β, transforming growth factor β.

16. **Ans. (d) Cytoplasm**
    [Harrison's Endocrinology 3rd ed pg 6, 7]
    See discussion of Chapter 1, Question 3.

17. **Ans. (d) mRNA**
    [Lippincott's Biochemistry- 5th ed pg 443-444; De Groot 7th ed pg 22-24]

    Post-translational Modifications
    - Proteolytic processing of larger precursor species to a final hormone
    - Alternative protein processing, a process by which a large precursor protein molecule (e.g. POMC) is fragmented into several functional units
    - Formation of disulfide bonds
    - Protein folding
    - Proteolytic cleavage
    - Covalent attachments—e.g. acetylation, addition and modification of carbohydrates, phosphates, and lipids
    - Unfolded protein response (UPR) pathway in the ER that adjusts the synthesis capacity of the ER relative to the amount of protein needed and keeps a check on the amount of proteins that are misfolded.

    Also see discussion of Chapter 2, Question 15.
    mRNA undergoes post-transcriptional modification.

18. **Ans. (d) Androgen receptor**
    [Williams 13th ed pg 11, 38, 217, 867, 1391]
    See discussion of Chapter 1, Question 9.

19. **Ans. (d) Insulin**
    [Harrison's Endocrinology 3rd ed pg 2; De Groot 6th ed pg 85]
    See discussion of Chapter 1, Question 15.

20. **Ans. (c) GH**
    [Harrison's Endocrinology 3rd ed pg 2; De Groot 6th ed pg 85]
    See discussion of Chapter 1, Question 15.

21. **Ans. (a) Insulin**

    [Williams pg 271, 511]

    In 15% of cases, Cushing's syndrome is associated with non-pituitary tumors secreting ACTH—the ectopic ACTH syndrome.

    Rarely, GH-secreting intramesenteric pancreatic islet cell tumor or a non-Hodgkin lymphoma may cause acromegaly.

22. **Ans. (a) Proinsulin to insulin**

    [Williams 13th ed pg 123, 124, 130, 138, 145, 146, 152, 495, 496, 750, 1390, 1636]

    Prohormone convertases are enzymes involved in post-translational processing of prohormones and neuropeptides, e.g. Prohormone convertases are involved in the conversion of:
    - TRH prohormone → TRH
    - CRH prohormone → CRH
    - GHRH prohormone → GHRH
    - Somatostatin prohormone → Somatostatin
    - GnRH prohormone → GnRH
    - POMC → ACTH, β-LPH and other related hormones
    - Proinsulin → Insulin
    - Proglucagon → Glucagon, GLP-1 and other related hormones

23. **Ans. (a) LH**

    [Harrison's Endocrinology 3rd ed pg 2; De Groot 6th ed pg 85]

    See discussion of Chapter 1, Question 15.

24. **Ans. (b) Situated at membrane**

    [De Groot 7th ed pg 11]

    G protein-coupled receptors (GPCRs)
    - Seven transmembrane domain G protein-coupled receptors (GPCRs) are membrane receptors
    - These receptors possess seven transmembrane-spanning regions composed of hydrophobic α-helical domains that are connected by extracellular and intracellular loops.
    - They bind a broad array of hormones. See discussion of Chapter 1, Question 15.
    - After the receptor binds a hormone, the transmembrane domains undergo conformational changes that alter interactions with intracellular G proteins.
    - The G proteins provide a link to intracellular signaling pathways such as adenyl cyclase, phospholipase C, mitogen-activated protein kinases (MAPK), and others.

    Also see discussion of Chapter 1, Question 2.

25. **Ans. (b) It is a steroid**

26. **Ans. (d) VDR**
    [Williams 13th ed pg 18, 19, 37; Harrison's Endocrinology 3rd ed pg 2; De Groot 6th ed pg 85]
    See discussion of Chapter 1, Questions 2 and 15.

27. **Ans. (d) CoR**
    [Williams 13th ed pg 347; Harrison's Endocrinology 3rd ed pg 6, 7]
    Thyroid hormone acts by binding to a specific nuclear TR, which, in turn, binds to DNA usually as a heterodimer with retinoid X receptor (RXR) at specific sequences (thyroid hormone response elements, or TREs).
    Co-repressor proteins bind to the receptor in the absence of ligand and silence gene transcription. Hormone binding induces conformational changes, triggering the release of co-repressors and inducing the recruitment of coactivators that stimulate transcription.

28. **Ans. (d) Thyroid stimulating hormone (TSH)**
    [Williams 13th ed pg 18, 19, 20, 123, 129, 137, 145, 152, 183, 188, 199, 207, 301, 492, 494, 595, 606, 704, 1256, 1267, 1269, 1270, 1703-1714; Clinical Chemistry, Immunology and Laboratory Quality Control: A Comprehensive Review for Board Preparation, Certification and Clinical Practice, pg 149]
    See discussion of Chapter 1, Question 1.

29. **Ans. (a) cAMP is formed**
    [Williams 13th ed pg 33]
    Adenylate cyclase catalyzes the conversion of ATP to cAMP.

30. **Ans. (d) Testosterone**
    [Williams 13th ed pg 18, 19, 37]
    See discussion of Chapter 1, Questions 1 and 2.

31. **Ans. All three (c), (d) and (e) are actions of glucocorticoids**
    [Williams 13th ed pg 503-505, 1340]
    Option (c) is more appropriate than options (d) and (e).

    Effects of Glucocorticoids
    Carbohydrate, Protein, and Lipid Metabolism
    - Stimulate glycogen synthesis.
    - Promote gluconeogenesis.
    - Inhibit glucose uptake and utilization in peripheral tissues (e.g. muscle, fat).
    - Activate lipolysis in adipose tissue, resulting in the release of free fatty acids into the circulation.
    - Stimulate adipocyte differentiation, promoting adipogenesis. Deposition of visceral or central adipose tissue.
    - Muscle protein synthesis is reduced.
    - Have a permissive effect on other hormones, including catecholamines and glucagon.

- *Result:* ↑ insulin resistance, ↑ blood glucose concentrations, protein and lipid catabolism. ↑ total cholesterol, ↑ triglycerides, ↓ HDL.

Skin, Muscle, and Connective Tissue
- Cause catabolic changes in muscle, skin, and connective tissue.
  - In the skin and connective tissue, inhibit epidermal cell division and DNA synthesis and reduce synthesis and production of collagen.
  - In muscle, cause atrophy for type II (phasic) muscle fibers.

Bone and Calcium Metabolism
- *Osteopenia and osteoporosis. Mechanism:*
  - Depletion of the osteoblastic cell population (most significant effect).
    - Inhibit the replication of osteoblast precursors and their differentiation into mature osteoblasts.
    - Induce apoptosis of osteoblasts and osteocytes, contributing to the decrease in bone-forming cells.
  - Inhibit osteoblast function.
  - Induce osteoclastogenesis and bone resorption.
- *Osteonecrosis (avascular necrosis). Mechanism:* Induce osteocyte apoptosis.
- Induce negative calcium balance by inhibiting intestinal calcium absorption and increasing renal calcium excretion.

Salt and Water Homeostasis and Blood Pressure Control
- *Increase blood pressure. Mechanisms:*
  - Increase sensitivity of vascular smooth muscles to pressor agents such as catecholamines and angiotensin II while reducing nitric oxide–mediated endothelial dilatation.
  - Angiotensinogen synthesis is increased.
  - Can act on the distal nephron in the kidney to cause sodium retention and potassium loss (mediated via the MR).
- Increase the glomerular filtration rate, proximal tubular epithelial sodium transport, and free water clearance.

Anti-inflammatory Actions and the Immune System
- *Glucocorticoids suppress immunologic responses. Mechanisms:*
  - Reduce lymphocyte counts acutely (T lymphocytes > B lymphocytes) by redistributing lymphocytes from the intravascular compartment to the spleen, lymph nodes, and bone marrow.
  - Neutrophil counts increase.
  - Eosinophil counts fall.
  - Direct actions on both T and B lymphocytes, including inhibition of immunoglobulin synthesis and stimulation of lymphocyte apoptosis.
  - Inhibit cytokine production from lymphocytes.
  - Inhibit monocyte differentiation into macrophages and macrophage phagocytosis and cytotoxic activity.
  - Prevent the actions of histamine and plasminogen activators.
  - Prostaglandin synthesis is impaired.

Central Nervous System and Mood
- Cause neuronal death, notably in the hippocampus.
- *Manifestations:* Depression, euphoria, psychosis, apathy, and lethargy.

Eye
Raise intraocular pressure through an increase in aqueous humor production and deposition of matrix within the trabecular meshwork, which inhibits aqueous drainage.

Gut
- *Increase risk of:*
  - Peptic ulcer disease.
  - Pancreatitis with fat necrosis.
- Control of epithelial ion transport in the gastrointestinal tract.

Growth and Development
- *Inhibit linear skeletal growth. Mechanism:*
  - Catabolic effects on connective tissue, muscle, and bone
  - Inhibition of the effects of IGF-1.
- *Role in normal fetal development:*
  - Stimulate lung maturation through the synthesis of surfactant proteins (SP-A, SP-B, and SP-C).
  - Stimulate conversion of noradrenaline to adrenaline in adrenal medulla and chromaffin tissue.

Endocrine Effects
- Suppress the secretion of thyroid-stimulating hormone (TSH, thyrotropin).
- Inhibit 5'deiodinase activity that mediates the conversion of thyroxine to active triiodothyronine.
- Inhibit gonadotropin-releasing hormone (GnRH) pulsatility and release of luteinizing hormone (LH) and follicle-stimulating hormone (FSH).

32. **Ans. (b) Calcitriol**
    [Williams 13th ed pg 1271, 1272]

33. **Ans. (e) All of the above are correct**
    [Williams 13th ed pg 214; De Groot 7th ed pg 1289]

    #### Effects of TSH on the Thyroid Gland
    - TSH affects thyroid gland growth.
    - *Effects of cell morphology:* TSH maintains trophic thyroid cell integrity.
    - Effect on thyroglobulin gene transcription: the transcriptional rate and possibly the mRNA stability are increased by TSH.
    - Effect on iodine metabolism: TSH stimulates iodide uptake and organification.
    - TSH acts on the iodinated thyroglobulin stored in the luminal colloid and stimulates its hydrolysis, resulting in the release of the constituent amino acids, including the iodothyronines T3 and T4.

The endpoint of TSH action is the production of thyroid hormones by the thyroid gland.

34. **Ans. (a) Target cells affected**
    [Greenspan's 9th ed]

    Relationship between Endocrine System and Nervous System
    Similarities between endocrine system and nervous system: Use of ligands and receptors to establish communication between cells,

    Differences between Endocrine System and Nervous System

	Nervous system	Endocrine system
Mechanism of communication		
	Highly compartmentalized, uses closed system of cables to connect cells at some distance from one another	Relies on circulating plasma to carry hormone to its targets in the periphery
Nature of the ligand–receptor interaction		
Ligand concentration	High (release of secretory granules into an incredibly small volume of the synaptic cleft)	Low (large volume of distribution in circulating plasma)
Affinity of receptor for ligand	Low	High (100–10,000 fold higher binding affinity)
Biological effects	Rapid response- virtually instantaneous (measured in seconds); Effects are short lived (Rapid dissociation of ligand from receptor)	Delayed response (measured in minutes to hours); Effects are long lasting
Area of signal distribution	Well-defined	Wide

    Thus, the systems are not only related but complementary in the roles that they play in contributing to normal physiological function.

35. **Ans. (e) Activation mutation of TSH receptor associated with non-autoimmune hypothyroidism**
    [Williams 12th ed pg 78; Williams 13th ed pg 10, 1297]
    See discussion of Chapter 2, Question 6.

36. **Ans. (c) JAK-STAT receptor**
    [Harrison's Endocrinology 3rd ed pg 2; De Groot 6th ed pg 85]
    See discussion of Chapter 1, Question 15.

37. **Ans. (d) Adrenergic receptor**
    [Williams 13th ed pg 37; Harrison's Endocrinology 3rd ed pg 2; De Groot 6th ed pg 85]

Nuclear Receptor Ligands and their Receptors

Ligand	Receptor
Classic Hormones	
Thyroid hormone	Thyroid hormone receptor (TR), subtypes α, β
Estrogen	Estrogen receptor (ER), subtypes α, β
Testosterone	Androgen receptor (AR)
Progesterone	Progesterone receptor (PR)
Aldosterone	Mineralocorticoid receptor (MR)
Cortisol	Glucocorticoid receptor (GR)
Vitamins	
1,25(OH)$_2$-Vitamin D$_3$	Vitamin D receptor (VDR)
All-*trans*-retinoic acid	Retinoic acid receptor, subtypes α, β, γ
9-*cis*-Retinoic acid	Retinoid X receptor (RXR), subtypes α, β, γ
Metabolic Intermediates and Products	
Fatty acids	Peroxisome proliferator-activated receptor (PPAR), subtypes α, δ, γ
Oxysterols	Liver X receptor (LXR), subtypes α, β
Bile acids	Bile acid receptor (BAR, also called FXR)
Heme	Rev-Erb subtypes α, β
Phospholipids	Liver receptor homologue-1 (LRH-1), Steroidogenic factor-1 (SF-1)
Xenobiotics	Pregnane X receptor (PXR), Constitutive androstane receptor (CAR)

Also, see discussion of Chapter 1, Question 15.

38. **Ans. (a) Glucocorticoid receptor**
    [Williams 13th ed pg 40]

    Most of the nuclear receptors reside in the nucleus, with or without their ligands. A major exception is the glucocorticoid receptor; in the absence of hormone, it is tethered in the cytoplasm to a complex of chaperone molecules, including heat shock proteins (HSPs). Hormone binding to the glucocorticoid receptor induces a conformational change that results in dissociation of the chaperone complex, allowing the hormone-activated glucocorticoid receptor to translocate to the nucleus by means of its nuclear localization signal (NLS).

39. **Ans. (c) PPAR**
    [Harrison's Endocrinology 3rd ed pg 2; De Groot 6th ed pg 85; Harrison's Endocrinology 2nd ed pg 7]

    See discussion of Chapter 1, Questions 3 and 15.

CHAPTER 2

Genetics of Endocrinology

QUESTIONS

1. **Brachydactyly is seen in:**
   a. Klinfelter syndrome
   b. Marfan syndrome
   c. Turner syndrome
   d. Prader-Willi syndrome

2. **Mitochondria all are true except:**
   a. Main site of protein synthesis
   b. Kreb cycle in inner membrane
   c. Circular DNA
   d. Maternal inheritance

3. **Ligand dependent suppression of gene activity called:**
   a. Repression
   b. Trans-repression
   c. Promoter
   d. Activator

4. **CTLA 4 a/w:**
   a. T2DM
   b. Graves'
   c. RTA
   d. Osteoporosis

5. **Graves' disease a/w:**
   a. HLA-DR1
   b. HLA-DR2
   c. HLA-DR3
   d. HLA-DR4

6. **Mutations associated with G-protein are seen in all except:**
   a. Nephrogenic DI
   b. Pseudohypoparathyroidism
   c. Sexual precocious puberty
   d. Neonatal hyperparathyroidism

7. **Gain of function mutation is seen in all except:**
   a. Jansen's disease
   b. Testotoxicosis
   c. Glucocorticoid resistance
   d. Familial non-autoimmune hyperthyroidism

8. **Loss of function mutation of GPCR results in all except:**
   a. ACTH receptor resistance
   b. Nephrogenic DI
   c. AD hypocalcemia
   d. Hypogonadotropic hypogonadism

9. **Role of Proto-oncogenes include all except:**
   a. Normal cell growth
   b. Derived from virus
   c. Present only in malignant tumors
   d. Transduce signals for growth factors

10. **Which one of the following best characterizes autosomal recessive disease?**
    a. Consanguineous marriage
    b. Oblique pedigree
    c. New mutations always manifest clinically
    d. None of the above

11. **Not true about nuclear DNA:**
    a. 50% code proteins
    b. Bind to histones
    c. Coding sequence interrupted by introns
    d. Base pairing by hydrogen bonding

12. **True about PCR is:**
    a. Amplification of DNA
    b. Heat labile polymerase is used
    c. Peptide primer is used
    d. DNTP addition not required

13. **Central dogma of molecular biology is:**
    a. DNA-RNA-Protein
    b. RNA-DNA-Protein
    c. DNA-Protein-RNA
    d. RNA-Protein-DNA

14. **Site of protein synthesis is:**
    a. Ribosome
    b. Nucleus
    c. Mitochondria
    d. Lysosome

15. **Post-transcriptional modifications are all except:**
    a. Acetylation
    b. Glycosylation
    c. Precipitation
    d. Phosphorylation

16. **Heteroplasmy occurs in relation to:**
    a. Mitochondrial disease
    b. Autosomal dominant disease
    c. Epigenetic disease
    d. Y-linked disease

ANSWERS

1. **Ans. (c) Turner's syndrome**
   [De Groot 7th ed pg 494, 997, 1149, 1153; Williams 13th ed pg 749; Sparling-Pediatric Endocrinology 4th ed pg 124, 746, 828, 985]

   Brachydactyly is seen in
   - Turner's syndrome
   - Pseudohypoparathyroidism/Albright's hereditary osteodystrophy (AHO)
   - Pseudopseudohypoparathyroidism
   - Bardet-Biedl syndrome
   - Kallmann syndrome (type 2)/Idiopathic hypogonadotropic hypogonadism due to FGFR1 mutation
   - Carpenter syndrome
   - Genitopatellar syndrome
   - Familial brachydactyly
   - Brachydactyly type E
   - Achondrodysostosis
   - Spondyloepimetaphyseal dysplasia/brachyolmia type 4.

2. **Ans. (a) Main site of protein synthesis**
   [Lippincott's Biochemistry 5th ed pg 445; Harper's biochemistry 28th ed pg 77]
   - Ribosomes are the main sites of protein synthesis
   - Human mitochondria contain two to ten copies of a small circular double-stranded DNA molecule. The majority of the peptides in mitochondria are coded by nuclear genes. The rest are coded by genes found in mitochondrial (mt) DNA. Because all mitochondria are contributed by the ovum during zygote formation—(mt) DNA is transmitted by maternal nonmendelian inheritance. Thus, in diseases resulting from mutations of mtDNA, an affected mother would pass the disease to all of her children but only her daughters would transmit the trait.

3. **Ans. (a) Repression**
   [Harper's biochemistry 28th ed pg 77]

   Transrepression is a process whereby one protein represses (i.e. inhibits) the activity of a second protein through a protein-protein interaction.

4. **Ans. (b) Graves'**
   [Williams 13th ed pg 1764]

   CTLA4 is associated with type 1 diabetes, Graves disease, Hypothyroidism, Celiac disease and Addison disease.

5. **Ans. (c) HLA-DR3**

6. **Ans. (b) Pseudohypoparathyroidism**
   [Williams 12th ed pg 78; Williams 13th ed pg 10, 1297]

   ### Diseases Caused by G-Protein-Coupled Receptor
   Loss-of-Function Mutations
   - V2 vasopressin receptor—Nephrogenic diabetes insipidus
   - ACTH receptor—Familial ACTH resistance
   - GHRH receptor—Familial GH deficiency
   - GnRH receptor—Hypogonadotropic hypogonadism
   - GPR54 receptor—Hypogonadotropic hypogonadism
   - Prokineticin receptor 2—Hypogonadotropic hypogonadism
   - FSH receptor—Hypergonadotropic ovarian dysgenesis
   - LH receptor—XY DSD
   - TSH receptor—Familial hypothyroidism
   - Ca^{2+} sensing receptor—Familial hypocalciuric hypercalcemia, Neonatal severe primary hyperparathyroidism
   - Melanocortin 4 receptor—Obesity
   - PTH/PTHrP receptor—Blomstrand chondrodysplasia

   Gain-of-Function Mutations
   - V2 vasopressin receptor—Nephrogenic inappropriate diuresis
   - LH receptor—Familial male precocious puberty
   - TSH receptor—Sporadic hyperfunctional thyroid nodules, Familial nonautoimmune hyperthyroidism
   - Ca^{2+} sensing receptor—Familial hypocalcemic hypercalciuria
   - PTH/PTHrP receptor—Jansen's metaphyseal chondrodysplasia

   Pseudohypoparathyroidism is caused by mutation in Gsα.

   Activating mutations in the Gsα protein can cause precocious puberty, hyperthyroidism, and acromegaly in McCune-Albright syndrome.

7. **Ans. (c) Glucocorticoid resistance**
   [Williams 12th ed pg 78]
   See discussion of Chapter 2, Question 6.

8. **Ans. (c) AD hypocalcemia**
   See discussion of Chapter 2, Question 6.

9. **Ans. (b) Derived from virus and (c) Present only in malignant tumors**
   [Robbins & Cotran Pathologic Basis of Disease 8th ed]

   Proto-oncogenes have multiple roles, participating in cellular functions related to growth and proliferation. Proteins encoded by proto-oncogenes may function as growth factors or their receptors, signal transducers, transcription factors, or cell cycle components. However, *mutations convert proto-oncogenes into constitutively active cellular oncogenes that are involved in tumor development because the oncoproteins they encode endow the cell with self-sufficiency in growth.*

10. **Ans. (a) Consanguineous marriage**
    [Robbins & Cotran Pathologic Basis of Disease 8th ed]

11. **Ans. (a) 50% code proteins**
    [Harper's Biochemistry 28th ed pg 302, 312, 317]
    Most of the DNA is non-protein-coding. ~1% of the human genome is composed of exonic DNA.

12. **Ans. (a) Amplification of DNA**
    [Harper's Biochemistry 28th ed pg 395]
    - The polymerase chain reaction (PCR) is a method of amplifying a target sequence of DNA.
    - *Steps:*
        - The DNA sample is first heated to separate the two strands of the template DNA containing the target sequence.
        - Two oligonucleotide primers added in vast excess hybridize to complementary sequences on opposite strands of DNA and flank the target sequence.
        - The two DNA strands each serve as a template for the synthesis of new DNA from the two primers. Each strand is copied by a heat-stable DNA polymerase, starting at the primer sites in the presence of all 4 dXTPs (dNTPs).
        - Repeated cycles result in the exponential amplification of DNA segments of defined length.

13. **Ans. (a) DNA-RNA-Protein**
    [Lippincott's Biochemistry 5th ed pg 395]
    The flow of information from DNA to RNA to protein is termed the "central dogma" of molecular biology.

14. **Ans. (a) Ribosome**
    [Lippincott's Biochemistry 5th ed pg 445]
    See discussion of Chapter 2, Question 2.

15. **Ans. (c) Precipitation**
    [Lippincott's Biochemistry 5th ed pg 443-444]
    Co- and post-translational modification of polypeptide chains include
    - Trimming
    - *Covalent attachments:*
        - Phosphorylation
        - Glycosylation
        - Hydroxylation
        - Carboxylation
        - Acetylation
        - Others (e.g. covalent binding of biotin, or lipids such as farnesyl groups).

- Protein folding
- Protein degradation.

16. **Ans. (a) Mitochondrial disease**
    [Robbins & Cotran Pathologic Basis of Disease 8th ed]
    Each mitochondrion contains numerous copies of mtDNA, and, typically, deleterious mutations of mtDNA affect some but not all of these copies. Thus, tissues/individuals may harbor both wild-type and mutant mtDNA, a situation called heteroplasmy. A minimum number of mutant mtDNA must be present in a cell or tissue before oxidative dysfunction gives rise to disease. This is called the "threshold effect." The clinical and pathologic appearance of the disease depends on whether the cells contain a large proportion of the mutated mitochondrial DNA or of normal mitochondria.

CHAPTER 3

Laboratory Techniques for Recognition of Endocrine Disorders

QUESTIONS

1. Radioisotope used in immunoassay:
   a. C-14
   b. I-125
   c. U
   d. Cobalt

2. Pooled serum is not used in:
   a. PRL
   b. Cortisol
   c. FSH/LH
   d. GH

3. Which of the following is not used for immunoassays?
   a. Radio-isotope
   b. Enzyme
   c. mRNA
   d. Chemiluminescent substance

4. Which subunit of peptide hormones interact with immunoassays?
   a. Alfa subunit
   b. Beta
   c. Gamma
   d. Delta

5. RIA uses:
   a. I-123
   b. I-125
   c. I-127
   d. I-131

6. Antibody labeling instead of Ag labeling:
   a. ELISA
   b. Radioimmunoassay
   c. Gel filtration
   d. None of the above

7. Monoclonal antibodies are used in:
   a. RIA
   b. HPCL
   c. Mass spectrometry
   d. Chemiluminescence

8. Final endpoint in ELISA is assessed by:
   a. Beta counter
   b. Gamma counter
   c. Fluorimeter
   d. Spectrophotometer/colorimeter

9. High dose Hook effect usually occurs with:
   a. RIA
   b. Immunometric assay
   c. Bioassay
   d. ELISA

ANSWERS

1. **Ans. (b) I-125**
   [Williams 13th ed pg 79, 80, 568; Chemistry and Applications of Iodine]
   There are 37 known isotopes of iodine, but only one, 127-I, is stable. The following isotopes are used as tracers and therapeutic agents in medicine:
   - *Iodine-127:* Nonradioactive. It is used in potassium iodide.
   - *Iodine-125 (half-life 59 days):* It is used as a gamma-emitting tag for proteins in biological assays.
   - *Iodine-123 (half-life 13 hours):* It is the isotope of choice for nuclear medicine imaging of the thyroid gland. Also used in MIBG scintigraphy.
   - *Iodine-131 (half-life 8 days):* It is a beta-emitting isotope. It is used to treat Graves' disease and thyroid cancers. It is also used as to kill tissues such as cancers that take up artificially iodinated molecules (example, MIBG).

2. **Ans. (d) GH**
   [Endocrine Abstracts (2013) 32 P888; Principles and Practice of Endocrinology and Metabolism pg 1118; J Clin Epidemiol. 1996 Mar;49(3):345-50; Send to Scand J Clin Lab Invest. 2008;68(6):508-12]

3. **Ans. (c) mRNA**
   [Williams 13th ed pg 80; Pediatric Endocrinology 4th ed pg 93]
   Immunoassays use radioactive, chemiluminescent, colorimetric (in ELISA), or fluorescent signals.

4. **Ans. (a) Alfa subunit**
   [Williams 13th ed pg 209, 212]
   The α-subunit is common to TSH, LH, FSH, and hCG, whereas the β-subunit is unique and confers specificity of action. Because of the high homology of the glycoprotein hormones, development of highly specific assays, especially those distinguishing free α-subunit from intact hormones, has been challenging.

5. **Ans. (b) I-125**
   [Williams 13th ed pg 79, 80]
   Although both I-125 and I-131 have been used to label the antigen in RIA. Option (b) is more appropriate than option (d).
   See discussion of Chapter 3, Question 1.

6. **Ans. (a) ELISA**
   [Williams 13th ed pg 80; Pediatric Endocrinology 4th ed pg 92, 93]
   There are two main immunoassay formats
   1. Competitive immunoassay
      - A primary antibody against the substance ("analyte") of interest is added to the patient's sample, together with a radiolabeled version

of the analyte ("tracer") that competes with the endogenous analyte for binding to the primary antibody.
- Any unbound tracer or analyte is washed away, and the amount of tracer in the precipitate is then quantified.
- The amount of signal detected decreases as the analyte in the patient's sample increases.
- *Example:* Radioimmunoassay (RIA); Nonisotopic signaling systems use colorimetric, fluorometric or chemiluminescent signals.

2. Immunometric (sandwich) assay
   - An antibody attached to a solid support is used to capture the analyte of interest, followed by the addition of a second, labeled antibody that binds to a different site on the analyte, creating an antibody-analyte-antibody sandwich.
   - After unbound detection antibody is washed away, that which remains generates a radioactive (immunoradiometric [IRMA]), chemiluminescent (immunochemiluminometric [ICMA]), colorimetric (enzyme-linked immunosorbent assay [ELISA]), or fluorescent (immunofluorescence assay [IFMA]) signal, depending on the label chosen.

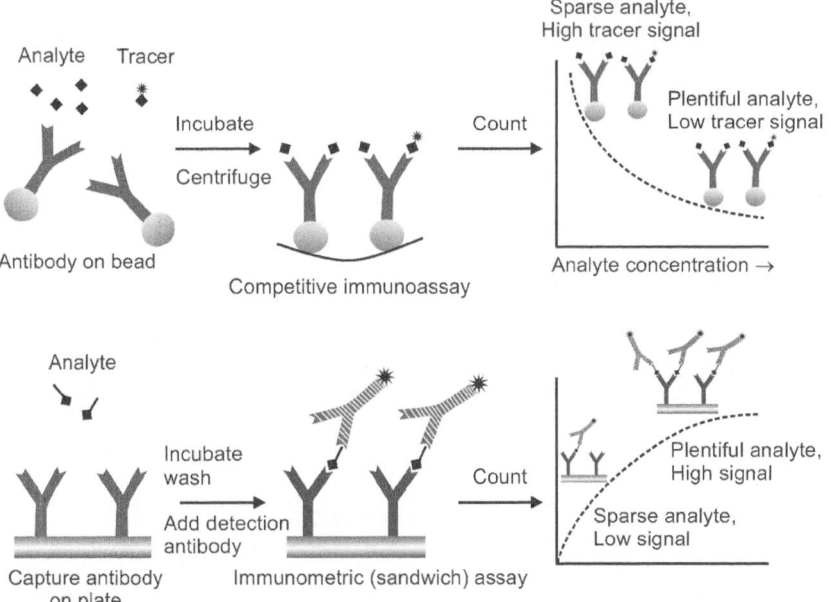

7. **Ans. (a) RIA and (d) Chemiluminescence**
   [Pediatric Endocrinology 4th ed pg 90, 93]

8. **Ans. (d) Spectrophotometer/colorimeter**
   [Pediatric Endocrinology 4th ed pg 93]
   See discussion of Chapter 3, Question 6.

9. **Ans. (b) Immunometric assay**
   [Pediatric Endocrinology 4th ed pg 93]

   Sandwich immunometric assays are vulnerable to the "hook" or "prozone" effect that can lead to falsely normal or low values in the presence of large amounts of the analyte. Generally, as analyte concentration increases, more antibody-analyte-antibody sandwiches are formed, leading to more signal detected. At extremely high analyte concentrations, however, it is possible for both capture and detection antibodies to be saturated with analyte prior to formation of a sandwich complex, leading to the detection antibody being washed away and the low signal being misinterpreted as a low concentration of analyte.

   This phenomenon is not seen with competitive immunoassays.

CHAPTER 4

Neuroendocrinology

QUESTIONS

1. Pituitary apoplexy can be caused by all except:
   a. Hypertension
   b. DM
   c. Sickle cell anemia
   d. Hypothyroidism

2. Earliest hormone to be involved in lymphocytic hypophysitis:
   a. ACTH
   b. TSH
   c. FSH
   d. LH

3. Prerequisite for prolactin test assay include all except:
   a. Fasting
   b. No galactorrhea for 3 days
   c. Abstinence for 3 days
   d. Follicular phase

4. Prerequisite for Growth hormone stimulation test, true is:
   a. Standing upright throughout
   b. Overnight fasting
   c. Clonidine 4 μg/day in adults
   d. Normal response >10 pg/mL

5. Pit-1 mutation does not decrease:
   a. GH
   b. TSH
   c. ACTH
   d. Prolactin

6. Lymphocytic hypophysitis, the most common hormone deficiency is:
   a. GH
   b. TSH
   c. ACTH
   d. LH

7. Septo-optic dysplasia:
   a. PIT-1
   b. HESX-1
   c. DAX
   d. PROP-1

8. Which of the following statements about LH is correct?
   a. Increased inhibin/activin in follicular phase
   b. After puberty LH pulses> FSH pulses
   c. Estrogen rise in late follicular phase cause LH surge
   d. Increase in LH in late follicular phase cause ovulation

9. Macroprolactinemia is a feature of:
   a. Microprolactinoma
   b. Macroprolactinoma
   c. Macromastia
   d. PRL Ab

10. Seen in hypothalamic lesions are all except:
    a. Anosmia
    b. Diabetes insipidus
    c. Autonomic dysfunction
    d. Obesity

11. All are non-endocrinological manifestation of hypothalamic disease except:
    a. Hyper sexuality
    b. Hyperphagia
    c. Rage behavior
    d. Increased dark adaptation time

12. The endocrine system:
    a. Releases chemicals into the bloodstream for distribution throughout the body
    b. Releases hormones that alter the metabolic activities of many different tissues and organs
    c. Produces effects that can last for hours, days, or even longer
    d. Can alter gene activity of cells
    e. All of the above

13. This hypophyseal structure receives signals from the hypothalamus via the hypophyseal portal vein:
    a. Follicles
    b. Adenohypophysis
    c. Neurohypophysis
    d. Pars intermedia
    e. Supraoptic nucleus

14. Lesions of which of the following hypothalamic nuclei cause loss of circadian rhythm?
    a. Ventromedial
    b. Dorsomedial
    c. Suprachiasmatic
    d. Supraoptic

15. Which of the following is a periodic disease of hypothalamic origin?
    a. Diencephalic epilepsy
    b. Kleine-Levin syndrome
    c. Periodic discharge syndrome of Wolf
    d. All of the above

16. Circadian rhythm means, change in hormone level:
    a. About a day
    b. Exactly a day
    c. Less than a day
    d. Longer than a day
17. Which of the following scientist is known as father of modern neuroendocrinology?
    a. Claude Bernard
    b. Geoffrey Harris
    c. Alfred Frohlich
    d. Andrew Schally
18. Rate limiting enzyme in the melatonin synthesis is:
    a. Hydroxyindole-O-methyl transferase
    b. Tryptophan hydroxylase
    c. Aromatic-l-amino acid decarboxylase
    d. Arylalkylamine-N-acetyltransferase

ANSWERS

1. **Ans. (d) Hypothyroidism**
   [Williams 13th ed pg 250]
   Pituitary apoplexy may result from:
   - Pituitary adenoma—spontaneous hemorrhage (pituitary tumor apoplexy)
   - Head trauma, with skull base fracture
   - Hypertension
   - Diabetes mellitus
   - Sickle cell anemia
   - Acute hypovolemic shock.

   Precipitating factors include:
   - Major surgery
   - Pregnancy
   - Gamma knife irradiation
   - Coagulopathy secondary to liver failure
   - *Drugs:* Anticoagulants, thyrotropin-releasing hormone (TRH), gonadotropin releasing hormone (GnRH) agonists, bromocriptine, cabergoline.

2. **Ans. (a) ACTH**
   [Williams 13th ed pg 248]
   In contrast to other forms of hypopituitarism, ACTH deficiency is most common in patients with lymphocytic hypophysitis, followed in frequency by TSH deficiency, gonadotropin deficiency, and GH or PRL deficiency. Diabetes insipidus can occur.

3. **Ans. (b) No galactorrhea for 3 days**

4. **Ans. (b) Overnight fasting**
   [Bart's endocrine e-protocol- pituitary function]
   Protocol for Clonidine Test for GH Reserve
   - *Precautions:* Systolic BP falls by 20–25 mm Hg in all subjects, patient should lie down for 2 hours after the test or until blood pressure is satisfactory.
   - *Preparation:* Fast from midnight.
   - *Procedure:*
     - IV cannula at 8.30 am and take basal GH at 8.30 am.
     - Clonidine 0.15 mg/m^2 orally at 9 am
     - Take further samples at 30, 45, 60, 90, 120 and 150 minutes for GH.
   - *Interpretation:* If the GH rises above 10 ng/mL, the GH reserve is probably normal.
   - The test is more accurate in children, not validated in adults.

5. **Ans. (c) ACTH**
   [Williams 13th ed pg 180]

Hereditary Pituitary Deficiency Caused by Transcription Factor Mutations

Gene	Pituitary deficiency
POU1F1 (Pit 1)	GH, PRL, ± TSH
PROP1	GH, PRL, TSH, LH, FSH, ± ACTH
HESX1	GH, PRL, TSH, LH, FSH, ACTH
PITX2	GH, PRL, TSH, FSH, LH
LHX3	GH, PRL, TSH, LH, FSH
LHX4	GH, TSH, ACTH
TBX19	ACTH
OTX2	GH, PRL, TSH, LH, FSH, ACTH
SOX2	GH, FSH, LH
SOX3	GH, TSH, ACTH, FSH, LH
IGSF1	GH, PRL, TSH
NR5A1	FSH, LH
NR0B1	FSH, LH

6. **Ans. (c) ACTH**
   [Williams 13th ed pg 248]
   See discussion of Chapter 4, Question 2.

7. **Ans. (b) *HESX1***
   [Williams 13th ed pg 990]
   Mutations in developmental transcription factors *HESX1*, *SOX2*, *SOX3*, and *OTX2* are implicated in the pathogeneses of septo-optic dysplasia.

8. **Ans. (c) Estrogen rise in late follicular phase cause LH surge and (d) Increase in LH in late follicular phase cause ovulation**
   [Williams 13th ed pg 590, 591, 593, 596, 1099]

9. **Ans. (d) PRL Ab**
   [Williams 13th ed pg 96]

10. **Ans. (a) Anosmia**
    [Williams 13th ed pg 166, 167, 307, 308]

    Clinical Features of Hypothalamic Syndromes
    Endocrine and Metabolic
    - Anterior pituitary dysfunction
      - Activating lesions
        * Central precocious puberty
        * Acromegaly
        * Cushing's disease
      - Lesions with hypothalamic loss-of-function
        * Hyperprolactinemia
        * Hypothalamic hypogonadism
        * Growth hormone deficiency
        * Hypothalamic hypoadrenalism
        * Hypothalamic hypothyroidism

- Disorders of water and electrolyte metabolism
  - Central diabetes insipidus
  - Syndrome of inappropriate secretion of antidiuretic hormone
- Disorders of food intake and weight control
  - Hypothalamic obesity.

Neurologic Manifestations of Nonendocrine Hypothalamic Disease Include
- Disorders of temperature regulation
  - Hyperthermia
  - Hypothermia
  - Poikilothermia
- Disorders of food intake
  - Hyperphagia (bulimia)
  - Anorexia nervosa, aphagia
  - Cachexia
- Disorders of water intake
  - Compulsive water drinking
  - Adipsia
  - Essential hypernatremia
- Disorders of sleep and consciousness
  - Narcolepsy/cataplexy
  - Somnolence
  - Sleep rhythm reversal
  - Akinetic mutism
  - Coma
  - Delirium
- Periodic disease of hypothalamic origin
  - Diencephalic epilepsy
  - Kleine-Levin syndrome
  - Periodic discharge syndrome of Wolff
- Disorders of psychic function
  - Rage behavior
  - Hallucinations
  - Hypersexuality
- Disorders of the autonomic nervous system
  - Pulmonary edema
  - Cardiac arrhythmias
  - Sphincter disturbance
- Miscellaneous
  - Diencephalic syndrome of infancy
  - Cerebral gigantism
- Congenital hypothalamic disease
  - Prader-Willi syndrome
  - Laurence-Moon-Biedl syndrome

11. **Ans. (d) Increased dark adaptation time**
    [Williams 13th ed pg 166, 167]
    See discussion of Chapter 4, Question 10.

12. **Ans. (e) All of the above**

13. **Ans. (b) Adenohypophysis**
    [Williams 13th ed pg 177]

14. **Ans. (c) Suprachiasmatic**
    [De Groot 7th ed pg 181]

15. **Ans. (d) All of the above**
    [Williams 13th ed pg 166, 167]
    See discussion of Chapter 4, Question 10.

16. **Ans. (a) About a day**
    [Williams 13th ed pg 122]

    Endocrine Rhythms
    - Circadian—About a day (24 hr)
    - Diurnal—Exactly a day
    - Ultradian—Less than a day (i.e. minutes or hours)
    - Infradian—Longer than a day (i.e. month or year)

17. **Ans. (b) Geoffrey Harris**
    [Williams 13th ed pg 122]

18. **Ans. (d) Arylalkylamine-N-acetyltransferase**
    Steps involved in Biosynthesis of melatonin from tryptophan in the pineal gland

    The rate-limiting step is catalyzed by the enzyme arylalkylamine N-acetyltransferase (AANAT).

CHAPTER 5

Pituitary Physiology and Diagnostic Evaluation

QUESTIONS

1. GH deficiency in adult manifests all except:
   a. DM
   b. Central obesity
   c. Atherosclerosis
   d. Decreased systolic blood pressure

2. Pit-1, which axis is not stimulated?
   a. Somatotroph
   b. Corticotroph
   c. Thyrotroph
   d. Lactotroph

3. All of the following suppresses prolactin levels except:
   a. T3 T4 and analogues
   b. Dopamine
   c. Glucocorticoids
   d. PPI

4. Hyperprolactinemia is seen in all except:
   a. Empty sella
   b. Lymphocytic hypophysitis
   c. Stalk section
   d. Hypothyroidism

5. Bromocriptine all are true except:
   a. Synthetic ergot analogue
   b. Bromocriptine resistance is known
   c. Dopamine agonist
   d. Causes perivascular fibrosis in prolactinomas

6. A 3-year-old girl presents with short stature, h/o secondary hypothyroidism at birth, adrenal axis normal and now has GH deficiency, diagnosis is:
   a. Laron's
   b. Multiple pituitary hormone deficiency
   c. Radiation induced hypopituitarism
   d. Craniopharyngioma

7. **Safest drug in pregnancy:**
   a. Bromocriptine
   b. Cabergoline
   c. Pergolide
   d. Quinagolide

8. **Prolactin levels in pregnancy:**
   a. Upto 50 mcg/L
   b. Upto 180
   c. Less than 150
   d. More than 300

9. **GnRH stimulation test all are true except:**
   a. Bolus of 25–100 mcg is enough
   b. LH rises in 20–30 mins
   c. LH rise > FSH rise
   d. FSH rise > LH rise

10. **Autoimmune endocrine disorder is all except:**
    a. Lymphocytic hypophysitis
    b. Xanthomatous hypophysitis
    c. Anti-sperm antibodies
    d. Granulomatous hypophysitis

11. **Deficiency of all seen in Prop-1 mutation except:**
    a. GH
    b. PRL
    c. TSH
    d. Oxytocin

12. **Peak ACTH after CRH stimulation test seen at:**
    a. 15 min
    b. 30 min
    c. 45 min
    d. 60 min

13. **All of the following are true about lactotrophs except:**
    a. 10–25% of pituitary cell population
    b. Arise from postmitotic somatotroph
    c. Lactotrophs are hyperfunctioning in Pit-1 mutation
    d. Lactotroph hypertrophy and hyperplasia occurs in pregnancy

14. **Earliest hormone to be expressed in the pituitary:**
    a. Corticotrophs
    b. Somatotrophs
    c. Lactotrophs
    d. Gonadotrophs

15. **Mutation of Pit-1 has effect in all except:**
    a. ACTH
    b. GH
    c. PRL
    d. TSH

16. **Non-ergot dopamine agonist is:**
    a. Leuprolide
    b. Quinagolide
    c. Pergolide
    d. Cabergoline

17. **Following causes increased PRL except:**
    a. Metoclopramide
    b. Rifampicin
    c. Hypothyroidism
    d. Seizure

18. Following pair is not homologous:
    a. PTH-PTHrP
    b. Insulin-calcitonin
    c. LH/FSH/TSH
    d. GH/PRL/hPL

19. In central hypothyroidism, TRH stimulation test is characterized by:
    a. Early response
    b. Delayed response
    c. Blunted nocturnal surge of TSH
    d. Blunted TSH surge during day

20. Most potent GH inhibitor is:
    a. Bromocriptine
    b. Somatostatin
    c. Cabergoline
    d. Methysergide

21. Tissue specific transcription factors for thyrotroph and lactotroph:
    a. DAX 1
    b. SF1
    c. Pit-1
    d. TEF
    e. PROP 1

22. Somatotroph and lactotroph/only somatotroph transcription factor:
    a. DAX-1
    b. SF1
    c. Pit-1
    d. TEF
    e. PROP 1

23. *HESX1* mutation is associated with:
    a. Septo-optic dysplasia
    b. Short stature
    c. Eugonadism
    d. DI
    e. Hyperprolactinemia

24. Drugs causing hyperprolactinemia include all except:
    a. Ranitidine
    b. Alpha-methyldopa
    c. Cabergoline
    d. Calcium channel blockers (CCBs)
    e. Verapamil

25. Systemic causes of hyperprolactinemia include all except:
    a. CRF
    b. Cirrhosis
    c. Hypothyroidism
    d. Hypertension

26. Which of the hormones has a binding protein in the circulation?
    a. LH
    b. FSH
    c. TSH
    d. GH

27. Hyperprolactinemia causes all except:
    a. Increased FSH
    b. Decreased FSH
    c. Increased ICT
    d. Visual field defects

28. ACTH is all except:
    a. Polypeptide
    b. Increased by stress
    c. Present in other tissues
    d. Correlate with cortisol level

29. Prolactin 35, presents with galactorrhea, MRI 1.1 cm adenoma, started on bromocriptine 1 mg BD, after 1 year, headache ↑↑↑, prolactin ↑↑. Most appropriate treatment:
    a. Change to cabergoline
    b. Transphenoidal sinus surgery
    c. Stereotactic radiosurgery
    d. Increase dose of bromocriptine

30. ACTH is affected in:
    a. LHX-3
    b. PIT-1
    c. PROP-1
    d. HESX-1

31. Treatment of choice for prolactinoma in pregnancy:
    a. Bromocriptine
    b. Cabergoline
    c. Pergolide
    d. Quinagolide

32. All the following receptors are associated with mutations except:
    a. TSH
    b. PTH
    c. Estrogen
    d. Vasopressin

33. Treatment of choice for pituitary microprolactinoma is:
    a. Observation
    b. Transsphenoidal surgery
    c. Pegvisomant
    d. Cabergoline

34. All of the following drugs can cause hyperprolactinemia except:
    a. Methyldopa
    b. Cimetidine
    c. Cabergoline
    d. Fluoxetine

35. Chromosome locus for prolactin is:
    a. 2
    b. 6
    c. 11
    d. 17

36. Lymphocytic hypophysitis:
    a. Disproportionate hormone deficiency
    b. Spontaneous recovery may occur
    c. Progressive mass effect uncommon
    d. Does not occur in males

37. All are used in therapy of prolactinoma except:
    a. Alpha methyldopa
    b. Cabergoline
    c. Lisuride
    d. Fluoxetine

38. Causes of increased GHRH secretion are all except:
    a. Bronchial carcinoids
    b. Optic glioma
    c. Pheochromocytoma
    d. Medullary thyroid carcinoma
    e. Follicular thyroid carcinoma

39. A 37-year-old female presents with galactorrhea. She has a history of dyspepsia for which she receives a combination of anti-ulcer therapy. Examination reveals a BMI of 23.5 kg/m² and a small amount of galactorrhea to expression. Investigations show a prolactin concentration of 850 mU/l (NR 50–500 mU/l), an oestradiol of 88 pmol/l (NR 130–500), a LH of 3.2 mU/l (NR 3.5–8) and a FSH of 2.8 mU/l (NR 3–8). What disorder should be considered?
    a. Addison's disease
    b. Hyperthyroidism
    c. MEN type 1
    d. Drug-induced hyperprolactinemia
    e. Hypothyroidism

40. Adult growth hormone deficiency is confirmed by:
    a. A low IGF-1 concentration
    b. An undetectable random Growth hormone concentration
    c. Suppression of GH below 2 mU/l (1.3 µg/L) with an oral glucose tolerance test
    d. A peak growth hormone concentration of 6 mU/l (2 µg/L) with insulin induced hypoglycemia
    e. A low IGF binding protein-3 (IGFBP3) concentration

41. Dopamine inhibits all except:
    a. Prolactin   b. TSH
    c. ACTH   d. FSH

42. Ghrelin does not stimulate:
    a. GH   b. Prolactin
    c. TSH   d. ACTH

43. A young lady, 4 weeks postpartum suddenly stopped lactation. The labor was prolonged requiring transfusion. ↓ Thyroxine, ↓ Cortisol. The next best step:
    a. Replacement thyroxine   b. Replacement of corticosteroids
    c. MRI of pituitary   d. Visual field assessment

44. Which of the following hormones is not a polypeptide?
    a. MSH   b. ACTH
    c. Melatonin   d. Growth hormone

45. Growth hormone acts directly on:
    a. Stimulation of protein synthesis
    b. Stimulation of cartilage formation
    c. Elevation of BSL
    d. Stimulation of bone formation

46. Hypopituitarism is characterized by:
    a. Infertility   b. Intolerance to heat
    c. Weight gain   d. Excessive growth of the soft tissue

47. Causes of hyperprolactinemia include all except:
    a. Chronic renal failure
    b. Hypothyroidism
    c. Pseudocyesis
    d. Levothyroxine treatment
    e. Pituitary apoplexy

48. Drugs used in prolactinoma include:
    a. Quinagolide
    b. Lisuride
    c. Fluoxetine
    d. Alpha-methyldopa
    e. Verapamil

49. All of the following are true about pituitary apoplexy except:
    a. Most commonly seen in preexisting adenoma
    b. Presence of ptosis is an indication for immediate surgery
    c. Ring enhancing lesion on MRI
    d. Medical treatment has good outcome
    e. Visual recovery inversely related to the time of surgery

50. Lymphocytic hypophysitis
    a. Does not occur in males
    b. Disproportionate deficiency in hormones
    c. Can have normal outcome
    d. Can present as sellar mass enlargement
    e. Diabetes insipidus

51. GH sufficiency is evaluated by:
    a. GHRH
    b. TRH
    c. Metyrapone
    d. Propranolol
    e. Pyridostigmine

52. Adult GH deficiency is characterized by all except:
    a. Increased HDL
    b. Decreased muscle mass
    c. Increased waist:hip ratio
    d. Evoked GH <3 ng/mL
    e. Decreased IGF1, decreased IGFBP3

ANSWERS

1. **Ans. (d) Decreased systolic blood pressure**
   [Williams 13th ed pg 194]

   Clinical Features of Adult Somatotropin Deficiency
   - Body composition
     - General and central adiposity
     - Reduced lean mass
     - Reduced bone mass
   - Function
     - Reduced exercise capacity
     - Muscle weakness
     - Impaired cardiac function
     - Hypohydrosis increase
   - Quality of life
     - Low mood
     - Fatigue
     - Low motivation
     - Reduced satisfaction
   - Cardiovascular risk profile
     - Abnormal lipid profile
     - Insulin resistance
     - Increased inflammatory markers
     - Intimal media thickening
   - Laboratory
     - Blunted peak GH to stimulation
     - Low IGF-1 (in 50–60%)
     - Hyperinsulinemia, Glucose intolerance
     - High LDL and low HDL cholesterol.

2. **Ans. (b) Corticotroph**
   [Williams 13th ed pg 179]

   Pit-1 is a transcription factor which determines somatotroph, lactotroph, and thyrotroph.

3. **Ans. (d) PPI**
   [Williams 13th ed pg 183, 186; Greenspan's 9th ed; De Groot 7th ed pg 96, 108]

   Regulation of Prolactin Secretion

Stimulate	Inhibit
Basic FGF	Dopamine
Epidermal growth factor	Endothelin-1
Vasoactive intestinal polypeptide (VIP)	TGF-β1
Prolactin-releasing peptide (PrRP)	Calcitonin

   Contd...

Contd...

Stimulate	Inhibit
TRH	Histamine
Estrogen	Somatostatin
Serotonin	Glucocorticoids
GH-releasing hormone (GHRH)	Thyroid hormone
Oxytocin	
Pituitary adenylate cyclase activating peptide (PACAP)	
Galanin	
Angiotensin II	

Etiology of Hyperprolactinemia

Physiologic	Pharmacologic
• Pregnancy	*Neuropeptides*
• Sucking	• Thyrotropin-releasing hormone
• Stress	*Dopamine receptor blockers*
• Sleep	• Phenothiazines: chlorpromazine, perphenazine
• Coitus	• Butyrophenones: haloperidol
• Exercise	• Thioxanthenes
Pathologic	• Metoclopramide
Hypothalamic-pituitary stalk damage	*Dopamine synthesis inhibitors*
• Tumors	• α-Methyldopa
• Craniopharyngioma	*Catecholamine depleters*
• Suprasellar pituitary mass extension	• Reserpine
• Meningioma	*Cholinergic agonists*
• Dysgerminoma	• Physostigmine
• Hypothalamic metastases	*Antihypertensives*
• Granulomas	• Labetolol
• Infiltrations	• Reserpine
• Rathke's cyst	• Verapamil
• Irradiation	*H2 antihistamines*
• Trauma: pituitary stalk section, sellar surgery, head trauma	• Cimetidine
Pituitary	• Ranitidine
• Prolactinoma	*Protease inhibitors*
• Acromegaly	*Estrogens*
• Macroadenoma (compressive)	• Oral contraceptives
• Idiopathic	• Oral contraceptive withdrawal
• Plurihormonal adenoma	*Anticonvulsants*
• Lymphocytic hypophysitis	• Phenytoin
• Parasellar mass	*Neuroleptics*
• Macroprolactinemia	• Chlorpromazine
Systemic disorders	• Risperidone
• Hypothyroidism	• Promazine
• Chronic renal failure	

Contd...

Contd...

• Polycystic ovary syndrome • Cirrhosis • Pseudocyesis • Epileptic seizures • Cranial irradiation • Chest: neurogenic, chest wall trauma, surgery, herpes zoster *Genetic* • Inactivating prolactin receptor mutation	• Promethazine • Trifluoperazine • Fluphenazine • Butaperazine • Perphenazine • Thiethylperazine • Thioridazine • Haloperidol • Pimozide • Thiothixene • Molindone *Dopamine receptor blockers* • Sulpiride • Metoclopramide • Domperidone *Opiates and Opiate Antagonists* • Heroin • Methadone • Apomorphine • Morphine *Antidepressants* • Tricyclic antidepressants: chlorimipramine, amitriptylin • Selective serotonin reuptake inhibitors: fluoxetine

4. **Ans. (a) Empty sella**
   [Williams 13th ed pg 186; Greenspan's 9th ed]
   See discussion of Chapter 5, Question 3.

5. **Ans. (a) Synthetic ergot analogue**
   [Williams 13th ed pg 262]
   Bromocriptine is a semisynthetic ergot alkaloid dopamine agonist.

6. **Ans. (b) Multiple pituitary hormone deficiency**

7. **Ans. (a) Bromocriptine**
   [Williams 13th ed pg 262]
   Bromocriptine therapy was not associated with increased abortions or terminations, prematurity, multiple births, or infant malformations above that expected in the control population. There is no compelling evidence that other dopamine agonists are less safe, but pregnancy exposure to the other agonist forms are less comprehensively documented.

8. **Ans. (b) Upto 180**
   [De Groot 7th ed pg 108]
   The referenced text states that there is a stepwise increase in serum PRL levels during pregnancy, achieving mean levels of 200 ng/mL at the end of pregnancy and up to 450 ng/mL in some cases.
   Thus, option (b) appears most appropriate.

Pituitary Physiology and Diagnostic Evaluation | 43

9. **Ans. (d) FSH rise > LH rise**
   [De Groot 7th ed pg 2683]

   ### Gonadotropin-releasing Hormone Stimulation Test
   - *Indication:* Suspected central precocious puberty (CPP); suspected pituitary gonadotropin deficiency; monitor long-acting GnRH analog therapy.

   ### Intravenous GnRH
   - *Medication:* 2.5 µg/kg, up to 100 µg maximum, rapid intravenous injection of GnRH
   - *Sampling:* Blood samples for measurements of serum LH and FSH concentrations are obtained immediately before and at 30, 45, and 60 minutes after GnRH injection. A single 30-minutes LH sample can be used to monitor GnRH analog therapy.
   - *Interpretation:* Prepubertally, levels increase two- to fourfold with a peak LH/FSH ratio approximating 0.7. Postpubertally, LH levels increase six- to tenfold and FSH four- to six-fold, with a mean peak LH/FSH ratio approximating 3.5. A cutoff of 15 U/L helped diagnose central precocious puberty (CPP) with >90% sensitivity and >80% specificity.

   ### Subcutaneous GnRH
   - *Medication:* 100 µg GnRH administered subcutaneously.
   - *Sampling:* Draw blood for serum LH and FSH measurements at –15 and 0 minute and at 40 minutes after GnRH.
   - *Interpretation:* LH and FSH values generally remain below 5 IU/L in normal prepubertal children; the FSH response usually exceeds the LH response. With the onset of puberty, there is a brisk LH response; values increase four- to six-fold above baseline. An ICMA LH value ≥10 IU/L after GnRH is strong evidence for CPP. Levels in the 5 to 10 IU/L range are suggestive of CPP.
   - *Comments:* The test does not reliably differentiate gonadotropin deficiency from constitutional delay in children with delayed puberty.

10. **Ans. (b) Xanthomatous hypophysitis**
    [Williams 13th ed pg 748, 749, 726; Endocrine Reviews 26(5):599, 600; Greenspan's 9th ed]

11. **Ans. (d) Oxytocin**
    [Williams 13th ed pg 180]
    See discussion of Chapter 4, Question 5.

12. **Ans. (b) 30 min**
    [Williams 13th ed pg 203]
    Administration of ovine or human CRH may invoke pituitary ACTH secretion may. CRH (100 µg or 1 µg/kg) is administered intravenously, and cortisol and ACTH are measured at –5, –1, 0, 15, 30, 60, 90, and 120 minutes. Normally, maximal ACTH responses (twofold to fourfold above baseline) are evoked at 30 minutes, and cortisol levels peak (over 20 µg/dL) at 60 minutes or increase more than 10 µg/dL above baseline.

13. **Ans. (c) Lactotrophs are hyperfunctioning in Pit-1 mutation**
    [Williams 13th ed pg 180, 182; De Groot 7th ed pg 107]
    - Lactotroph cells account for about 15% to 25% of functioning anterior pituitary cells.
    - The majority of PRL-producing cells arise from postmitotic somatotrophs.
    - Occasional mammosomatotroph cells co-secrete both PRL and GH, often stored within the same granule.
    - Pit-1 mutation lead to prolactin deficiency (also deficiency of GH and TSH) (See discussion of Chapter 4, Question 5)
    - During pregnancy, lactotrophs undergo hypertrophy and hyperplasia.

14. **Ans. (a) Corticotrophs**
    [Williams 13th ed pg 179]
    - At 6 weeks, corticotroph cells are identifiable, and immunoreactive ACTH is detectable by 7 weeks.
    - At 8 weeks, somatotroph cells are evident with immunoreactive GH expression.
    - At 12 weeks, differentiated thyrotrophs and gonadotrophs express immunoreactive β-subunits for TSH, LH, and FSH, respectively.
    - After 24 weeks, fully differentiated PRL-expressing lactotrophs are evident (Prior to that, immunoreactive PRL is only detectable in mixed mammosomatotrophs, also expressing GH.

15. **Ans. (a) ACTH**
    [Williams 13th ed pg 180]
    See discussion of Chapter 4, Question 5.

16. **Ans. (b) Quinagolide**
    [Goodman & Gilman's Pharmacological Basis of Therapeutics- 12th ed; De Groot 7th ed pg 121; Pituitary Tumors in Pregnancy pg 75]

    Dopamine Receptor Agonists
    - *Bromocriptine:* A semisynthetic ergot alkaloid that interacts with D_2 receptors.
    - *Cabergoline:* A synthetic ergot derivative with a longer $t_{1/2}$, higher affinity, and greater selectivity for the D_2 receptor (approximately four times more potent) than bromocriptine.
    - *Quinagolide:* A non-ergot D_2 agonist.
    - *Pergolide:* An ergot derivative.
    - *Lisuride:* An ergot derivative.

17. **Ans. (b) Rifampicin**
    [Williams 13th ed pg 186; Greenspan's 9th ed]
    See discussion of Chapter 5, Question 3.

18. **Ans. (b) Insulin-calcitonin**

19. **Ans. (b) Delayed response and (c) Blunted nocturnal surge of TSH**
    [Williams 13th ed pg 161, 1807]
    - TRH stimulation test has been used for the differentiation of hypothalamic disease from pituitary disease. The typical pituitary response to TRH administration in patients with TRH deficiency is an enhanced and somewhat delayed peak, whereas the response with pituitary failure is subnormal or absent. In practice, the test is of limited value as the responses to TRH in hypothalamic and pituitary disease overlap so much that they cannot be used reliably for a differential diagnosis.
    - A delayed TSH response to TRH and a diminished nocturnal TSH surge are suggestive of dysfunction of the hypothalamic control of the thyroid axis and may represent a diagnosis of hidden central hypothyroidism.

20. **Ans. (b) Somatostatin**
    [Greenspan's 9th ed]

    The secretion of GH is predominantly mediated by two hypothalamic hormones: GHRH and somatostatin (GH-inhibiting hormone). These hypothalamic influences are regulated by an integrated system of neural, metabolic, and hormonal factors.

Factors affecting GH secretion	
Increase	*Decrease*
Physiologic Sleep Exercise Stress (physical or psychologic) Postprandial • Hyperaminoacidemia • Hypoglycemia (relative)	Postprandial hyperglycemia Elevated free fatty acids
Pharmacologic Hypoglycemia • Absolute: insulin or 2-deoxyglucose • Relative: postglucagon Hormones • GHRH • Ghrelin • Peptide (ACTH, α-MSH, vasopressin) • Estrogen Neurotransmitters, etc. • Alpha-adrenergic agonists (clonidine) • Beta-adrenergic antagonists (propranolol) • Serotonin precursors • Dopamine agonists (levodopa, apomorphine, bromocriptine) • GABA agonists (muscimol) • Potassium infusion • Pyrogens (pseudomonas endotoxin)	Hormones • Somatostatin • Growth hormone • Progesterone • Glucocorticoids Neurotransmitters, etc. • Alpha-adrenergic antagonists (phentolamine) • Beta-adrenergic agonists (isoproterenol) • Serotonin agonists (methysergide) • Dopamine antagonists (phenothiazines)

    Contd...

Contd...

Increase	Decrease
Pathologic Protein depletion and starvation Anorexia nervosa Ectopic production of GHRH Chronic renal failure Acromegaly • TRH • GnRH	Obesity Acromegaly; dopamine agonists Hypothyroidism Hyperthyroidism

21. **Ans. (c) Pit-1**
    [Williams 13th ed pg 179]

22. **Ans. (c) Pit-1**
    [Williams 13th ed pg 179]

23. **Ans. (a) Septo-optic dysplasia**
    [Williams 13th ed pg 990]
    See discussion of Chapter 4, Question 7.

24. **Ans. (c) Cabergoline**
    [Williams 13th ed pg 186]
    See discussion of Chapter 5, Question 3.

25. **Ans. (d) Hypertension**
    [Williams 13th ed pg 186]
    See discussion of Chapter 5, Question 3.

26. **Ans. (d) GH**
    [Williams 13th ed pg 190]

27. **Ans. (a) Increased FSH**
    [Williams 13th ed pg 261, 617]

28. **Ans. (d) Correlate with cortisol level**
    [Williams 13th ed pg 199, 201, 202; Greenspan's 9th ed]
    Episodic release of ACTH is independent of circulating cortisol levels (i.e. the magnitude of an ACTH impulse is not related to preceding plasma cortisol levels).

29. **Ans. (a) Change to cabergoline**
    [J Clin Endocrinol Metab, February 2011, 96(2):277-280]

30. **Ans. (d) *HESX1***
    [Williams 13th ed pg 180]
    See discussion of Chapter 4, Question 5.

31. **Ans. (a) Bromocriptine**
    [J Clin Endocrinol Metab, February 2011, 96(2):282]

32. **Ans. (c) Estrogen**
    [Williams 12th ed pg 78; Williams 13th ed pg 10, 1297]
    See discussion of Chapter 2, Question 6.

33. **Ans. (d) Cabergoline**
    [Williams 13th ed pg 262]

34. **Ans. (b) Cabergoline**
    [Williams 13th ed pg 186]
    See discussion of Chapter 5, Question 3.

35. **Ans. (b) 6**
    [Williams 13th ed pg 182]

36. **Ans. (b) Spontaneous recovery may occur**
    [Williams 13th ed pg 248, 249]

37. **Ans. (a) Alpha-methyldopa and (d) Fluoxetine**
    [Pituitary Tumors in Pregnancy pg 75]

38. **Ans. (e) Follicular thyroid carcinoma**
    [Williams 13th ed pg 270; Am J Med Genet A. 2017 Sep;173(9):2353-2358]

    GHRH hypersecretion may be seen in:
    - Hypothalamic tumor (e.g. hamartomas, choristomas, gliomas, and gangliocytomas)
    - Bronchial carcinoid
    - Pancreatic islet cell tumor
    - Small cell lung cancer
    - Adrenal adenoma
    - Medullary thyroid carcinoma
    - Pheochromocytoma
    - Endometrial cancer
    - Breast cancer.

39. **Ans. (d) Drug-induced hyperprolactinemia**
    [Williams 13th ed pg 186, 187, 261, 617]

40. **Ans. (d) A peak growth hormone concentration of 6 mU/L (2 µg/L) with insulin induced hypoglycemia**
    [Williams 13th ed pg 193-195]

41. **Ans. (c) ACTH**
    [Greenspan's 9th ed; Central Regulation of the Endocrine System pg 530]
    Dopamine ↑es GH, ↓es prolactin, ↓es TSH.

42. **Ans. (c) TSH**
    [Williams 13th ed pg 597]
    Ghrelin is a potent GH secretagogue. In addition, ghrelin acutely increases circulating PRL, ACTH, cortisol, and aldosterone levels.

43. **Ans. (b) Replacement of corticosteroids**
    [Williams 13th ed pg 250; De Groot 7th ed pg 197]

44. **Ans. (c) Melatonin**
    [Williams 13th ed pg 18, 19, 20, 123, 129, 137, 145, 152, 183, 188, 199-201, 207, 301, 492, 494-496, 595, 606, 704, 1256, 1267, 1269, 1270, 1703-1714; Clinical Chemistry, Immunology and Laboratory Quality Control: A Comprehensive Review for Board Preparation, Certification and Clinical Practice, pg 149]

45. **Ans. (a) Stimulation of protein synthesis**
    [Williams 13th ed pg 191]

46. **Ans. (a) Infertility**
    [De Groot 7th ed pg 194, 195]

47. **Ans. (d) Levothyroxine treatment**
    [Williams 13th ed pg 186; Endocrine Emergencies Recognition and Treatment pg 176, 181]
    See discussion of Chapter 5, Question 3.

48. **Ans. (a) Quinagolide**
    [Pituitary Tumors in Pregnancy pg 75; De Groot 7th ed pg 121]
    Option (a) is more appropriate than option (b).

49. **Ans. (b) Presence of ptosis is an indication for immediate surgery**
    [De Groot 7th ed pg 194; Clinical Endocrinology, 74, 13-15; Williams 13th pg 251; Endocrine Emergencies Recognition and Treatment pg 187, 188]

    MRI Findings in Hemorrhage
    - *Days 1–2 (acute phase):* Hyperintense on T1-weighted images and hypointense on T2-weighted. (MRI may fail to demonstrate hemorrhage during the acute phase 1).
    - *Days 3–15 (subacute phase):* Both T1 and T2-weighted signals appear bright.
    - *Days >15:* A fluid–fluid level may be observed in the mass due to sedimentation of blood products.

    MRI Findings in Infarct
    - Pituitary infarction without hemorrhage is low signal intensity with associated rim enhancement on T1 and T2-weighted MRI sequences.

50. **Ans. Both (c) Can have normal outcome and (e) Diabetes insipidus**
    [Williams 13th ed pg 249]

Pituitary Physiology and Diagnostic Evaluation | **49**

Diabetes insipidus, which is encountered in up to 20% of patients, has been attributed to posterior pituitary or stalk infiltration of the inflammatory process.

51. **Ans. (a) GHRH**
    [Williams 13th ed pg 194, 195, 1018, 1019]
    See discussions of Chapter 5, Question 52 and Chapter 17, Question 12. Although propranolol an pyridostigmine (in combination with GHRH) have also been mentioned among agents used for GH provocative testing, GHRH appears to be the most appropriate answer.

52. **Ans. (a) Increased HDL**
    [Williams 13th ed pg 194, 195; The Somatotrophic Axis in Brain Function pg 238]
    - The diagnosis of adult GHD is established by provocative testing of GH secretion.
    - Provocative tests include ITT, arginine, glucagon, clonidine, L-dopa, growth hormone–releasing peptide (GHRP), and GHRH, alone or in combination with arginine or pyridostigmine.
    - As provocative tests vary in the ability to evoke GH release, different diagnostic thresholds are used for different tests.
    - Validated diagnostic tests for the diagnosis of growth hormone deficiency in adults

Test	GH Threshold (µg/L)
Insulin-induced hypoglycemia	<5
Arginine-GHRH	<9
GHRP 6-GHRH	<15
GHRP 2-GHRH	<17
GHRP 2	<15
Glucagon	<3
Low IGF-1 and ≥3 PHDs	N/A

    - ITT is the gold standard test for GHD. Normal subjects respond to insulin-induced hypoglycemia with peak GH concentrations of > 5 µg/L. Severe GHD is defined by a peak GH response to hypoglycemia of less than 3 µg/L.
    - Also see discussion of Chapter 5, Question 1.

CHAPTER 6

Pituitary Masses and Tumors

QUESTIONS

1. Patient of macroprolactinoma on cabergoline treatment presented with headache, GTCS and altered sensorium, diagnosis is:
   a. Apoplexy
   b. Temporal lobe involvement
   c. Cavernous sinus involvement
   d. Optic chiasmal compression

2. Pegvisomant treatment monitoring by:
   a. Serial basal GH
   b. IGF serial measurement
   c. Post glucose GH levels
   d. Glucose clamp

3. A 14-year-old male with GH secreting pituitary adenoma—which of the following are not helpful in diagnosis?
   a. HT > 35D
   b. HT > 25D midparental
   c. MRI with adenoma
   d. IGF↑

4. Craniopharyngioma true is:
   a. Isolated peak 5–15 years
   b. Bimodal peak 5–15 and >50 years
   c. After 50 years
   d. Never occurs in 1st decade

5. GH level for acromegaly diagnosis after glucose suppression test:
   a. >1 mcg/L
   b. <1 mcg/L
   c. >4 mcg/L
   d. <4 mcg/L

6. Features of florid acromegaly are all except:
   a. Galactorrhea
   b. Visual field abnormalities
   c. Seborrhea
   d. Hypothyroidism

7. Bilateral adrenal hyperplasia due to a pituitary tumor, treatment can be all except:
   a. Octreotide
   b. Trans-sphenoidal surgery
   c. Bilateral adrenalectomy
   d. Radiotherapy

8. Rarest pituitary tumor is
   a. Corticotroph
   b. Lactotroph
   c. Nonfunctioning
   d. Somatotroph

9. True about suprasellar meningioma are all except:
   a. Isointense on T1 and T2
   b. 1/5th of all meningioma
   c. Calcification is seen
   d. Avascular hence easily removed during surgery

10. A 10-year-old child obesity growth failure, polyuria and suprasellar calcification, diagnosis:
    a. Hypothyroid
    b. Cushing
    c. Exogenous obesity
    d. Craniopharyngioma

11. Pegvisomant prevents:
    a. Release of GH from somatotrophs
    b. GHRH to GH
    c. Dimerization of GH receptor
    d. Tumor growth

12. Most common presentation of lymphocytic hypophysitis:
    a. DI
    b. Headache
    c. Visual symptoms
    d. Galactorrhea

13. Headache with pituitary tumor 1.5 mm, treatment should be:
    a. Gamma knife
    b. Trans-sphenoidal surgery
    c. Bromocriptine
    d. Somatostatin analogue

14. Most common presentation of gonadotroph adenoma:
    a. Clinically nonfunctioning adenoma
    b. Hypergonadism
    c. Hypogonadism
    d. Galactorrhea

15. Posterior pituitary radiation all of the following are seen except:
    a. Secondary malignancy
    b. Decreased cerebrovascular disease
    c. Optic neuritis
    d. Brain necrosis
    e. Hypopituitarism on follow-up

16. What is neuroimaging modality of choice for craniopharyngioma:
    a. CT head with contrast
    b. CT head without contrast
    c. MRI head with gadolinium contrast (w12th p1112)
    d. MRI head with and without gadolinium contrast

17. Which of the following is false
    a. Posterior pituitary appears white on T1 weighted images
    b. Sphenoid air has no signal
    c. Bone has high signal intensity
    d. CSF on T1 weighted image is black

18. Blood supply of anterior pituitary:
    a. Superior hypophyseal artery
    b. Inferior hypophyseal artery
    c. Hypothalamic portal plexus
    d. Internal capillary plexus (gomitoli)

19. Acromegaly:
    a. Post-glucose GH >1.0
    b. Random GH >1.0
    c. ↓IGF-1
    d. Fasting GH >1.0

20. Low IGF-1 is seen all except:
    a. Hypocortisolism
    b. Malnutrition
    c. Liver disease
    d. Uncontrolled DM
    e. Hypothyroidism

21. MC pituitary adenoma secretes:
    a. GH
    b. Prolactin
    c. ACTH
    d. TSH

22. Not true about pituitary adenoma:
    a. Hypointense on T1W MRI
    b. Hyperintense on T2W MRI
    c. No contrast enhancement with gadolinium
    d. Stalk deviation is seen

23. Which of the following is not seen in pituitary apoplexy?
    a. Fever
    b. Hypertension
    c. Bilateral visual disturbances
    d. Headache

24. Which is not true about acromegaly?
    a. Carney complex—autosomal dominant
    b. Gsα protein mutations
    c. Raised ICT is proportional to prolactin levels
    d. May be associated with MEN1

25. Tall stature with DM; which of the following tests is most useful?
    a. ACTH
    b. Somatomedin
    c. Cortisol
    d. TSH

26. All of the following are true about pituitary apoplexy except:
    a. Spontaneous in pre-existing adenoma
    b. Visual recovery inversely correlated with time lapsed before surgery
    c. Ptosis is an emergent indication for surgery
    d. Ring enhancing lesion

27. **Best therapy of macrosomatotropinoma:**
    a. Octreotide followed by surgery
    b. Surgery followed by octreotide
    c. Octreotide with pegvisomant
    d. Surgery with pegvisomant
    e. Surgery with octreotide with pegvisomant

28. **Sellar mass associated with:**
    a. Early loss of blue vision
    b. Binasal hemianopia
    c. Personality disorder
    d. Precocious puberty

29. **Oral therapy with which of the following may cause galactorrhea?**
    a. Bromocriptine
    b. Cabergoline
    c. Spironolactone
    d. Cimetidine
    e. Domperidone

30. **A 53-year-old male is suspected of having acromegaly. Which of the following is the best investigation to confirm the diagnosis?**
    a. 9 am growth hormone concentrations
    b. An insulin tolerance test with growth hormone concentrations
    c. Glucose tolerance test with growth hormone concentrations
    d. Growth hormone releasing hormone test
    e. Insulin-like growth factor-1 (IGF-1)

31. **A 56-year-old male presents with a 5-year history of increased sweats and change in shoe size. Examination reveals prognathism and macroglossia, with large hands. Blood pressure is 180/94 mm Hg but visual field examination is full to confrontation. Which of the following tests would be diagnostic?**
    a. Oral glucose tolerance test
    b. TRH test
    c. Insulin tolerance test
    d. Pituitary MRI
    e. IGF-1 concentration

32. **Which of the following is associated with a GH secreting pituitary tumor?**
    a. Gs-alpha subunit mutation
    b. Pit-1 mutation
    c. H-ras mutation
    d. Rb-1 mutation

33. **In acromegaly, visceralomegaly is not found in:**
    a. Liver
    b. Spleen
    c. Prostate
    d. Adrenal

34. **Which of the following statements is most appropriate about craniopharyngioma?**
    a. 10% are sellar
    b. Diabetes insipidus is first manifestation
    c. GH and gonadotropin deficiency are most
    d. Usually present after 50 years of age

35. **All of the following are true about treatment of craniopharyngioma except:**
    a. The dose of thyroxine is adjusted to achieve a TSH between 3 and 5
    b. Cortisol before T4 treatment
    c. Cortisol treatment can precipitate diabetes insipidus
    d. One of the side effects of surgery is obesity

36. **The best test to confirm acromegaly:**
    a. IGF-1
    b. Fasting GH level
    c. Response to TRH
    d. GH level during sleep
    e. GH level after infusion of arginine

37. **Optimal therapy for macrosomatotropinoma can be:**
    a. Surgery followed by octreotide
    b. Octreotide followed by surgery
    c. Surgery followed by pegvisomant
    d. Octreotide and pegvisomant
    e. Surgery and cabergoline

38. **Which one of the following is not true regarding lymphocytic hypophysitis?**
    a. Has an equal incidence in males and females
    b. Child could presents with diabetes insipidus
    c. Can only be diagnosed on biopsy
    d. Should be suspected in a peripartum females presenting with a pituitary mass
    e. May be managed conservatively

ANSWERS

1. **Ans. (a) Apoplexy**
   [Williams 13th ed pg 251]

2. **Ans. (b) IGF serial measurement**
   [Williams 13th ed pg 282; J Clin Endocrinol Metab, November 2014, 99(11):3942]
   - Pegvisomant is a GH-receptor antagonist, which competes with endogenous GH for binding at its receptor and blocks subsequent IGF-1 generation.
   - The antagonist does not target the GH-secreting pituitary tumor, and GH hypersecretion persists during drug administration.
   - Therefore measuring GH is not an efficacy marker.
   - IGF-1 measurement is the appropriate marker of patient responsiveness.

3. **Ans. (d) IGF↑**
   [Williams 13th ed pg 272]
   - Pituitary gigantism should be considered in children who are more than 3 standard deviations above normal mean height for age, or more than 2 standard deviations over their adjusted mean parental height.
   - The biochemical diagnosis is similar to that for acromegaly (i.e. GH levels are in excess of 1 μg/L after a glucose load and serum IGF-1 concentrations are elevated).
   - In children undergoing pubertal growth spurts, GH responses to glucose may be paradoxical and serum IGF-1 concentrations are often physiologically elevated.
   - Thus, the diagnosis requires clear-cut MRI evidence for a pituitary lesion.
   - Thus option (d) is the most appropriate response.

4. **Ans. (b) Bimodal peak 5–15 and >50 years**
   [Williams 13th ed pg 246]
   Bimodal age distribution, occurring in children between 5 and 14 years old and adults from 50 to 74 years of age.

5. **Ans. (a) >1 mcg/L**
   [J Clin Endocrinol Metab, November 2014, 99(11):3933]
   In patients with elevated or equivocal serum IGF-1 levels, the diagnosis of acromegaly is confirmed by lack of suppression of GH to<1 μg/L following documented hyperglycemia during an oral glucose load.

6. **Ans. (d) Hypothyroidism**
   [Williams 13th ed pg 272-275]

   Clinical Features of Acromegaly*
   - Local tumor effects
   - Pituitary enlargement

- Visual field defects
- Cranial nerve palsy
- Headache

Somatic Effects
- Acral enlargement
  - Thickening of soft tissues in hands and feet
- Musculoskeletal
  - Gigantism
  - Prognathism, maxillary widening, teeth separation
  - Jaw malocclusion
  - Arthralgias and arthritis
  - Carpal tunnel syndrome
  - Acroparesthesia
  - Proximal myopathy
  - Hypertrophy of frontal bones, cranial ridges
  - Facial coarsening, large fleshy lips and nose
- Skin
  - Hyperhidrosis
  - Oily
  - Skin tags
- Colon
  - Polyps
- Cardiovascular
  - Left ventricular hypertrophy
  - Asymmetric septal hypertrophy
  - Cardiomyopathy
  - Hypertension
  - Congestive heart failure
- Pulmonary
  - Sleep disturbances
  - Sleep apnea—central and obstructive
  - Narcolepsy
- Visceromegaly
  - Tongue
  - Thyroid
  - Salivary gland
  - Liver
  - Spleen
  - Kidney
  - Prostate

Endocrine-Metabolic Effects
- Reproductive
  - Menstrual abnormalities
  - Galactorrhea
  - Decreased libido, impotence, low sex hormone—blinding globulin

- Multiple endocrine neoplasia type 1 (MEN1)
  - Hyperparathyroidism
  - Pancreatic islet cell tumors
- Carbohydrates
  - Impaired glucose tolerance
  - Insulin resistance and hyperinsulinemia
  - Diabetes mellitus
- Lipids
  - Hypertriglyceridemia
- Minerals
  - Hypercalciuria, increased 1,25-hydroxyvitamin D3
  - Urinary hydroxyproline
- Electrolytes
  - Low renin
  - Increased aldosterone
- Thyroid
  - Low thyroxine-binding globulin
  - Goiter (diffuse/nodular toxic or nontoxic)
  - Graves' disease

Others
- Voice deepening
- Raynaud's phenomenon
- Exophthalmos, open-angle glaucoma
- Psychiatric
- ↓ quality of life.

7. **Ans. (a) Octreotide**
   [Williams 13th ed pg 510, 511; J Clin Endocrinol Metab, August 2015, 100(8):2808, 2820-2822; Endocrine Reviews, August 2015, 36(4):427-458]

   Cushing disease is characterized by bilateral adrenocortical hyperplasia due to ACTH secreting pituitary adenoma.

   Treatment Options of Cushing Disease
   - *First line treatment:*
     - Trans-sphenoidal surgery
   - *Second line therapeutic options:*
     - Repeat trans-sphenoidal surgery,
     - Radiotherapy,
     - Medical therapy (see discussion of Chapter 9, Question 8)
     - Bilateral adrenalectomy.

8. **Ans. (a) Corticotroph**
   [Williams 13th ed pg 258; Greenspan's 9th ed]

   Prolactinomas are the most common type, accounting for about 60% of primary pituitary tumors; GH hypersecretion occurs in approximately 20%; and ACTH excess in 10%. Hypersecretion of TSH, the gonadotropins, or alpha subunits is unusual. Nonfunctional tumors represent 10% of all pituitary adenomas, and some of these may in fact be gonadotropin-secreting or alpha subunit-secreting adenomas.

9. **Ans. (d) Avascular hence easily removed during surgery**
   [Williams 13th ed pg 246]

   Meningiomas
   - Meningiomas arise from arachnoid and meningioendothelial cells
   - Those occurring in the sellar and parasellar region account for about one fifth of all meningiomas
   - Well circumscribed
   - Secondary hyperprolactinemia occurs in up to half of these patients, who
   - Usually present with local mass effects—headache, visual disturbances, optic atrophy
   - On MRI, meningiomas are isodense on both T1- and T2-weighted imaging
   - Dural calcification may be evident on CT scanning
   - Because of their rich vascularization, these tumors pose an intraoperative risk for hemorrhage and a resultant higher surgical mortality rate.

10. **Ans. (d) Craniopharyngioma**
    [Williams 13th ed pg 246]

11. **Ans. (c) Dimerization of GH receptor**
    [De Groot 7th ed pg 224]

12. **Ans. (b) Headache**
    [Oxford Textbook of Endocrinology and Diabetes 2nd ed pg 248]

13. **Ans. (b) Trans-sphenoidal surgery**

14. **Ans. (a) Clinically nonfunctioning adenoma**
    [Williams 13th ed pg 265]
    - Most nonfunctioning or hormonally silent tumors arise from gonadotroph cells
    - Gonadotroph cell tumors most frequently present as clinically nonfunctioning masses
    - They usually express gonadotropin subunits detectable by immunohistochemistry and are not associated with elevated serum gonadotropins.

15. **Ans. (b) Decreased cerebrovascular disease**
    [Williams 13th ed pg 243, 244]

    Posterior Pituitary Radiation-Side Effects
    - *Hypopituitarism:* Within 10 years after radiation, up to 80% of patients may have gonadotroph, somatotroph, thyrotroph, or corticotroph deficits
    - Second brain tumors; occurs in <5%, e.g. Glioma

- Cerebrovascular disease
- Visual damage
- Brain necrosis
- Cognitive dysfunction

16. **Ans. (d) MRI head with and without gadolinium contrast**
    [Williams 13th ed pg 1132]

17. **Ans. (c) Bone has high signal intensity**
    [Williams 13th ed pg 235; www.mayfieldclinic.com/PE-MRI.htm; http://casemed.case.edu/clerkships/neurology/Web%20Neurorad/MRI%20Basics.htm]
    - The posterior pituitary lobe exhibits a discrete bright spot of high signal intensity on T1-weighted images
    - Air and hard bone do not give an MRI signal so these areas appear black.
    - Appearance of various tissues on MRI

Tissue	T1-weighted	T2-weighted
CSF	Dark	Bright
Brain-cortex	Gray	Light gray
Brain-white matter	Light	Dark gray
Fat (e.g. subcutaneous tissue, within bone marrow)	Bright	Light
Air (e.g. pharynx, sphenoid sinus)	Very dark	Very dark
Muscle	Gray	Dark gray
Inflammation	Dark	Bright

18. **Ans. (c) Hypothalamic portal plexus**
    [Williams 13th ed pg 177, 178]
    - The superior hypophyseal artery (branch from the internal carotid arteries) supply the hypothalamus, where they form a capillary network in the median eminence.
    - Long and short hypophyseal portal vessels originate from infundibular plexuses and the stalk, respectively.
    - These vessels form the hypothalamic-portal circulation, the predominant blood supply to the anterior pituitary gland.
    - A contractile internal capillary plexus (gomitoli) is derived from stalk branches of the superior hypophysial arteries.
    - Systemic arterial blood supply is maintained by inferior hypophyseal arterial branches, which predominantly supply the posterior pituitary.

19. **Ans. (a) Post-glucose GH >1.0**
    [J Clin Endocrinol Metab, November 2014, 99(11):3933]
    See discussion of Chapter 6, Question 5.

20. **Ans. (a) Hypocortisolism**
    [Williams 13th ed pg 195]

21. **Ans. (b) Prolactin**
    [Williams 13th ed pg 258; Greenspan's 9th ed]
    See discussion of Chapter 6, Question 8.

22. **Ans. (c) No contrast enhancement with gadolinium**
    [Williams 13th ed pg 236; Grainger and Allison's Diagnostic Radiology 5th ed]

23. **Ans. (b) Hypertension**
    [Endocrine Emergencies Recognition and Treatment pg 179]

    Pituitary Apoplexy Pathophysiology and Correlating Clinical Manifestations
    Leakage of blood or necrotic tissue into:
    - Subarachnoid space and/or basal cisterns: Features of subarachnoid hemorrhage or meningitis including hyperpyrexia, headache, nausea and/or vomiting, nuchal rigidity, altered consciousness
    - Surrounding brain parenchyma: Altered consciousness, seizures
    - Pituitary damage: Hypopituitarism, resolution of preexisting hyperfunctioning endocrinopathy.

    Pressure or compression on:
    - *Cavernous sinus:* Chemosis, proptosis
    - *Cranial nerve III:* Ptosis, mydriasis, diplopia due to medial rectus, superior rectus, and inferior oblique palsies
    - *Cranial nerve IV:* Head-tilt or diplopia due to superior oblique palsy
    - *Cranial nerve V (first and second divisions):* Facial paresthesia, loss of corneal reflex
    - *Cranial nerve VI:* Diplopia due to lateral rectus palsy
    - *Internal carotid and its branches:* Hemiplegia, unilateral focal hemispheric signs, altered consciousness, seizures
    - *Hypothalamus:* Hyperpyrexia, altered consciousness, impaired water balance, sympathetic dysregulation
    - *Optic tracts and/or chiasm:* Impaired visual acuity, visual field defects
    - *Sympathetic chain:* Horner's syndrome—ptosis, miosis, anhidrosis, loss of ciliospinal reflex, conjunctival erythema.

24. **Ans. (c) Raised ICT is proportional to prolactin levels**
    [Williams 13th ed pg 257, 269]

    Familial syndromes causing acromegaly
    - Multiple endocrine neoplasia type I
    - McCune—Albright syndrome
    - Familial acromegaly
    - Carney complex.

25. **Ans. (b) Somatomedin**
    Somatomedin = IGF

26. **Ans. (c) Ptosis is an emergent indication for surgery**
    [De Groot 7th ed pg 194; Clinical Endocrinology, 74, 13-15; Williams 13th 251; Endocrine Emergencies Recognition and Treatment pg 187, 188]
    See discussion of Chapter 5, Question 49.

27. (b) Surgery followed by octreotide
[J Clin Endocrinol Metab, November 2014, 99(11):3934-3935]

28. Ans. (c) Personality disorder
[Williams 13th ed pg 233]

Local Effects of an Expanding Pituitary, Parasellar, or Hypothalamic Mass

Impacted structure	Clinical effect
Pituitary	Growth failure, adult hyposomatotropism, hypogonadism, hypothyroidism, hypoadrenalism
Optic tract	Loss of red perception, bitemporal hemianopia, superior or bitemporal field defect, scotoma, blindness
Hypothalamus	Temperature dysregulation, obesity, diabetes insipidus; thirst, sleep; appetite, behavioral, and autonomic nervous system dysfunctions
Cavernous sinus	Ptosis, diplopia, ophthalmoplegia, facial numbness
Temporal lobe	Uncinate seizures
Frontal lobe	Personality disorder, anosmia
Central	Headache, hydrocephalus, psychosis, dementia, laughing seizures

29. Ans. (e) Domperidone
[Williams 13th ed pg 186; De Groot 7th ed pg 108]

See discussion of Chapter 5, Question 3.

Domperidone is a dopamine antagonist producing large rises in prolactin concentrations. Spironolactone has no effect on prolactin and Cimetidine produces hyperprolactinaemia only when given IV. Both bromocriptine and cabergoline are dopamine agonists and reduce prolactin.

Thus, option (e) is a better choice than option (d).

30. Ans. (c) Glucose tolerance test with growth hormone concentrations
[J Clin Endocrinol Metab, November 2014, 99(11):3933]

See discussion of Chapter 6, Question 5.

Although IGF-1 concentrations are elevated these are not diagnostic and may fall during illness.

31. (a) Oral glucose tolerance test
[J Clin Endocrinol Metab, November 2014, 99(11):3933]

See discussion of Chapter 6, Question 5.

32. Ans. (a) Gs-alpha subunit mutation
[Williams 13th ed pg 269]

33. **Ans. (d) Adrenal**
    [Williams 13th ed pg 272-275]
    See discussion of Chapter 6, Question 6.

34. **Ans. (c) GH and gonadotropin deficiency are most**
    [Williams 13th ed pg 162, 163, 245, 246, 996, 1131, 1132]
    Option (c) is a better choice than option (b).

    Craniopharyngioma
    - Result from metaplastic changes in rests of squamous epithelial cell rests that originate in Rathke's pouch and the craniopharyngeal duct during fetal development.
    - This tumor is a congenital malformation present at birth and gradually grows over the ensuing years.
    - Over 60% arise from within the sella, and others arise from parasellar cell rests.
    - Benign neoplasms.
    - Constitutes about 3% of all intracranial tumors and up to 10-15% of childhood brain tumors.
    - Most common pediatric tumor occurring in the sellar and parasellar area.
    - Most common brain tumor associated with hypothalamic-pituitary dysfunction.
    - They show a bimodal age distribution, occurring in children between 5 and 14 years old and adults from 50 to 74 years of age. Symptoms usually arise before the age of 20 years. Roughly 25% are diagnosed in patients over the age of 25.
    - *Variants:*
        - *Adamantinomatous:* More common variant (about 70% of cases) in children; usually contain both a cystic component (filled with a fluid which ranges from the consistency of machine oil to a shimmering, cholesterol-laden liquid) and a solid component (characterized by organized epithelial cells); have dysregulation of the Wingless-type MMTV integration site family signaling pathway (Wnt signaling pathway) and a mutation in the β-catenin gene *(CTNNB);* have a greater propensity to relapse
        - *Papillary:* More common variant in adults; typically papillary in nature, solid, and less likely to be calcified or cystic; has BRAF mutations; less aggressive.
    - They may also contain calcifications (about 70% of patients).
    - *Clinical features:*
        - Features of mass intracranial lesion and increased intracranial pressure: most common presentations, especially in children; include headache, projectile vomiting, papilledema, and somnolence;

weakness of one or more limbs, visual and olfactory hallucinations, seizures and dementia have been reported
- Visual defects from compression of the optic chiasm or nerves: especially in adults; asymmetric visual disturbances, visual field defects (including bilateral temporal field deficits), papilledema, and optic atrophy.
- If cavernous sinus invasion is present, other cranial nerves may also be involved.
- *Endocrine dysfunction:* Seen in 80%-90% of patients; 50%-80% have abnormalities of at least one anterior pituitary hormone at diagnosis- the most frequent hormone deficiencies are GH and gonadotropins, TSH and ACTH deficiency are also common; diabetes insipidus is present in 25% to 50% of patients and is often the first manifestation.
- The serum concentration of prolactin is normal or increased. Pituitary stalk compression or damage to hypothalamic dopaminergic neurons results in hyperprolactinemia.
- Delayed bone age is common and may point to the onset of tumor growth.
- *Imaging:*
  - MRI is the imaging modality of choice. A recommended examination includes T1-weighted thin sagittal and coronal sections through the sella and suprasellar regions, obtained before and after contrast administration. Cystic and solid components can be identified by MRI, and anatomic relationships can be delineated. The presence of hydrocephalus can be detected. T2-weighted and fluid attenuation inversion recovery (FLAIR) images are useful to further delineate cysts and are hyperintense.
  - Computed tomography scans can be useful to determine the presence of calcification (most children and about half of all adults exhibit characteristic flocculent or convex calcifications).
- *Treatment:*
  - Treatment may involve radical surgery, radiotherapy, or a combination of these modalities.
  - Smaller craniopharyngiomas, usually intrasellar, can be treated by trans-sphenoidal microsurgery, but larger or suprasellar masses usually require craniotomy and may result in partial or almost complete removal of the lesion. Postoperative irradiation is commonly used, especially if tumor resection was incomplete.
  - *Side effects of surgery:* Postoperative obesity (associated with increased appetite, as well as altered food intake-regulating hormones leptin and ghrelin), visual problems, anterior pituitary hormone deficits, diabetes insipidus, aberrant sleep patterns and even narcolepsy and daytime somnolence.
- *Outcome:* Although survival rates are high (92%) recurrences and progressions are frequent. Postoperative recurrence may occur in about 20% of patients.

35. **Ans. (a) The dose of thyroxine is adjusted to achieve a TSH between 3 and 5**

36. **Ans. (a) IGF-1**
    [J Clin Endocrinol Metab, November 2014, 99(11):3933]
    See discussion of Chapter 6, Question 5.
    Although the most appropriate answer amongst the options is Ser. IGF-1 levels although glucose suppressed GH levels < 1 mcg/L is the confirmatory test.

37. **Ans. (a) Surgery followed by octreotide**
    [J Clin Endocrinol Metab, November 2014, 99(11):3934-3935]

38. **Ans. (a) Has an equal incidence in males and females**
    [Williams 13th ed pg 248, 249; De Groot 7th ed pg 194]

CHAPTER 7

Posterior Pituitary

QUESTIONS

1. SIADH is characterized by all except:
   a. Hypouricemia
   b. Decreased urine osmolality
   c. Euvolemic hyponatremia
   d. Decreased ECF osmolality

2. Which of the following criteria (urine osmolarity after fluid deprivation: urine osmolarity after desmopressin) after water deprivation test is diagnostic of central DI?
   a. <300:>750
   b. >750:>750
   c. 300–750:<750
   d. >300:<300

3. Desmopressin as compared to AVP (Renal antidiuretic; vasopressor effect)
   a. Increased; decreased
   b. Equal; equal
   c. Decreased; increased
   d. Decreased; decreased

4. SIADH is associated with all except:
   a. Encephalitis, meningitis
   b. Bronchogenic ca
   c. Urine osmolarity< plasma osmolarity
   d. Clinical euvolemia

5. Features of SIADH are all except:
   a. M/C cause of euvolemic hypo-osmolarity
   b. Dehydration
   c. Does not cause edema
   d. Natriuresis

6. m/c mutation in male congenital nephrogenic DI:
   a. V1
   b. V2
   c. AP2
   d. All are equally prevalent

7. **Drug of choice for DI in pregnancy:**
   a. AVP
   b. Lysine-VP
   c. DDAVP (Desmopressin)
   d. Carbamazepine

8. **Not used in DI:**
   a. Clofibrate
   b. Carbamazepine
   c. Lithium
   d. Chlorpropamide

9. **SIADH is seen in:**
   a. Hypothyroidism
   b. Ca lung
   c. INH
   d. Rifampicin

10. **Nephrogenic DI is a feature of all except:**
    a. Hypocalcemia including primary hypoparathyroidism
    b. Hypokalemia
    c. Cushing's syndrome
    d. Lithium

11. **All of the following are true about SIADH except:**
    a. No edema with postural hypotension
    b. Edema with postural hypotension
    c. Decrease uric acid, BUN
    d. Increased urine sodium

12. **Management of SIADH includes:**
    a. Daily Na⁺ measurement
    b. Daily weight measurement
    c. Water intake 300–1000 ml
    d. Desmopressin nasal spray

13. **DIDMOAD syndrome include:**
    a. DM
    b. DI
    c. Optic atrophy
    d. All of the above

14. **Drugs causing SIADH are all except:**
    a. Vincristine
    b. Chlorpropamide
    c. Carbamazepine
    d. Rifampicin

15. **Drugs causing DI include all except:**
    a. Lithium
    b. Amphotericin B
    c. Ciprofloxacin
    d. Aminoglycoside

16. **DI is not associated with which of the following congenital malformation:**
    a. Septo-optic dysplasia
    b. Holoprosencephaly
    c. Ectopic pituitary
    d. Renal cyst
    e. PCKD

17. **Vasopressin is most sensitive to:**
    a. Osmolality
    b. Nausea
    c. BP
    d. Blood volume

18. **Most severe osteogenesis imperfecta:**
    a. Ia
    b. V
    c. Ib
    d. III
    e. IV

19. **Uric acid in all except:**
    a. Metobolic syndrome
    b. SIADH
    c. Obesity
    d. Pre-eclampsia

20. **Serum Na^{2+} 128, Blood sugar 630 mg/dl, causes of $\downarrow Na^+$:**
    a. Pseudohyponatremia
    b. Dilutional hyponatremia
    c. Depletional hyponatremia
    d. None of the above

21. **Case of ca breast with depression; presented with Polyuria and dehydration; lab inv. reveal Na-149, K-3.6, urine osmolality-150 mOsmol/L; diagnosis is:**
    a. Psychogenic polydipsia
    b. Nephrogenic DI
    c. Central DI
    d. SIADH

22. **Case of oat cell ca with altered sensorium; lab inv. reveal hyponatremia, high urine osmolality; possible diagnosis is:**
    a. SIAD
    b. Cushing's syndrome
    c. DI

23. **Nonrenal actions of AVP include all except:**
    a. Stimulates ACTH
    b. Glycogenolysis
    c. Smooth muscle contraction
    d. Stimulates thirst

24. **Drugs causing nephrogenic DI include all except:**
    a. Lithium
    b. Carbamazepine
    c. Foscarnet
    d. Rifampicin

25. **Vasopressin is the same hormone as:**
    a. Cortisol
    b. Epinephrine
    c. ADH
    d. hGH
    e. Oxytocin

26 **Oxytocin is secreted by the:**
    a. Adenohypophysis
    b. Neurohypophysis
    c. Zona glomerulosa
    d. Pars intermedia
    e. Cervix

27. **Thirst is stimulated by:**
    a. Increase in plasma osmolality and volume
    b. Increase in plasma osmolality and decrease in volume
    c. Decrease in osmolality and increase in volume
    d. Decrease in plasma osmolality and volume

28. **Which one of the following couldn't cause inappropriate secretion of vasopressin from posterior pituitary gland?**
    a. Pulmonary TB
    b. Addison's disease
    c. Post operative
    d. Bronchial ca
    e. Lymphoma

29. **Which of the following is a feature of SIADH, except?**
    a. Increased urinary osmolality compared with plasma osmolality
    b. Hyponatremia
    c. Decreased serum osmolality
    d. Increased renal sodium excretion
    e. Responds to chlorpropromide

ANSWERS

1. **Ans. (b) Decreased urine osmolality**
   [Williams 13th ed pg 316, 317]

2. **Ans. (a) <300:>750**
   [Indian Journal of Endocrinology and Metabolism, Jan-Feb 2016, Vol 20, Issue 1 pg 13]
   Interpretation of the water deprivation test and the desmopressin challenge test in the diagnosis of diabetes insipidus

Diagnosis	Urine osmolality (mOsm/kg)	
	After fluid deprivation	After desmopressin
Central diabetes insipidus (CDI)	<300	>750
Nephrogenic diabetes insipidus (NDI)	<300	<300
Primary polydipsia (PP)	>750	–
Consider partial CDI or partial NDI or PP	300–750	<750

3. **Ans. (a) Increased; decreased**
   [Williams 13th ed pg 310]
   Desmopressin, a synthetic analogue of vasopressin characterized by
   - Markedly ↓ed pressor activity
   - ↑ed half-life
   - ↑ed specificity for antidiuresis (2000 times)

4. **Ans. (c) Urine osmolarity< plasma osmolarity**
   [Williams 13th ed pg 316-318; European Journal of Endocrinology (2014) 170, G15, G16]

   Common Causes of the Syndrome of Inappropriate Antidiuretic Hormone Secretion (SIADH)
   - Tumors
     - Pulmonary/mediastinal (bronchogenic carcinoma, mesothelioma, thymoma)
     - Nonchest (duodenal carcinoma, pancreatic carcinoma, ureteral/prostate carcinoma, uterine carcinoma, nasopharyngeal carcinoma, leukemia, lymphomas)
   - Central nervous system disorders
     - Mass lesions (tumors, brain abscesses, subdural hematoma)
     - Inflammatory diseases (encephalitis, meningitis, systemic lupus erythematosus, acute intermittent porphyria, multiple sclerosis)
     - Degenerative/demyelinative diseases (Guillain-Barré syndrome, spinal cord lesions)

- Miscellaneous (subarachnoid hemorrhage, head trauma, acute psychosis, delirium tremens, pituitary stalk section, transsphenoidal adenomectomy, hydrocephalus)
- Drug-Related
  - Stimulated release of AVP (nicotine, phenothiazines, tricyclics)
  - Direct renal effects or potentiation of AVP antidiuretic effects (dDAVP, oxytocin, prostaglandin synthesis inhibitors)
  - Mixed or uncertain actions (ACE inhibitors, carbamazepine and oxcarbazepine, chlorpropamide, clofibrate, clozapine, cyclophosphamide, 3,4-methylenedioxymethamphetamine [ecstasy], omeprazole; serotonin reuptake inhibitors, vincristine)
- Pulmonary
  - Infections (tuberculosis, acute bacterial and viral pneumonia, aspergillosis, empyema)
  - Mechanical/ventilatory causes (acute respiratory failure, COPD, positive-pressure ventilation)
- *Other causes:*
  - Acquired immunodeficiency syndrome (AIDS) and AIDS-related complex
  - Prolonged strenuous exercise (marathon, triathlon, ultramarathon, hot-weather hiking)
  - Senile atrophy
  - Idiopathic

Clinical Criteria to Diagnose SIADH
- Decreased effective osmolality of the ECF (plasma osmolality <275 mOsm/kg H_2O)
- Inappropriate urinary concentration at some level of hypo-osmolality (urine osmolality >100 mOsm/kg H_2O)
- Clinical euvolemia
- Elevated urinary sodium excretion with normal salt and water intake (Urine sodium concentration >30 mmol/L)
- Absence of other potential causes of euvolemic hypo-osmolality, notably, hypothyroidism, hypocortisolism, and diuretic use

Other supportive criteria
- Inappropriately elevated plasma vasopressin level in relation to plasma osmolality
- Hypouricemia (serum uric acid <4 mg/dL)
- Serum urea <21.6 mg/dL
- Failure to correct hyponatraemia after 0.9% saline infusion
- Fractional sodium excretion >0.5%
- Fractional urea excretion >55%
- Fractional uric acid excretion >12%
- Correction of hyponatremia through fluid restriction

Posterior Pituitary | **71**

5. **Ans. (b) Dehydration**
   [Williams 13th ed pg 316, 317]

6. **Ans. (b) V2**
   [Williams 13th ed pg 312]

   Causes of Congenital Nephrogenic DI
   - Mutation of the V2 receptor:
     - X-linked recessive
     - Accounts for 90% of the cases
   - Mutation of the aquaporin-2 water channels
     - Autosomal recessive, may be autosomal dominant.

7. **Ans. (c) DDAVP (Desmopressin)**
   [Williams 13th ed pg 311]

8. **Ans. (c) Lithium**
   [Williams 13th ed pg 309]

   Therapeutic Agents for Treatment of Diabetes Insipidus
   - Water
   - *Water-retaining agents:*
     - L-Arginine vasopressin
     - Desmopressin, 1-(3-mercaptopropionic acid)-8-D-arginine vasopressin
     - Chlorpropamide
     - Carbamazepine*
     - Clofibrate*
     - Indomethacin.
   - *Natriuretic agents:*
     - Thiazide diuretics
     - Amiloride
     - Indapamide.

9. **Ans. (b) Ca lung**
   [Williams 13th ed pg 316-318; European Journal of Endocrinology (2014) 170, G16]
   See discussion of Chapter 7, Question 4.
   Other potential causes of euvolemic hypoosmolality like hypothyroidism should be ruled out before the diagnosis of SIADH can be made.

10. **Ans. (a) Hypocalcemia including primary hypoparathyroidism**
    [Harrison's Endocrinology 3rd ed pg 53 Greenspan's 9th ed; Williams 13th ed pg 504]

Causes of Acquired Nephrogenic Diabetes Insipidus
- Drugs
  - Lithium
  - Demeclocycline
  - Methoxyflurane
  - Amphotericin B
  - Aminoglycosides
  - Cisplatin
  - Rifampin
  - Foscarnet
- Metabolic
  - Hypercalcemia, hypercalciuria
  - Hypokalemia
- Obstruction (ureter or urethra)
- Vascular
  - Sickle cell disease and trait
  - Ischemia (acute tubular necrosis)
- Granulomas
  - Neurosarcoid
- Neoplasms
  - Sarcoma
- Infiltration
  - Amyloidosis
- Pregnancy
- PCKD
- Idiopathic

Glucocorticcoids can cause free water clearance by antagonism of the action of vasopressin.

11. **Ans. (b) Edema with postural hypotension**
    [Williams 13th ed pg 316, 317]
    See discussion of Chapter 7, Question 4.

12. **Ans. (a) Daily Na⁺ measurement**
    [Williams 13th ed pg 322, 324]

13. **Ans. (d) All of the above**
    [Williams 13th ed pg 1773]
    DIDMOAD syndrome include diabetes insipidus, diabetes mellitus, progressive bilateral optic atrophy, and sensorineural deafness.

14. **Ans. (d) Rifampicin**
    [Williams 13th ed pg 318; European Journal of Endocrinology (2014) 170, G16]
    See discussion of Chapter 7, Question 4.

15. **Ans. (c) Ciprofloxacin**
    [Harrison's Endocrinology 3rd ed pg 53]
    See discussion of Chapter 7, Question 10.

16. **Ans. (d) Renal cyst**
    [Harrison's Endocrinology 3rd ed pg 53]

    ### Causes of Pituitary Diabetes Insipidus
    Acquired
    - Head trauma (closed and penetrating)
    - Neoplasms
      - Primary
        - Craniopharyngioma
        - Pituitary adenoma (suprasellar)
        - Dysgerminoma
        - Meningioma
      - Metastatic (lung, breast)
      - Hematologic (lymphoma, leukemia)
    - Granulomas
      - Neurosarcoid
      - Histiocytosis
      - Xanthoma disseminatum
    - Infectious
      - Chronic meningitis
      - Viral encephalitis
      - Toxoplasmosis
    - Inflammatory
      - Lymphocytic infundibuloneurohypophysitis
      - Wegener's granulomatosis
      - Lupus erythematosus
      - Scleroderma
    - Chemical toxins
      - Tetrodotoxin
      - Snake venom
    - Vascular
      - Sheehan's syndrome
      - Aneurysm (internal carotid)
      - Aortocoronary bypass
      - Hypoxic encephalopathy
    - Pregnancy (vasopressinase)
    - Idiopathic

    Congenital Malformations
    - Septo-optic dysplasia
    - Midline craniofacial defects
    - Holoprosencephaly
    - Hypogenesis, ectopia of pituitary

Genetic
- Autosomal dominant (AVP-neurophysin gene)
- Autosomal recessive (AVP-neurophysin gene)
- Autosomal recessive—Wolfram (4p – WFS 1 gene)
- X-linked recessive (Xq28)
- Deletion chromosome 7q

Also see discussion of Chapter 7, Question 10.

17. **Ans. (a) Osmolality**
    [Williams 13th ed pg 302, 303]

18. **Ans. (d) III**
    [De Groot 7th ed pg 1180, 1181; Harrison's Principles of Internal Medicine pg 2508; http://www.oif.org/site/PageServer?pagename=AOI_Types]
    - OI Type I is the mildest and most common form
    - OI Type II is the most severe form
    - OI Type III is the most severe type among children who survive the neonatal period.

    Also see discussion of Chapter 19, Question 29.

19. **Ans. (b) SIADH**
    [Williams 13th ed pg 317, Harrison's Principles of Internal Medicine 19th ed pg 431 e-2]

    SIADH is characterized by hypouricemia.

    Causes of Hyperuricemia
    Urate Overproduction
    - Primary idiopathic
    - HPRT deficiency
    - PRPP synthetase overactivity
    - Hemolytic process
    - Lymphoproliferative diseases
    - Myeloproliferative diseases
    - Polycythemia vera
    - Psoriasis
    - Paget's disease
    - Glycogenosis III, V and VII
    - Rhabdomyolysis
    - Exercise
    - Alcohol
    - Obesity
    - Purine-rich diet

    Decreased Uric Acid Excretion
    - Primary idiopathic
    - Renal insufficiency
    - Polycystic kidney disease

- Diabetes insipidus
- Hypertension
- Acidosis
  - Lactic acidosis
  - Diabetic ketoacidosis
- Starvation ketosis
- Berylliosis
- Sarcoidosis
- Lead intoxication
- Hyperparathyroidism
- Hypothyroidism
- Toxemia of pregnancy
- Bartter's syndrome
- Down syndrome
- Drug ingestion
  - Salicylates (<2 g/d)
  - Diuretics
  - Alcohol
  - Levodopa
  - Ethambutol
  - Pyrazinamide
  - Nicotinic acid
  - Cyclosporine

Combined Mechanism
- Glucose-6-phosphatase deficiency
- Fructose-1-phosphate aldolase deficiency
- Alcohol
- Shock

20. **Ans. (b) Dilutional hyponatremia**
    [European Journal of Endocrinology (2014) 170, G12]
    In hyperglycemia-induced hyponatremia, hyponatremia is caused by dilution due to hyperosmolality.

21. **Ans. (c) Central DI**

22. **Ans. (a) SIAD**
    [Williams 13th ed pg 316-318]
    See discussion of Chapter 7, Question 4.

23. **Ans. (d) Stimulates thirst**
    [Harrison's Endocrinology 3rd ed pg 51, 52; Williams 13th ed pg 302]
    - The most important physiologic action of AVP is to reducing water excretion by promoting concentration of urine. This is achieved by increasing the hydro-osmotic permeability of cells that line the distal tubule and medullary collecting ducts of the kidney

- At high concentrations, AVP also—
  - Causes contraction of smooth muscle in blood vessels and in the gastrointestinal tract,
  - Induces of glycogenolysis in the liver,
  - Potentiates adrenocorticotropic hormone (ACTH) release by corticotropin-releasing factor,
  - Stimulate factor VIII and von Willebrand factor production.

24. **Ans. (b) Carbamazepine**
    [Williams 13th ed pg 318; European Journal of Endocrinology (2014) 170, G16; Harrison's Endocrinology 3rd ed pg 53; Greenspan's 9th ed]
    See discussions of Chapter 7, Questions 4, 8 and 10.

25. **Ans. (c) ADH**
    [Williams 13th ed pg 301]

26. **Ans. (b) Neurohypophysis**
    [Williams 13th ed pg 300]

27. **Ans. (b) Increase in plasma osmolality and decrease in volume**
    [Williams 13th ed pg 302, 304; Harrison's Endocrinology 3rd ed pg 52]
    - Vasopressin can be stimulated by
      - Increases in osmolality of the ECF,
      - Decreases in intravascular volume or pressure,
      - Nausea,
      - Acute hypoglycemia,
      - Glucocorticoid deficiency,
      - Smoking,
      - Hyperangiotensinemia.
    - Similar to vasopressin, thirst can be stimulated by increases in osmolality of the ECF or by decreases in intravascular volume.

28. **Ans. (b) Addison's disease**
    [Williams 13th ed pg 318; European Journal of Endocrinology (2014) 170, G16]
    See discussion of Chapter 7, Question 4.
    Other potential causes of euvolemic hypoosmolality like hypocortisolism should be ruled out before a diagnosis of SIADH can be made.

29. **Ans. (e) Responds to chlorpropromide**
    [Williams 13th ed pg 316-318; European Journal of Endocrinology (2014) 170, G15, G16]
    See discussion of Chapter 7, Question 4.

CHAPTER 8

Thyroid

QUESTIONS

1. Iodine in thyroid storm is used:
   a. Before antithyroid drugs
   b. After antithyroid drugs
   c. Never used
   d. Can be used before or after antithyroid drugs

2. Thyrotoxic crisis can be precipitated by all except:
   a. Vigorous palpation   b. Radioiodine
   c. Sedative   d. DKA

3. After radioiodine therapy with I131, a lady can safely conceive after a minimum time gap of:
   a. 2 weeks   b. 2 months
   c. 6 weeks   d. 6 months

4. Indirectly support diagnosis of myxedema are:
   a. Hypernatremia   b. Increased CPK
   c. Hypocholesterolemia   d. All

5. D/D between subacute thyroiditis and thyrotoxicosis factitia:
   a. Thyroid scan   b. USG neck
   c. S. Thyroglobulin   d. Anti TPO antibody

6. Pt. of AF started on Amiodarone therapy. After a few weeks total T4 elevated, free T4 elevated, free T3 normal, TSH normal. Diagnosis is:
   a. Type 1 AIT
   b. Type 2 AIT
   c. Displacement of thyroid hormone from binding proteins by amiodarone
   d. Expected normal response

7. In Amiodarone, content of iodine is:
   a. 17%
   b. 27%
   c. 37%
   d. 47%
8. Thyroid stores are sufficient to maintain euthyroid state for:
   a. 25 d
   b. 50 d
   c. 75 d
   d. 100 d
9. TBG binding increase in all except:
   a. Active acromegaly
   b. Estrogen Rx
   c. Pregnancy
   d. Tamoxifen
10. Amino acid in thyroid hormone is:
    a. Tyrosine
    b. Phenylalanine
    c. Lysine
    d. Isoleucine
11. S/E of Thionamide are all except:
    a. Skin rash
    b. Hepatotoxicity
    c. Arthralgia
    d. Leucocytosis
12. Thyroxine dose in children < 1 yr:
    a. 1–5 mcg/kg/day
    b. 5–10 mcg/kg/day
    c. 11–15 mcg/kg/day
    d. 16–20 mcg/kg/day
13. S/E of thyroxine therapy are all except:
    a. Benign intracranial hypertension in children
    b. Acute psychosis in children
    c. SIADH
    d. Osteoporosis with over treatment
14. True about PTC histopathology are all except:
    a. Nuclear enlargement
    b. Dark chromatin
    c. Nuclear grooving
    d. Nuclear crowding
15. All of the following are indicative of aggressiveness except:
    a. Psammoma body
    b. Age > 45 years
    c. LN involvement
    d. Multifocality
16. Amiodarone induced thyroiditis is associated with all except:
    a. Increased IL6
    b. Increased CRP
    c. Increased vascularity
    d. TPO -ve
17. Mother with Graves' disease. Test to prevent neonatal hyperthyroidism:
    a. Antibody to TSHR
    b. T3/T4
    c. Anti TPO
    d. Ser. TSH
18. Graves' disease is associated with all except:
    a. Soft/firm goitre
    b. Pressure symptom
    c. Ophthalmopathy
    d. Bruit

19. **Goitre with decreased RAIU all except:**
    a. Subacute thyroiditis
    b. Graves' disease
    c. Amiodarone induced thyrotoxicosis
    d. Chronic Lymphocytic thyroiditis

20. **Subacute thyroiditis is associated with all except:**
    a. ↑ESR
    b. ↑thyroglobulin
    c. Anti-TPO antibodies
    d. Upto 50% of patients develop residual hypothyroidism

21. **Cross placenta:**
    a. T3   b. T4
    c. TSH   d. TRH

22. **Sheehan's syndrome monitoring treatment:**
    a. Total T3   b. Total T4
    c. Free T3/T4   d. TSH

23. **Struma ovarii:**
    a. Thyrotoxicosis
    b. Goitre
    c. Increased uptake of Radioiodine
    d. Ovarian cancer

24. **Deiodinase contains:**
    a. Magnesium   b. Chromium
    c. Selenium   d. Iodine

25. **Thyrotoxic periodic paralysis is characterized by all except:**
    a. Intermittent
    b. Precipitated by carbohydrate load
    c. Increased CPK enzyme of muscle origin
    d. More common in Caucasians than Asians

26. **Least lymph node involve out in which thyroid Ca:**
    a. Papillary   b. Follicular
    c. Medullary   d. Anaplastic

27. **Indication of therapy in subclinical hypothyroid include all except:**
    a. Obesity
    b. Anti TPO Antibody positive
    c. Irregular cycle
    d. Infertility

28. **Familial dysalbuminemic hyperthyroxinemia is characterized by all except:**
    a. T3 normal   b. FT4 normal
    c. AD condition   d. TBG increased

29. **True about TBG are all except:**
    a. T4 has 15–20 times more affinity than T3
    b. Increased TBG seen in hepatic failure
    c. T4 binds to prealbumen
    d. Estrogen, acute hepatitis increase levels of TBG

30. **Low RAIU is seen in all except:**
    a. Graves' disease
    b. Hashimoto's thyroiditis
    c. Amiodarone induced thyroiditis
    d. Chronic lymphocytic thyroiditis

31. **Consumption hypothyroidism is due to:**
    a. Increased D3 in hemangioma
    b. Overexpression of D1
    c. Central in nature
    d. Increased intake of soya products causing decreased T4 absorption

32. **Iodine is not used in treatment:**
    a. Endemic goitre
    b. Dehalogenase deficiency
    c. TSH receptor defect
    d. NIS defect

33. **In which condition thyroid is visible on Tc scan but not on radio-iodine scan:**
    a. NIS defect
    b. Organification defect
    c. Thyroglobulin synthesis defect
    d. None of the above

34. **Characteristic histopathologic finding in subacute thyroiditis:**
    a. Fibrous tissue
    b. Multinucleate cells
    c. Neutrophil sheets
    d. Lymphocyte sheets

35. **NIS is seen in all except:**
    a. Lactating breast
    b. Salivary glands
    c. Colon
    d. Placenta

36. **"Struma Ovarii", all except:**
    a. Ovarian teratoma
    b. Thyrotoxicosis
    c. Low RAIU seen
    d. Goitre

37. **In papillary ca thyroid, post thyroidectomy with radio ablation, thyroglobulin level should be:**
    a. <1 ng/mL
    b. <2 ng/mL
    c. <5 ng/mL
    d. <10 ng/mL

38. **All are true in subacute thyroiditis except:**
    a. Increased T4
    b. Increased ESR
    c. Increased thyroglobulin
    d. Anti TPO +ve

39. **In endemic goiter/MNG, I2 causes hyperthyroidism, this is called:**
    a. Jod-Basedow effect
    b. Wolff-Chaikoff block
    c. Graves' effect
    d. Stunning

40. Medullary ca thyroid, most common mutation is:
    a. RET
    b. RAS
    c. Rb
    d. p53
41. Which of the following is on the other arm heterodimer in thyroid nuclear receptor?
    a. RXR
    b. VDR
    c. c-myc
    d. LXR
42. Radiological manifestation of congenital hypothyroidism all except:
    a. Delayed closure of anterior fontanelle
    b. Slipped capital femoral epiphyses
    c. Deciduous teeth
    d. Epiphyseal dysgenesis
43. Thyroiditis is caused by all except:
    a. Bromocriptine therapy
    b. Bacteria
    c. Fungus
    d. Viruses
44. Iodine therapy is useful in all except:
    a. TSH receptor mutation
    b. Mild NIS defect
    c. Dehalogenase enzyme deficiency
    d. Endemic goiter
45. Most sensitive test for detection of TSH-R stimulating antibodies:
    a. Human thyroid follicular cell
    b. HELA transfected with TSH-R
    c. CHO transfected with TSH-R
    d. FRTL-5
46. Graves' disease associated with all except:
    a. Decreased RAIU
    b. Soft and diffuse goiter
    c. Surgery for pressure effects
    d. Clinically infiltrative ophthalmopathy seen in 50%
47. False about TBG:
    a. T4 binds 20 times more than T3
    b. TBG increases in pregnancy and acute hepatitis
    c. Hepatic failure increases TBG
    d. Salicylates, phenytoin, furosemide competes with T4 for binding to TBG
48. Dehalogenases contain:
    a. Bromide
    b. Selenium
    c. Chromium
    d. Mg
49. Which is not true?
    a. T4 bind to TBG 10–15 times more than T3
    b. T3 affinity with receptor 10–15 times more than T4
    c. t1/2 of T4 is 6.7 days
    d. fT4–0.2%; fT3–0.03%

50. **Propranolol does not help in which manifestation of hyperthyroidism?**
    a. SVT
    b. Sweating
    c. Lid retraction
    d. Oxygen consumption rate

51. **5'-deiodinase converts:**
    a. T4→T3
    b. T4→rT3
    c. rT3→T4
    d. T3→T4

52. **↑T3 and ↑T4 in all except:**
    a. Increased TBG
    b. Thyroid hormone resistance
    c. Severe hyperthyroidism
    d. Phenytoin

53. **↓T3 and ↓T4 in all except:**
    a. Decreased TBG
    b. Carbamazepine
    c. Severe systemic illness
    d. OCP intake

54. **Increased T4 and decreased T3 in all except:**
    a. Dysalbuminemic hyperthyroxinemia
    b. Amiodarone
    c. Oral cholecystographic agents
    d. None of the above

55. **TPO is:**
    a. Hemeprotein
    b. Selenoprotein
    c. Cuproprotein
    d. Albumenprotein

56. **Ideal treatment of choice for toxic adenoma:**
    a. Subtotal thyroidectomy
    b. Block replacement
    c. Radioiodine
    d. Hemithyroidectomy

57. **Thyroid changes in pregnancy, true all except:**
    a. Increased TBG
    b. Decreased D3 (type-3 deiodinase)
    c. Increased hCG
    d. Increase in the thyroid gland size by 18%

58. **Thyroid scan safe in:**
    a. Low dose I-131
    b. High dose I-131
    c. Low dose I-123
    d. Fluoroscan

59. **Superior thyroid artery arises from:**
    a. External carotid artery
    b. Common carotid
    c. Internal carotid
    d. Subclavian

60. **Increased in thyrotoxicosis all except:**
    a. Lp (a)
    b. Ferritin
    c. SHBG
    d. vWF

61. **T½ of thyroxine is:**
    a. 1 day
    b. 4 days
    c. 7 days
    d. 14 days

62. Stored thyroid stores sufficient for:
    a. 10 days   b. 30 days
    c. 50 days   d. 40 days

63. Which of the following is immunogenic?
    a. GH   b. Cholesterol
    c. Serotonin   d. Thyroxine

64. False +ve hypothyroidism is seen in:
    a. Cushing's   b. Addisons'
    c. Acromegaly   d. T2DM

65. Seen in craniosynostosis:
    a. Ectopic thyroid
    b. Thyroid hormone dysfunction
    c. Atrophic thyroid
    d. Excess T4 treatment

66. Decreased uptake in all except:
    a. Subacute thyroiditis
    b. Primary hypothyroidism
    c. Chronic diarrhea
    d. Exogenous thyroid administration

67. Increased uptake in all except:
    a. Jod-Basedow
    b. Trophoblastic tumors
    c. TSH secreting melanoma
    d. Graves

68. Freely permeable through placenta:
    a. Iodine   b. TSH
    c. T4   d. PTU

69. Starting dose of carbimazole in newborns:
    a. 1 mg/kg   b. 2 mg/kg
    c. 3 mg/kg   d. 4 mg/kg

70. 3rd generation TSH bioassay measure:
    a. 0.4   b. 0.04
    c. 0.004   d. 0.0004

71. In Graves' disease seen is all except:
    a. Urinary incontinence
    b. Oliguria
    c. Hypoglycemia
    d. Pernicious anemia

72. Goitre is absent in Graves' disease in:
    a. 3%   b. 10%
    c. 20%   d. 50%

73. Blood manifestations of Graves' disease all except:
    a. Megaloblastic anemia
    b. NCNC anemia
    c. Iron deficiency anemia
    d. Leucopenia

74. False elevation of TSH is seen in:
    a. AGH deficiency
    b. Addison's disease
    c. Cushing's disease
    d. Type 1 DM

75. Hashitoxicity characterized by all except:
    a. Decreased RAIU
    b. Increased ESR is a must
    c. Normal ESR
    d. Remains 1–2 m

76. Thyroxin (T4) requirement is increased in all except:
    a. Pregnancy
    b. Malabsorption
    c. Decreased ATT
    d. Elderly

77. Hyperthyroidism is seen in all except:
    a. Thyroiditis
    b. Dyshormonogenesis
    c. Graves' disease
    d. Jod-Basedow effect

78. Treatment of Graves ophthalmopathy:
    a. Steroids
    b. Cyclosporine
    c. Octreotide
    d. Calcitonin

79. A 22-year-old female with a small goitre with features of thyrotoxicosis for last 2 months the next diagnosis will be:
    a. TPO Ab
    b. RAIU
    c. USG
    d. Thyroid scan

80. True about calcitonin in MCT all except:
    a. Basal calcitonin is raised
    b. Positive immunoreactivity for CEA + calcitonin
    c. CEA raised indicate malignancy
    d. Serum levels can guide regarding need for lymph node dissection

81. Drugs that inhibit binding of thyroxin to TBG all except:
    a. Furosemide
    b. Phenytoin
    c. Clofibrate
    d. Mefenamic acid

82. Earliest function that appear in fetal thyroid:
    a. Tg
    b. Colloid store
    c. Iodine trapping
    d. T3 synthesis

83. Differentiation and development of thyroid:
    a. NIS
    b. TTF1
    c. TTF2
    d. PAX8
    e. THOX

84. **Low T4, normal TSH:**
    a. Sick euthyroid syndrome
    b. Hyperalbuminemia
    c. Thyroprivic hypothyroidism
    d. Thyrotropoprivic hypothyroidism

85. **Post-thyroidectomy detectable level of TG found in:**
    a. Anti TG Ab
    b. Ineffective T4 suppression
    c. Residual tissue
    d. TBG excess
    e. Ineffective NIS

86. **Drugs inhibiting T4 to T3 conversion are all except:**
    a. Glucocorticoids
    b. Phenytoin
    c. PTU
    d. Amiodarone

87. **↓ S TSH in sick euthyroid syndrome:**
    a. IL-12
    b. IL-18
    c. Stress cortisol response
    d. ↑rT3
    e. ↓rT3

88. **Apart from thyroid dysfunction most common side effect of amiodarone is:**
    a. Diarrhea
    b. Proteinuria
    c. Corneal microdeposits
    d. Lymphocytic hypophysitis

89. **Iodine therapy is indicated in all except:**
    a. Endemic goitre
    b. Dehalogenase effect(w12th p424)
    c. Mild NIS mutation(w12th p423)
    d. Thyroid hormone receptor mutation

90. **Which nutritional deficiency is associated with congenital hypothyroidism?**
    a. Zn
    b. Selenium
    c. Calcium
    d. Molybdenum

91. **Indications for surgery in Graves' disease include all except:**
    a. Active Graves' orbitopathy
    b. Large goiter
    c. Elderly
    d. Women desiring fertility

92. **Thyrotoxicosis in pregnancy all except:**
    a. Carbimazole is used
    b. TSH should be maintained between 3-5
    c. FT4 should be maintained in high normal range
    d. TRAb concentration can predict risk of development of fetal hyperthyroidism

93. **↑T3/T4 with ↑TSH is seen in all except:**
    a. TR mutation
    b. Secondary hyperthyroid
    c. Wrong lab report
    d. Primary hypothyroidism

94. **Transient hyperthyroidism -> hypothyroidism all except:**
    a. Subacute thyroiditis
    b. Silent thyroiditis
    c. Postpartum thyroiditis
    d. Hashimoto's thyroiditis

95. **Central hypothyroid true all except**
    a. Myxedema is presentation
    b. Myxedema coma never seen
    c. Decreased T3/T4, mild increase in TSH
    d. Pituitary adenoma may be a cause

96. **Monitoring of thyroid hormone maintenance:**
    a. 3 months
    b. 6 months
    c. 1 year
    d. 2 years

97. **rT3 true is**
    a. ↑ in Sick-euthyroid syndrome
    b. ↓ in Sick-euthyroid syndrome
    c. ↓ in 1° hypothyroidism
    d. ↓ during amiodarone use

98. **Thyroxine maintenance in pregnancy is monitored with:**
    a. FT4
    b. TSH
    c. FT4 & TSH
    d. T3

99. **Thianamides in hyperthyroidism used due to all except:**
    a. Inhibit autoimmunity
    b. Inhibits T4 to T3 conversion
    c. Inhibit organification
    d. Remission of space occupying lesion

ANSWERS

1. **Ans. (b) After antithyroid drugs**
   [Werner & Ingbar's The Thyroid 10th ed pg 484]
   Inorganic iodide is administered to inhibit release of already synthesized T4 and T3 from the thyroid.
   Thionamide antithyroid drugs should be given about an hour before iodide is given, because influx of iodide into the thyroid can increase T4 and T3 synthesis and therefore increase the stores of the two hormones, thereby prolonging the period of thyrotoxicosis.

2. **Ans. (c) Sedative**
   [Werner & Ingbar's The Thyroid 10th ed pg 483; Williams 13th ed pg 394]

3. **Ans. (d) 6 months**
   [Williams 13th ed pg 391]

4. **Ans. (c) Increased CPK**
   [Werner & Ingbar's The Thyroid 10th ed pg 603]

5. **Ans. (c) S. Thyroglobulin**
   [Williams 13th ed pg 407, 408]

6. **Ans. (d) Expected normal response**
   [Williams 13th ed pg 403, 404; Werner & Ingbar's The Thyroid 10th ed pg 197, 198]

7. **Ans. (c) 37%**
   [Williams 13th ed pg 403]
   Amiodarone contains 37% iodine by weight.
   About 6 mg of iodide are released per day of the 75 mg of iodine present in a 200 mg tablet.

8. **Ans. b. 50 d**
   [Williams 13th ed pg 339]

9. **Ans. (a) Active acromegaly**
   [Greenspan's 9th ed; Endocrine Secrets 6th ed pg 337; Werner & Ingbar's The Thyroid 10th ed pg 292]
   Causes of Abnormal Serum Thyroxine Determinations in Euthyroid Individuals
   - Euthyroid hyperthyroxinemia
     – ↑Plasma protein binding
       • ↑Thyroxine-binding globulin (TBG)
         ▹ Inherited
         ▹ Estrogen effect (pregnancy, estrogen therapy, estrogen-containing oral contraceptives)

- Hepatitis
- *Drugs:* tamoxifen, 5-fluorouracil, clofibrate, methadone, heroin, mitotane
  - ↑Transthyretin binding
    - Inherited
    - Paraneoplastic production by hepatic and pancreatic tumors
  - ↑ Albumin binding
    - Inherited (familial dysalbuminemic hyperthyroxinemia)
- ↓T4-to-T3 conversion[a]
  - Systemic illness
  - *Medications:* amiodarone, radiocontrast agents, glucocorticoids, propranolol
- Thyroxine therapy in hypothyroidism[a]
- Generalized resistance to thyroid hormone[a]
- Anti-T4 antibody (assay interference)
- Euthyroid Hypothyroxinemia
  - ↓Thyroxine-binding globulin
    - ↓TBG production
      - Inherited
      - Androgens
      - Glucocorticoids
      - Drugs: danazol, L-asparaginase
    - ↑TBG clearance
      - Nephrotic syndrome
      - Severe liver disease
      - Protein-losing gastroenteropathy
  - Systemic illness[b] (↓TBG levels, ↓ binding affinity of TBG for thyroid hormones)
  - Medications:
    - NSAIDs (fenamates e.g. mefenamic acid, phenylbutazone), furosemide, heparin (Displacement of thyroid hormones from TBG)
    - Phenytoin, carbamazepine[b] (Displacement of thyroid hormones from TBG; ↑ hepatic metabolism of T4, ↓ TSH responses to TRH)
  - Exogenous thyromimetic compounds (T3 [Cytomel])[b]
  - Iodine deficiency (with normal serum T3)[b]

NB: [a]Both total and free T4 elevated; [b]Both total and free T4 low.

10. Ans. (a) Tyrosine
    [Williams 13th ed pg 336]

11. Ans. (d) Leucocytosis
    [Williams 13th ed pg 386, 387]

12. Ans. (c) 11–15 mcg/kg/day
    [Werner & Ingbar's The Thyroid 10th ed pg 795]

13. **Ans. (c) SIADH**
    [Werner & Ingbar's The Thyroid 10th ed pg 800; Williams 13th ed pg 439]
    Administration of excessive doses of Levothyroxine also increases cardiac wall thickness and contractility and, in elderly patients, increases the risk of atrial fibrillation.

14. **Ans. (b) Dark chromatin**
    [Williams 13th ed pg 462]
    - PTCs appear as firm, unencapsulated or partially encapsulated tumors.
    - PTCs may be partly necrotic
    - Some are cystic
    - Typically, PTC shows a predominance of papillary structures, consisting of a fibrovascular core lined by a single layer of epithelial cells
    - The papillae are usually admixed with neoplastic follicles having characteristic nuclear features
    - Characteristic nuclear changes:
        - Nuclei are larger than in normal follicular cells and overlap
        - May be fissured like coffee beans
        - Chromatin is hypodense (ground-glass nuclei)
        - Limits are irregular
        - Frequently contain an inclusion corresponding to a cytoplasmic invagination.
    - Psammoma bodies are often present in the core of papillae or in the tumor stroma; they are microscopic structures of calcified layers
    - Subtypes:
        - *Follicular variant of PTC:* The lining cells of the neoplastic follicles have the same nuclear features as seen in typical PTC; there is follicular predominance over the papillae; the encapsulated follicular variant is associated with a favourable outcome.
        - *Diffuse sclerosing variant:* Characterized by diffuse involvement of one or both thyroid lobes, widespread lymphatic permeation, prominent fibrosis, and lymphoid infiltration; controversy exists regarding outcome for the diffuse sclerosing variant.
        - *Tall cell variant:* Characterized by well-formed papillae that are covered by cells twice as tall as they are wide; aggressive.
        - *Columnar cell variant:* Characterized by presence of prominent nuclear stratification of elongated cells; aggressive.
        - *Hobnail variant:* Micropapillary pattern; poor prognostic finding.
    - Presence of necrosis and a high mitotic rate are associated with an aggressive behavior.

15. **Ans. (a) Psammoma body**
    [De Groot 7th ed pg 1620]

    Factors Associated with Adverse Prognosis
    - Older age
    - Distant metastases

- Less well-differentiated histologic variant
- Follicular, widely invasive, tall cells, columnar cells, oxyphilic cells, Hürthle cells, insular
- Large tumor size
- Extrathyroidal invasion
- Multicentricity
- Lymph node metastases
- High tumor grade and DNA aploidy
- Male gender
- BRAF (V600E) mutation.

16. **Ans. (b) Increased CRP**
    [J Clin Endocrinol Metab. 1994 Feb;78(2):423; Thyroid. 2003 Jul;13(7):643; Eur Thyroid J 2018;7:59]
    - Serum IL-6 values in AIT patients with no apparent thyroid abnormalities were markedly higher. Values in AIT patients with nodular goiter and/or thyroid autoimmune disease, although slightly higher than healthy controls, did not significantly differ from those in patients with spontaneous hyperthyroidism due to Graves' disease or toxic adenoma/nodular goiter.
    - The occurrence of positive CRP values did not differ significantly between patients with type I and type II AIT and controls.
    - AIT 1 is associated with increased vascularity, while AIT 2 is characterized by absence of hypervascularity.
    - Anti-thyroid antibodies, such as anti-thyroid peroxidase antibodies, are often positive in AIT 1 and negative in AIT 2.

17. **Ans. (a) Antibody to TSHR**
    [Thyroid. Volume 26, Number 10, 2016 pg 1385]

18. **Ans. (b) Pressure symptom**
    [Williams 13th ed pg 382, 383; De Groot 7th ed pg 1448, 1449]

19. **Ans. (b) Graves' disease**
    [Williams 13th ed pg 363, 384, 404-406]
    (See discussion of Chapter 8, Questions 66 and 67)

20. **Ans. (d) Upto 50% patients develop residual hypothyroidism**
    [Williams 13th ed pg 406-408]

    The disease usually subsides within a few months leaving no residual deficiency of thyroid function in 90% of patients.

21. **Ans. (d) TRH**
    [Pediatric Endocrinology: Mechanisms, Manifestations, and Management pg 493]

    The placenta is impermeable to maternal TSH and is partially permeable to maternal T4 and T3. Maternal TRH and iodide freely cross the placenta.

22. **Ans. (c) Free T3/T4**
    [Williams 13th ed pg 214, 250]
    - Option (c) is more appropriate than option (b).
    - During pregnancy, the pituitary gland normally enlarges in response to estrogen stimulation. The hypervascular gland is particularly vulnerable to arterial pressure changes and prone to hemorrhage. Sheehan syndrome is classically described after severe postpartum hemorrhage. The presentation varies from development of hypovolemic shock resulting in adenohypophyseal vessel vasospasm and pituitary necrosis to the gradual onset of partial to complete pituitary insufficiency.
    - The dose of T4 in hypopituitary patients is titrated to achieve midnormal serum free T4 levels. Measurement of TSH levels is not useful in determining thyroid hormone replacement because the damaged thyrotroph is unlikely to adequately reflect appropriate feedback suppression. As many women with pituitary failure also likely receive estrogen replacement, free instead of total T4 level is measured to avoid the confounding effects of increased TBG levels.

23. **Ans. (a) Thyrotoxicosis**
    [Williams 13th ed pg 408, 409]
    Struma Ovarii
    - Thyroid tissue may be present in teratomas. Occasionally such foci are hyperfunctional- thyrotoxicosis may occur in as many as 8% to 10% of patients.
    - *Clinical presentation:*
        - Thyrotoxicosis
        - No goiter
        - Lower abdominal symptoms such as pain or a mass. Rarely ascites is present
    - *Laboratory studies:*
        - ↓TSH, ↑free T4
        - RAIU is low
        - Tg may be elevated, particularly if the teratoma is malignant and has metastasized to the peritoneum
        - Abdominal CT scan or MRI shows a multilocular ovarian mass or masses
    - *Treatment:*
        - The patient should be rendered euthyroid if thyrotoxicosis is significant followed by removal of the involved ovary or ovaries
        - Therapeutic radioiodine will be required for metastatic disease after ablation of the normal thyroid gland.

24. **Ans. (c) Selenium**
    [Williams 13th ed pg 344]

25. **Ans. (d) More common in Caucasians than Asians**
    [Williams 13th ed pg 371; Journal of Thyroid Research Volume 2014, Article ID 649502]

26. **Ans. (b) Follicular**
    [De Groot 7th ed pg 1615

27. **Ans. (a) Obesity**
    [ESI Manual of Clinical Endocrinology 2nd edition pg 330; De Groot 7th ed pg 1555]

    Indication of therapy in subclinical hypothyroid
    - TSH > 10 mU/L
    - Symptoms suggestive of hypothyroidism
    - Positive TPO-Ab
    - Evidence of atherosclerotic cardiovascular disease, heart failure, or associated risk factors for these diseases
    - Pregnancy
    - Patients planning to become pregnant
    - Infertility.

    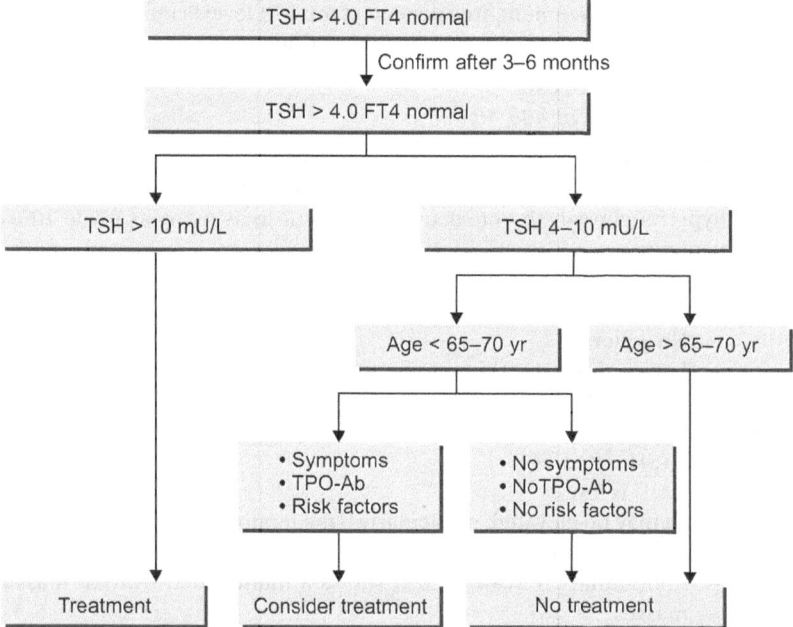

    Flow diagram for the management of subclinical hypothyroidism.

28. **Ans. (d) TBG increased**
    [Williams 13th ed pg 342]

    ### Familial Dysalbuminemic Hyperthyroxinemia (FDH)
    - Autosomal dominant disorder
    - The plasma contains high amounts of a usually minor albumin variant that binds T4 (but not T3) with increased avidity
    - ↑ total T4
    - Free T4, and total and free T3 remain normal
    - Patient is clinically euthyroid.

Thyroid | **93**

29. **Ans. (b) Increased TBG seen in hepatic failure**
    [Greenspan's 9th ed; Endocrine Secrets 6th ed pg 337; Williams 13th ed pg 341; Harrison's Endocrinology 3rd ed pg 66]
    Also See discussion of Chapter 8, Question 9.

30. **Ans. (a) Graves' disease**
    [Williams 13th ed pg 363, 384, 404-406]
    See discussion of Chapter 8, Questions 66 and 67.

31. **Ans. (a) Increased D3 in hemangioma**
    [Williams 13th ed pg 345]

32. **Ans. (c) TSH receptor defect**
    [Werner & Ingbar's The Thyroid 10th ed pg 235, 236, 537, 547, 548; De Groot 7th ed pg 1641]

33. **Ans. (d) None of the above**
    [Werner & Ingbar's The Thyroid, 10th ed pg 537; Eur J Nucl Med Mol Imaging. 2002 Aug;29 Suppl 2:S435]
    Rapid and high uptake of thyroid radioiodine uptake is seen in iodide organification defect and thyroglobulin synthesis defect.
    NIS defect is associated with absence of radioiodine or pertechnetate uptake in the thyroid.

34. **Ans. (b) Multinucleate cells**
    [Williams 13th ed pg 406]

35. **Ans. (c) Colon**
    [Williams 13th ed pg 337; De Groot 7th ed pg 1641]
    NIS is expressed in Thyroid cell (basolateral membrane).
    NIS has also been identified in other iodide-concentrating cells:
    - Salivary glands
    - Lacrimal gland
    - Nasopharynx
    - Lactating mammary glands, mammary carcinoma cells
    - Choroid plexus
    - Gastric mucosa
    - Small intestinal mucosa
    - Placenta (cytotrophoblast and syncytiotrophoblast)
    - Uterus
    - Ovary
    - Testis
    - Thymus
    - Skin
    - Lung tissue
    - Ciliary body.

36. **Ans. (d) Goitre**
   [Williams 13th ed pg 408, 409]

37. **Ans. (a) <1 ng/mL**
   [Thyroid. 2016 Jan;26(1):66]
   Criteria for absence of persistent tumor (excellent response):
   In patients who have undergone total or near-total thyroidectomy and RAI treatment (remnant ablation, adjuvant therapy or therapy), disease-free status comprises all of the following:
   - No clinical evidence of tumor
   - No imaging evidence of tumor by RAI imaging and/or neck US
   - Low serum Tg levels during TSH suppression (Tg <0.2 ng/mL) or after stimulation (Tg <1 ng/mL) in the absence of interfering antibodies.

38. **Ans. (d) Anti TPO +ve**
   [De Groot 7th ed pg 1531]
   Serum thyroid peroxidase antibody concentrations are usually normal.

39. **Ans. (a) Jod-Basedow effect**
   [Williams 13th ed pg 351, 388, 403]
   - *Jod-Basedow effect:* Administration of supplemental iodine to subjects with endemic iodine deficiency goiter can result in iodine-induced hyperthyroidism. This response termed the Jod-Basedow effect.
   - *Wolff-Chaikoff effect:* High doses of iodine in excess of several milli grams can acutely inhibit organic binding (Wolff-Chaikoff effect). The mechanism for organification inhibition may involve inhibitory effects of high iodide concentrations on TPO and THOX2. This is a transient phenomenon.

40. **Ans. (a) RET**
   [Williams 13th ed pg 471]

41. **Ans. (a) RXR**
   [Harrison's Endocrinology 3rd ed pg 6]
   See discussion of Chapter 1, Question 3.

42. **Ans. (b) Slipped capital femoral epiphyses**
   [Williams 13th ed pg 424; https://www.accessdata.fda.gov/drugsatfda_docs/label/2008/021342s008s014lbl.pdf]

43. **Ans. (a) Bromocriptine therapy**
   [Williams 13th ed pg 405, 408]

   Causes of Thyroiditis
   - *Autoimmune thyroiditis:* Hashimoto thyroiditis; there are typically no local symptoms of thyroid inflammation, leading to the terms silent or painless thyroiditis, also referred to as lymphocytic thyroiditis or hashitoxicosis

- Viral thyroiditis (also termed subacute, de Quervain, or granulomatous thyroiditis)
- *Acute thyroiditis:* Due to bacterial or fungal infections
- *Drug-induced thyroiditis:*
  - Amiodarone
  - Lithium
  - IL-2
  - Interferon-α
  - Granulocyte/macrophage colony-stimulating factor (GM-CSF)
  - Lleuprolide
- Multitargeting kinase inhibitors, e.g. sunitinib, sorafenib.

44. **Ans. (a) TSH receptor mutation**
[Werner & Ingbar's The Thyroid 10th ed pg 235, 236, 537, 547, 548; De Groot 7th ed pg 1641]

45. **Ans. (c) CHO transfected with TSH-R**
[Williams 13th ed pg 385; De Groot 7th ed pg 1374, 1375]

Two types of tests may be employed for the detection of TRAbs.
- *Protein-binding inhibition assays:*
  - Assesses the capacity of patient serum or IgG
    - To inhibit the binding of labeled TSH to solubilized TSHRs, or
    - To compete with a monoclonal antibody to the TSH binding site on the TSHR.
  - Low cost, good precision, sensitivity > 95%.
- *Bioassay:*
  - Assesses the capacity of the patient's serum or IgG to stimulate adenylate cyclase in thyroid epithelial cells or mammalian cells expressing recombinant TSHR
  - Expensive, poor precision, but positive in the vast majority of patients
  - Cells lines that have been used: human thyroid cell cultures, cultured rat thyroid cell line FRTL5, cell lines that express the recombinant TSH receptor
  - The recombinant human TSH receptor assay is more sensitive than the formerly used TSAb assays.
- One of the major drawbacks with the bioassays mentioned earlier is that they are unsuitable for use as routine laboratory tools. This problem has been largely circumvented, with the advent of a luminescence-linked bioassay for TSAbs. This assay uses Chinese hamster ovary cells stably transfected with the human TSH receptor and a cAMP-dependent luciferase reporter.

46. **Ans. (a) Decreased RAIU**
[Williams 13th ed pg 383, 384, 391, 392]

47. **Ans. (c)** Hepatic failure increases TBG
    [Greenspan's 9th ed; Endocrine Secrets 6th ed pg 337; Williams 13th ed pg 341; Harrison's Endocrinology 3rd ed pg 66]
    See discussion of Chapter 8, Questions 9 and 29.

48. **Ans. (b)** Selenium
    [Williams 13th ed pg 344]

49. **Ans. (d)** fT4–0.2%; fT3–0.03%
    [Williams 13th ed pg 345, 348]
    - T3 has 10- to 15-fold lower affinity for TBG than T4
    - T3 has a 15-fold higher binding affinity for TRs than does T4, explaining its function as the active thyroid hormone.
    - Half-life of T3 is 0.75 days and that of T4 is 6.7 days
    - Fraction of total hormone in free form ($\times 10^{-2}$) for T3 is 0.3 and that for T4 is 0.02

50. **Ans. (d)** Oxygen consumption rate
    [Williams 13th ed pg 389; Werner & Ingbar's The Thyroid 10th ed pg 502; Advances in Graves' Disease and Other Hyperthyroid Disorders pg 153]
    - Beta blockers provide relief from symptoms of thyrotoxicosis: anxiety, tachycardia, palpitations, tremor, excessive sweating, heat intolerance, eye lid retraction.
    - They improve negative nitrogen balance, heart rate, cardiac output, oxygen consumption.
    - However they do not normalize the metabolic rate.
    - Beta blockers also reduce blood pressure in hypertensive patients but have no effect in patients with normal blood pressure.

51. **Ans. (a)** T4 → T3
    [Harrison's Endocrinology 3rd ed pg 62]

52. **Ans. (d) Phenytoin**
    [Greenspan's 9th ed; Endocrine Secrets 6th ed pg 337]
    See discussion of Chapter 8, Question 9.

53. **Ans. (d) OCP intake**
    [Greenspan's 9th ed; Endocrine Secrets 6th ed pg 337]
    See discussion of Chapter 8, Question 9.

54. **Ans. (a) Dysalbuminemic hyperthyroxinemia**
    [Werner & Ingbar's The Thyroid 10th ed pg 195, 197, 198; Williams 13th ed pg 342]
    See discussion of Chapter 8, Question 28.

55. **Ans. (a) Hemeprotein**
    [Williams 13th ed pg 338]

56. **Ans. (c) Radioiodine**
    [Harrison's Endocrinology 3rd ed pg 91]

57. **Ans. (b) Decreased D3 (type-3 deiodinase)**
    [Williams 13th ed pg 352]

58. **Ans. (c) Low dose I-123**
    [Williams 13th ed pg 363]

59. **Ans. (a) External carotid artery**
    [Williams 13th ed pg 335]
    Two pairs of vessels constitute the major arterial blood supply:
    1. Superior thyroid artery, arising from the external carotid artery
    2. Inferior thyroid artery, arising from the subclavian artery.

60. **Ans. (a) Lp (a)**
    [Williams 13th ed pg 362]

    Biochemical Markers of Thyroid Status
    - Thyrotoxicosis
        - Increased
            - Osteocalcin
            - Urine pyridinium collagen cross-links
            - Alkaline phosphatase (bone or liver)
            - Atrial natriuretic hormone
            - Sex hormone–binding globulin
            - Ferritin
            - von Willebrand factor
        - Decreased
            - Low-density lipoprotein cholesterol
            - Lipoprotein(a)
    - Hypothyroidism
        - Increased
            - Creatine kinase (MM isoform)
            - Low-density lipoprotein cholesterol

- Lipoprotein(a)
- Plasma norepinephrine
- Decreased
  - Vasopressin

61. Ans. (c) 7 days
    [Williams 13th ed pg 436]

62. Ans. (c) 50 days
    [Williams 13th ed pg 339]

63. Ans. (a) GH
    [Safety of Biologics Therapy pg 350]

64. Ans. (b) Addisons'
    [Williams 13th ed pg 355, 530]

65. Ans. (d) Excess T4 treatment
    [https://www.accessdata.fda.gov/drugsatfda_docslabel/2008/021342s008s0 14lbl.pdf]
    Overtreatment has been associated with craniosynostosis in infants.

66. Ans. (c) Chronic diarrhea
    [Williams 13th ed pg 363]

    Factors that Influence 24-hour Thyroid Iodide Uptake
    - Factors that increase uptake
      - Increased hormone synthesis
        - Hyperthyroidism
        - Response to glandular hormone depletion
          - Recovery from thyroid suppression (by exogenous hormone)
          - Recovery from subacute thyroiditis
          - Antithyroid agents
        - Excessive hormone losses
          - Nephrotic syndrome
          - Chronic diarrheal states
          - Soybean ingestion
      - Normal hormone synthesis
        - Iodine deficiency
          - Dietary insufficiency
          - Excessive loss (dehalogenase defect, pregnancy)
        - Hormone biosynthetic defects
    - Factors that decrease uptake
      - Decreased hormone synthesis
        - Primary hypofunction
          - Primary hypothyroidism
          - Antithyroid agents
          - Hormone biosynthetic defects

- ➢ Hashimoto disease
- ➢ Subacute thyroiditis
- ♦ Secondary hypofunction
- ♦ Exogenous thyroid hormones
- – Not reflecting decreased hormone synthesis
  - ♦ Increased availability of iodine
    - ➢ Diet or drugs
    - ➢ Cardiac or renal insufficiency
  - ♦ Increased hormone release
- ▪ Very severe hyperthyroidism (rare)

67. **Ans. (a) Jod-Basedow**
[Werner & Ingbar's The Thyroid 10th ed pg 261]

Differential diagnosis of thyrotoxicosis- increased or decreased RAIU
- ▪ Increased uptake
  - – Graves' disease
  - – Multinodular toxic goiter
  - – Solitary autonomously functioning nodule
  - – Hydatidiform mole, trophoblastic tumors, choriocarcinoma
  - – Metastatic thyroid cancer
- ▪ Decreased uptake
  - – Subacute thyroiditis granulomatous thyroiditis (de Quervain's)
  - – Silent thyroiditis
  - – Postpartum thyroiditis
  - – Iodine- induced thyrotoxicosis (Jod-Basedow phenomenon)
  - – Amiodarone-induced thyrotoxicosis
  - – Thyrotoxicosis factitia
  - – Struma ovarii (decreased over the thyroid, increased in ovarian tumor in the pelvis)

68. **Ans. (a) Iodine**
[De Groot 7th ed pg 2536]

69. **Ans. (a) 1 mg/kg**
[Werner & Ingbar's The Thyroid 10th ed pg 804]

Dose of methimazole in the neonatal period: 0.25-1 mg/kd/day in 2-3 divided doses

70. **Ans. (b) 0.04**
[https://www.medscape.com/viewarticle/452667_3]

Most TSH methods now claim a detection limit of 0.02 mIU/L or less ("third generation" assays)

71. **Ans. (b) Oliguria**
[Williams 13th ed pg 372; J Res Med Sci. 2013 Feb; 18(2): 167; Tietz Textbook of Clinical Chemistry and Molecular Diagnostics pg 716]

- Thyrotoxicosis produces mild polyuria, which may lead to nocturia. Patients may exhibit urgency, urge incontinence, and enuresis (either primary or secondary).
- Anti-insulin antibodies causing hypoglycemia have been reported in Graves' disease
- Approximately 3% of patients with Graves' disease have pernicious anemia, and a further 3% have antibodies to intrinsic factor but normal absorption of vitamin B12. Autoantibodies against gastric parietal cells may also be present.

72. **Ans. (d) 50%**
    [Williams 13th ed pg 382]

73. **Ans. (c) Iron deficiency anemia**
    [De Groot 7th ed pg 1450]

    Manifestations of Graves's Hyperthyroidism on Hematopoietic system
    - Mild leukopenia with relative lymphocytosis
    - Normocytic anemia
    - Pernicious anemia
    - Aplastic anemia
    - Autoimmune thrombocytopenic purpura
    - Increases in factor VIII levels and fibrinogen.

74. **Ans. (b) Addison's disease**
    [Williams 13th ed pg 355, 530]

75. **Ans. (b) Increased ESR is a must**
    [Williams 13th ed pg 405, 406]

76. **Ans. (d) Elderly**
    [Williams 13th ed pg 438]

    Conditions that Alter Levothyroxine Requirements
    - Increased levothyroxine requirements
        - Pregnancy
        - Gastrointestinal disorders
            - Mucosal diseases of the small bowel (e.g. sprue)
            - After jejunoileal bypass and small bowel resection
            - Impaired gastric acid secretion (e.g. atrophic gastritis)
            - Diabetic diarrhea
        - Therapy with certain pharmacologic agents
            - Drugs that interfere with levothyroxine absorption
                - Cholestyramine
                - Sucralfate
                - Aluminum hydroxide
                - Calcium carbonate
                - Ferrous sulfate

- Drugs that increase the cytochrome P450 enzyme (CYP3A4)
  - Rifampin
  - Carbamazepine
  - Estrogen
  - Phenytoin
  - Sertraline
  - ? Statins
- Drugs that block T4 to T3 conversion
  - Amiodarone
- Conditions that may block deiodinase synthesis
  - Selenium deficiency
  - Cirrhosis
- Decreased levothyroxine requirements
  - Aging (65 years and older)
  - Androgen therapy in women.

77. Ans. (b) Dyshormonogenesis
[Williams 13th ed pg 403, 3770]

Causes of Hyperthyroidism
- Excessive TSH-receptor stimulation
  - Graves disease (TRAbs)
  - Pregnancy-associated transient hyperthyroidism (hCG)
  - Trophoblastic disease (hCG)
  - Familial gestational hyperthyroidism (mutant TSH receptor)
  - TSH-producing pituitary adenoma
- Autonomous thyroid hormone secretion
  - Multinodular toxic goiter (somatic mutations)
  - Solitary toxic thyroid adenoma (somatic mutation)
  - Congenital activating TSH-receptor mutation (genomic mutation)
- Destruction of follicles with release of hormone
  - Subacute de Quervain thyroiditis (virus infection)
  - Painless thyroiditis/postpartum thyroiditis
  - (hashitoxicosis—autoimmune)
  - Acute thyroiditis (bacterial infection)
  - Drug-induced thyroiditis (amiodarone, interferon-γ)
- Extrathyroidal sources of thyroid hormone
  - Iatrogenic overreplacement with thyroid hormone
  - Excessive self-administered thyroid medication
  - Food and supplements containing excessive thyroid hormone
  - Functional thyroid cancer metastases
  - Struma ovarii.

Also see discussion of Chapter 8, Question 39.

78. Ans. (a) Steroids
[Williams 13th ed pg 393]

79. **Ans. (b) RAIU**
    [Williams 13th ed pg 384, 385]

80. **Ans. (c) CEA raised indicate malignancy**
    [Williams 13th ed pg 471, 472, 479]
    Serum CEA levels are higher in more aggressive MTC.

81. **Ans. (c) Clofibrate**
    [Greenspan's 9th ed; Endocrine Secrets 6th ed pg 337; Werner & Ingbar's The Thyroid 10th ed pg 292]
    See discussion of Chapter 8, Question 9.

82. **Ans. (a) Tg**
    [Williams 13th ed pg 325]
    - Future follicular cells acquire the capacity to form thyroglobulin (Tg) as early as the 29th day of gestation
    - Thyroxine-binding globulin (TBG) is detectable in the serum by the 10th gestational week
    - Capacities to concentrate iodide and synthesize thyroxine (T4) are delayed until about the 11th week
    - The capacity of the pituitary to synthesize and secrete TSH is not apparent until the 14th week.

83. **Ans. (b) TTF1, (c) TTF2 and (d) PAX8**
    [Williams 13th ed pg 336]
    A number of transcription factors, including thyroid transcription factors TTF1 (NKX2-1) and TTF2 (FOXE1), PAX8, and hepatocyte nuclear factor 3 (HNF-3 [FOXE2]), as well as TSH, are necessary to achieve functional differentiation of the thyroid follicular cells and the onset of hormonogenesis.

84. **Ans. (d) Thyrotropoprivic hypothyroidism**
    [Williams 13th ed pg 424; De Groot 7th ed pg 1358]

    Conditions that may be associated with Low T4, normal TSH
    - Low TBG (congenital or acquired)
    - Endogenous T4 antibodies
    - Iodine deficiency
    - Desiccated thyroid or T3 replacement
    - Treated thyrotoxicosis
    - Drugs competing with T4 binding to serum proteins
    - Central hypothyroidism.

85. **Ans. (c) Residual tissue**
    [Williams 13th ed pg 476]

86. **Ans. (b) Phenytoin**
    [Williams 13th ed pg 346, 347; Werner & Ingbar's The Thyroid 10th ed pg 194]

Drugs inhibiting T4 to T3 conversion
- Propyl thiouracil
- Amiodarone
- Glucocorticoids (high doses)
- Iodinated contrast agents
- Propranolol.

87. Ans. (c) Stress cortisol response
[Werner & Ingbar's The Thyroid 10th ed pg 208]

	Changes in NTIS	Causes of NTIS
Hypothalamus TRH Pituitary TSH Thyroid T4 T3 Blood TBG–T4 T3 Liver T4 T3 rT3 T3 T4S T3 TR	↑ D2 activity ↓ D3 activity ↓ TRH production	↓ serum leptin (starvation) ↑ cytokines ↑ serum cortisol
	↓ nocturnal TSH surge ↓ serum TSH (severe NTI)	↓ TRH production ↑ cytokines ↑ serum cortisol
	↓ T4 – PR (severe NTI)	↓ serum TSH
	↓ serum T3, ↑ rT3 ↑ serum T4 and fT4 ↓ serumT4 and fT4 ↓ TBG binding	↓ T3-PR, ↓ rT3 MCR, ~ ↓ D1 activity ↑ T4 –MCR ~ ↓ T4 uptake ↓ T4-PR (severe NTI) ↓ TBG binding ↓ TBG, serum inhibitors
	↓ tissue T4 uptake	↑ serum IS, NEFA, bilirubin ↓ tissue ATP content
	↓ D1 activity ↑ D3 activity ↑ serum T4S, T3S	↓ T4 tissue uptake, ↓ GSH, ↓ Se ↑ cytokines ↑ conjugation ~ ↓ D1 activity
	↓ TR-binding capacity	↑cytokines

A schematic diagram of the nonthyroidal illness syndrome (NTIS): GSH, Glutathione; IS, indoxyl sulfate; MCR, metabolic clearance rate; NEFA, non-esterified fatty acids; PR, production rate.

88. Ans. (c) Corneal microdeposits
[Katzung- Basic and Clinical Pharmacology 11th ed]

89. Ans. (d) Thyroid hormone receptor mutation
[Werner & Ingbar's The Thyroid 10th ed pg 235, 236, 537, 547, 548; De Groot 7th ed pg 1641]

90. Ans. (b) Selenium
[Williams 13th ed pg 866]

91. Ans. (c) Elderly
[Thyroid. Volume 26, Number 10, 2016 pg 1351, 1352]

Clinical situations that favor surgery as treatment for Graves' hyperthyroidism
- Women planning a pregnancy in <6 months
- Symptomatic compression or large goiters (≥80 g)
- Relatively low uptake of RAI
- When thyroid malignancy is documented or suspected (e.g. suspicious or indeterminate cytology)
- Large thyroid nodules especially if greater than 4 cm or if non-functioning/hypofunctioning on ^{123}I or ^{99m}Tc pertechnetate scanning
- Coexisting hyperparathyroidism requiring surgery; especially if TRAb levels are particularly high
- Patients with moderate to severe active GO.

Contraindications to a surgery as treatment for Graves' hyperthyroidism:
- Substantial comorbidity such as cardiopulmonary disease, end-stage cancer
- Lack of access to a high-volume thyroid surgeon
- Pregnancy is a relative contraindication, and surgery should only be used when rapid control of hyperthyroidism is required and antithyroid medications cannot be used. Thyroidectomy is best avoided in the first and third trimesters of pregnancy. Second trimester is the safest time.

92. **Ans. (b) TSH should be maintained between 3-5**
    [Williams 13th ed pg 397, 398]
    - Medical therapy is the method of choice in pregnancy.
    - PTU should be reserved for the first trimester of pregnancy. Subsequently, methimazole could be prescribed.
    - The maternal serum free T4 level should be maintained at or just above the upper normal nonpregnant range, and no attempt should be made to normalize the serum TSH concentration.

93. **Ans. (d) Primary hypothyroid**
    [Williams 13th ed pg 424]

94. **Ans. (a) Subacute thyroiditis**
    [Williams 13th ed pg 398, 399, 405-407; Werner & Ingbar's The Thyroid 10th ed pg 416, 422]

    Although all the mentioned conditions may be associated with transient thyrotoxicosis followed by development of hypothyroidism, the incidence of permanent hypothyroidism is relatively rare in subacute thyroiditis, occurring in only upto 5% patients.

95. **Ans. (b) Myxedema coma never seen**
    [Werner & Ingbar's The Thyroid 10th ed pg 561, 564; Endocrinol Metab Clin N Am 35 (2006) 689]

    In 5% of cases of myxedema coma are seen in patient with central hypothyroidism.

96. **Ans. (c) 1 year**
    [Williams 13th ed pg 438]

97. **Ans. (a) ↑ in Sick-euthyroid syndrome**
    [Werner & Ingbar's The Thyroid 10th ed pg 208]
    See discussion of Chapter 8, Question 87.

98. **Ans. (b) TSH**
    [Werner & Ingbar's The Thyroid 10th ed pg 827]

99. **Ans. (b) Inhibits T4 to T3 conversion**
    [Werner & Ingbar's The Thyroid 10th ed pg 493]

    Mechanism of action of thionamides
    - Intrathyroidal actions
        - Inhibition of iodine oxidation and organification
        - Inhibition of iodotyrosine coupling
        - Possible alteration of the structure of thyroglobulin
        - Possible inhibition of thyroglobulin biosynthesis
    - Extrathyroidal actions
        - Inhibition of conversion of T4 to T3 (by PTU, but not MMI)
    - Immunosuppressive actions (intrathyroidal/extrathyroidal).

CHAPTER 9

Adrenal Cortex

QUESTIONS

1. Adrenomedullin—all except:
   a. Hypertension
   b. Vasodilator
   c. Related to calcitonin
   d. Role in osteoblast formation

2. Commonest cause of acute adrenal insufficiency is:
   a. Steroid withdrawal
   b. Tuberculosis
   c. Hemorrhage
   d. Autoimmune adrenalitis

3. Addison's disease presents with all except:
   a. Hyperkalemia
   b. Eosinophilia
   c. Decreased hematocrit
   d. Hyperpigmentation

4. Central hypoadrenalism presents with:
   a. Hypotension
   b. Hyponatremia
   c. Hypopigmentation
   d. Hypoglycemia

5. An 8-year-old boy with Addison's disease with serum calcium 6.5 mg/dL with PO_4 5.8 mg/dL, PTH decrease:
   a. Ca only
   b. Ca + hydrochlorothiazide
   c. Ca + calcitriol
   d. Both b and c equally effective

6. A 40-year-old lady presented with Addison's biochemistry, with BP -90/50 mm Hg, RBS-79 mg/dL, TLC-6400/mm^3, Na$^+$-128, K$^+$-5.8, given normal saline of 2 liters, but with no improvement, next line of management is:
   a. ACTH stimulation test
   b. Dopamine infusion
   c. Random cortisol sample followed by Inj. hydrocortisone
   d. IV colloids

7. True about corticosteroid are all except:
   a. Glucocorticoid : mineralocorticoid ratio of hydrocortisone is 1:1
   b. Dexamethasone 40:<0.01
   c. Prednisolone 4:0.25
   d. Dexamethasone T½ 12 hrs

8. FDA approved drug for Cushing's syndrome with hyperglycemia is:
   a. Etomidate   b. Ketoconazole
   c. Mifepristone   d. Metyrapone

9. Most common cause of adrenal insufficiency in <7 years male:
   a. Congenital adrenal hypoplasia
   b. Addison's disease
   c. Metastasis
   d. Adrenoleukodystrophy

10. Hypokalemia in ectopic Cushing's syndrome is due to:
    a. 11βHSD inhibition   b. 11βHSD mismatch
    c. Kaliuretic effect   d. Increased aldosterone level

11. All of the following are used in treatment of Cushing's syndrome except:
    a. Aminoglutethimide   b. Ketoconazole
    c. Fluconazole   d. Metyrapone

12. Dexamethasone/Hydrocortisone:
    a. 20:1   b. 30:1
    c. 40:1   d. 50:1

13. Characteristic feature of Cushing's syndrome:
    a. Myopathy and bruising   b. DM and hypertension
    c. Hypertension and striae d. DM and striae

14. Addison's pigmentation:
    a. Exposed areas and on old scar
    b. Covered areas and old scar
    c. Exposed areas and new scar
    d. Covered areas and new scar

15. True regarding 21 hydroxylase deficiency is all except:
    a. Most common cause of CAH
    b. 21 hydroxylase is located on ER
    c. >90% due to de novo mutation
    d. 2 genes for 21 hydroxylase, one function and other is silent

16. In which of CAH, female phenotype in genetic male:
    a. StAR deficiency   b. 21 hydroxylase deficiency
    c. 11 hydroxylase deficiency d. Oxidoreductase deficiency

17. Pseudo-Cushing is not seen in:
    a. Depression   b. Iatrogenic
    c. Alcohol   d. Obesity

18. Commonest presentation of adrenal carcinoma:
    a. Abdominal lump
    b. Increase secretion of glucocorticoid and androgen
    c. Incidentally detected in routine examination
    d. Aldosterone hypersecretion
19. Following has the highest mineralocorticoid activity:
    a. Dexamethasone
    b. Prednisolone
    c. Hydrocortisone
    d. Methyl prednisolone
20. Following has the longest T½:
    a. Cortisone
    b. Dexamethasone
    c. Triamcinolone
    d. Methyl prednisolone
21. Following precautions are taken to minimize the complication of chronic glucocorticoid therapy except:
    a. Na^+ restriction
    b. K^+ restriction
    c. Colon restriction
    d. Ca^+ restriction
22. Features of Cushing's syndrome include all except:
    a. Proximal muscle weakness
    b. Moon facies
    c. Petechiae
    d. Alopecia
    e. Thick skin
23. True about steroid is:
    a. All steroids have nitrogen
    b. All steroids have high affinity for water
    c. All steroids have fatty acid and glycerol
    d. None has very high caloric value
24. Best screening test for Cushing's syndrome in pregnant females is:
    a. 24 hr UFC
    b. Midnight cortisol
    c. Dexamethasone suppression test
    d. Basal cortisol
25. All of the following drugs are indicated in Rx of Cushing's syndrome except:
    a. Cyproheptadine
    b. Aminoglutethimide
    c. Ketoconazole
    d. Fluconazole
26. Which of the following causes underandrogenization in karyotypic males with adrenal insufficiency?
    a. 21αhydroxylase deficiency
    b. 11βhydroxylase deficiency
    c. P 450 oxidoreductase deficiency
    d. Lipoid CAH (StAR deficiency)

27. **Which of the following is false about pseudo-Cushing's syndrome?**
    a. Seen in alcoholism
    b. Overnight dexamethasone suppression test is negative
    c. Low dose dexamethasone test cannot differentiate from true Cushing's syndrome
    d. Insulin-induced hypoglycemia is useful

28. **True about salivary cortisol:**
    a. Represent free cortisol
    b. Represent albumin bound cortisol
    c. Depends on salivary flow
    d. Only cotton pad to be kept in mouth

29. **CRH stimulation detects:**
    a. 1°/2° adrenal insufficiency
    b. Ectopic ACTH syndrome
    c. Adrenal cause of Cushing's syndrome
    d. All of the above

30. **Follow-up of Addison's disease on replacement therapy is by:**
    a. 8 AM cortisol
    b. 8 AM ACTH
    c. Clinical
    d. Midnight cortisol

31. **ACTH stimulation used in all except:**
    a. Hypoaldosteronemia
    b. CAH
    c. Adrenal insufficiency
    d. HPA axis suppression

32. **Young type 1 DM started having hyperpigmention, BP-99/50 mm Hg, next investigation to be done is:**
    a. ACTH stimulation test
    b. GAD Ab
    c. IA2 Ab
    d. ZnT 8 Ab

33. **Most potent anti-inflammatory drug:**
    a. Dexamethasone
    b. Prednisolone
    c. Methyl prednisolone
    d. Triamcinolone

34. **Which is not true about Cushing's syndrome?**
    a. Urinary free cortisol is diagnostic
    b. Petrosal venous sinus sampling will lateralize the pituitary adenoma
    c. Following pituitary surgery, postoperative glucocorticoid replacement is indicated
    d. Salivary cortisol is a convenient method for diagnosis

35. **Drugs used for Rx of Cushing's syndrome:**
    a. Cyproheptadine
    b. Ketoconazole
    c. Aminoglutethimide
    d. Fluconazole

36. **Pseudo-Cushing's syndrome; all true except:**
    a. Alcoholism
    b. Overnight dexamethasone suppression used to differentiate from true Cushing's
    c. Loperamide test useful
    d. Insulin induced hypoglycemia useful
    e. High dose dexamethasone will suppress Cushing

37. **Features of primary cortisol resistance include all except:**
    a. Virilization
    b. Hypertension
    c. Cushingoid stigmata
    d. Hypokalemia

38. **Steroids with long duration of action:**
    a. Prednisolone
    b. Methyl prednisolone
    c. Triamcinolone
    d. Dexamethasone

39. **Which of the following antibodies are typically found in autoimmune adrenalitis (Addison's disease)?**
    a. Anti-rho antibody
    b. Anti-peroxidase antibody
    c. Anti-21 hydroxylase antibody
    d. Anti-nuclear antibody
    e. Anti-tryptophan hydroxylase antibody

40. **Which of the following doses of prednisolone is equivalent in its glucocorticoid potency to 20 mg of hydrocortisone?**
    a. 2 mg
    b. 5 mg
    c. 10 mg
    d. 15 mg
    e. 20 mg

41. **Following enzyme deficiency causes hypertension:**
    a. 11βhydroxylase
    b. 21αhydroxylase
    c. 3β HSD
    d. StAR

Adrenal Cortex | **111**

ANSWERS

1. **Ans. (a) Hypertension**
   [De Groot 7th ed pg 1010]

   Adrenomedullin
   - Peptide related to calcitonin
   - ≈ 50 amino acids
   - A potent dilator of many vascular beds
   - Protective against conditions such as cardiac hypertrophy, perivascular fibrosis, renal damage, and pulmonary hypertension.
   - Can stimulate osteoblast proliferation at low concentration.

2. **Ans. (b) Tuberculosis**
   [Harrison's Endocrinology 3rd ed pg 118-121, Williams 13th ed pg 524-526]
   See discussion of Chapter 9, Question 9.

3. **Ans. (c) Decreased hematocrit**
   [Williams 13th ed pg 528; De Groot 7th ed pg 1769, 1770]

   Clinical Features of Primary Adrenal Insufficiency
   - Symptoms
     - Weakness, tiredness, fatigue
     - Anorexia
     - Gastrointestinal symptoms (Nausea, Vomiting, Constipation, Abdominal pain, Diarrhea)
     - Salt craving
     - Postural dizziness
     - Muscle or joint pains
   - Signs
     - Weight loss
     - Hyperpigmentation
     - Hypotension (<110 mm Hg systolic)
     - Vitiligo
     - Auricular calcification
   - Laboratory findings
     - Electrolyte disturbances (Hyponatremia, Hyperkalemia, Hypercalcemia)
     - Azotemia
     - Anemia
     - Eosinophilia

   Most of the features are same for primary and secondary adrenal insufficiency. However, certain characteristic features distinguish between the two.

   Features specific to primary disease are:
   - Presence of both glucocorticoid and mineralocorticoid deficiency (in secondary adrenal insufficiency the mineralocorticoid function is

often preserved). This accounts for differences in salt and water balance between the two groups. Thus, salt craving and postural dizziness are characteristic of primary adrenal failure
- Hyperpigmentation of the skin and mucosa, caused by enhanced stimulation of the skin MC1 receptor by ACTH and possibly other pro-opiomelanocortin-related peptides. It is the most specific sign of primary adrenal insufficiency (absent in secondary adrenal insufficiency)
- Vitiligo in autoimmune adrenal insufficiency
- Adrenal calcification.

4. **Ans. (c) Hypopigmentation**
   [Williams 13th ed pg 528; De Groot 7th ed pg 1769, 1770]
   See discussion of Chapter 9, Question 3.

5. **Ans. (c) Ca + calcitriol**
   [Williams 13th ed pg 524, 525, 1303]
   50% of patients with autoimmune adrenal insufficiency have associated autoimmune diseases
   - Thyroid disease (most common)—hypothyroidism, thyrotoxicosis, nontoxic goiter
   - Gonadal failure—ovarian/testicular
   - Type 1 diabetes mellitus
   - Hypoparathyroidism
   - Pernicious anemia

   The boy in the given case has associated hypoparathyroidism
   Treatment of hypoparathyroidism:
   - Oral calcium and 1α-hydroxylated vitamin D metabolites (e.g. Calcitriol) are the mainstay of therapy of hypoparathyroidism.
   - *Role of thiazide diuretics:* Thiazide diuretic can be added to the therapeutic regimen to decrease renal calcium losses in cases where difficulty is encountered in attaining the therapeutic goal to maintain serum calcium in the low normal range without causing frank hypercalciuria.
   - *Other therapeutic modalities:* PTH has been used experimentally for the treatment of hypoparathyroidism. This therapy controls hypocalcemia with lower urine calcium excretion than with calcium and calcitriol therapy.

6. **Ans. (c) Random cortisol sample followed by Inj. hydrocortisone**
   [Williams 13th ed pg 531]
   The lady in the given case has presented with Acute Adrenal Insufficiency. Acute adrenal insufficiency is a life-threatening emergency, and treatment should not be delayed while waiting for definitive proof of diagnosis
   Treatment of Acute Adrenal Insufficiency (Adrenal Crisis):
   - Emergency Measures
     - Establish intravenous access.

- Draw blood for electrolytes, glucose, cortisol and ACTH. Do not wait for laboratory results.
- Infuse 2–3 L of 154 0.9% saline (NaCl) solution, or 5% dextrose in 0.9% saline solution, as quickly as possible (1 L in first hour).
- Inject intravenous hydrocortisone (100 mg immediately and every 6 hr).
- Use supportive measures as needed.

- Subacute measures after stabilization of the patient
  - Continue intravenous 154 mmol/L NaCl (0.9% saline) solution at a slower rate for next 24–48 hr.
  - Search for and treat possible infectious precipitating causes of the adrenal crisis.
  - Perform a short ACTH stimulation test to confirm the diagnosis of adrenal insufficiency.
  - Determine the type of adrenal insufficiency and its cause.
  - Taper glucocorticoids to maintenance dosage over 1–3 days.
  - Begin mineralocorticoid replacement with fludrocortisone (0.1 mg by mouth daily) when saline infusion is stopped.

7. **Ans. (d) Dexamethasone T½ 12 hrs**
   [Harrison's Endocrinology 2nd ed pg 131, De Groot 7th ed pg 1742, 1743]

	Estimated Potency	
Glucocorticoid Preparations	**Glucocorticoid**	**Mineralocorticoid**
Short-Acting		
Hydrocortisone/Cortisol	1	1
Cortisone	0.8	0.8
Intermediate-Acting		
Prednisone	4	0.25
Prednisolone	4	0.25
Methylprednisolone	5	<0.01
Triamcinolone	5	<0.01
Long-Acting		
Paramethasone	10	<0.01
Betamethasone	25	<0.01
Dexamethasone	30–40	<0.01

- The relative potencies of the glucocorticoids correlate with their affinities for the glucocorticoid receptor.
- The observed potency of a glucocorticoid, however, is determined not only by the intrinsic biological potency but also by the duration of action.
- The T½ of cortisol in the circulation is 80 to 115 minutes. The T½ values of other commonly used agents are as follows: Cortisone,

0.5 hour; prednisone, 3.4 to 3.8 hours; prednisolone, 2.1 to 3.5 hours; methylprednisolone, 1.3 to 3.1 hours; and dexamethasone, 1.8 to 4.7 hours.
- Little correlation exists between the circulating half-life (T½) of a glucocorticoid and its duration of action or its potency. Also, the many actions of glucocorticoids do not have an equal duration.
- This is consistent with the mechanism of action of steroid hormones. A glucocorticoid continues to act inside the cell after it has disappeared from the circulation. Moreover, the events initiated by a glucocorticoid may continue to occur, or a product of these events (such as a specific protein) may be present, after the disappearance of the glucocorticoid from the circulation.
- The commonly used glucocorticoids are classified as short-acting, intermediate-acting, and long-acting on the basis of the duration of adrenocorticotropic hormone (ACTH) suppression after a single dose, equivalent in anti-inflammatory activity to 50 mg of prednisone.

8. **Ans. (c) Mifepristone**
[J Clin Endocrinol Metab, August 2015, 100(8):2820-2822; Endocrine Reviews, August 2015, 36(4):427-458]

Drugs that have been evaluated for medical treatment of Cushing's syndrome can be classified as follows:

Adrenal Directed Therapy
- Block cortisol production through the inhibition of enzymes involved in steroidogenesis
- Include
  - Adrenostatic drugs, or steroidogenesis inhibitors, which inhibit one or more enzymes responsible for the adrenal steroidogenesis
  - Adrenolytic drugs, which, beyond the effect on steroidogenesis inhibition, induce cell death at the level of the adrenal gland
  a. *Ketoconazole:*
     - Inhibits side-chain cleavage, 17,20-lyase, and 11-β hydroxylase enzymes
     - Adverse effects: mild asymptomatic elevation in serum transaminases (10–15% of cases), idiosyncratic severe hepatic dyscrasia (1 in 15 000 individuals), male hypogonadism
  b. *Metyrapone:*
     - Inhibits 11-β hydroxylase
  c. *Etomidate:*
     - Inhibits 11β-hydroxylase and cholesterol side chain cleavage
     - Most potent adrenostatic agent
     - For severe hypercortisolism in seriously ill patients
     - Needs iv infusion and monitoring in ICU

d. *Mitotane:*
   - Inhibits CYP11A1 (P450 side-chain cleavage) and has a direct cytotoxic action on the adrenal cortex
   - Adrenostatic and adrenolytic properties
   - Primarily used to treat adrenal carcinoma
   - Has sustained effects because of its storage in adipose tissue
   - Teratogen.
e. *Aminoglutethimide:*
   - Block cholesterol side-chain cleavage, 11β-hydroxylase and 18-hydroxylase
   - No longer used because of an unfavorable adverse event profile
f. *Trilostane:*
   - Inhibit 3β-hydroxysteroid dehydrogenase/Δ5-Δ4-isomerase
   - No longer used because of limited efficacy.

Medical Pituitary-directed Therapy
- Inhibit tumoral ACTH secretion and, secondarily, cortisol production
- Two main categories of drugs
  - Neuromodulatory drugs, which directly influence the HPA axis
  - Nuclear receptor ligands, which indirectly influence the HPA axis

A. Neuromodulatory drugs
  1. Serotonin antagonists
     - Limited use because of variable efficacy and the occurrence of serious adverse effects
     a. Cyproheptadine
        - Antiserotonergic, antihistaminic, and anticholinergic
     b. Metergoline
        - Selective antiserotonergic agent
     c. Ritanserine
        - More selective serotonin antagonist
     d. Ketanserine
        - More selective serotonin antagonist
  2. GABA agonists
     a. Valproic acid
        - Limited value because of scant efficacy and serious adverse effects
  3. Dopamine agonists
     a. Cabergoline.
        - High affinity for the dopamine receptor subtype 2
        - Adverse effects: nausea, dizziness, asthenia, valvulopathy
     b. Bromocriptine
        - Limited use because of variability in responsiveness, lack of control during long-term treatment, and adverse effects

4. Somatostatin analogs.
    a. Pasireotide
        - Somatostatin receptor (SST) agonist that binds to somatostatin receptor subtypes 1,2,3 and 5 with substantially high affinity for SST1 and SST5 (Corticotroph tumors have a high expression of SST5)
        - Adverse effects: hyperglycemia, diarrhea, prolonged QTc interval, thyroid abnormalities, transient ↑ LFTs, gallstones, and GH deficiency
        [Octreotide has been found to be ineffective in the majority of patients with CD]
B. Nuclear receptor ligands
    1. PPAR-γ agonists
        - Inadequate in the long-term treatment of CD
        a. Rosiglitazone
        b. Pioglitazone
    2. Retinoic acid receptor agonists
        - Retinoic acid
            - Limited data

Glucocorticoid Receptor Directed Drugs
- Peripherally block the activation of the glucocorticoid receptor, without influencing pituitary and adrenal hormone production.
    a. Mifepristone
        - Glucocorticoid receptor antagonist and antiprogestin
        - Approved by FDA for the control of diabetes or glucose intolerance secondary to hypercortisolism in patients who failed surgery or are not surgical candidates.
        - Abortifacient

NB: The drugs presently in use for the treatment of Cushing's syndrome include Ketoconazole, Metyrapone, Etomidate, Mitotane, Cabergoline, Pasireotide and Mifepristone.

9. **Ans. (d) Adrenoleukodystrophy**
[Harrison's Endocrinology 3rd ed pg 118-121, Williams 13th ed pg 524-526]
- Most common cause of adrenal insufficiency: suppression of the HPA axis as a consequence of exogenous glucocorticoid
- Most common cause of primary adrenal insufficiency worldwide: infectious diseases (most commonly tuberculosis)
- Most common cause of primary adrenal insufficiency in western world: autoimmune adrenalitis
- Most common cause of primary adrenal insufficiency in male child younger than 7 years: adrenoleukodystrophy

Adrenal Cortex | **117**

- Most common cause of secondary adrenal insufficiency—excluding iatrogenic suppression: pituitary or hypothalamic tumors (or their treatment by surgery or irradiation)
- Acute adrenal insufficiency is more frequently observed in patients with primary adrenal insufficiency.

10. **Ans. (b) 11βHSD mismatch**
    [Williams 13th ed pg 494, 516, 574]
    Glucocorticoids and mineralocorticoids bind equally to the mineralocorticoid receptor. Specificity of action is provided in many tissues by the presence of a glucocorticoid inactivating enzyme, 11β-hydroxysteroid dehydrogenase 2 (HSD11B2) which converts cortisol to cortisone and prevents glucocorticoids from interacting with the receptor. Patients with ectopic Cushing's syndrome usually have high rates of cortisol secretion. Cortisol saturates the renal HSD11B2 enzyme, resulting in cortisol-induced mineralocorticoid hypertension and hypokalemia. In addition, these patients have higher levels of the ACTH dependent mineralocorticoid, 11-deoxycorticosterone which contributes to hypokalemia.

11. **Ans. (c) Fluconazole**
    [J Clin Endocrinol Metab, August 2015, 100(8):2820–2822; Endocrine Reviews, August 2015, 36(4):427-458]
    See discussion of Chapter 9, Question 8.

12. **Ans. (b) 30:1**
    [De Groot 7th ed pg 1743]
    See discussion of Chapter 9, Question 7.
    Although, as per the above-mentioned discussion, both options (b) and (c) appear to be correct, option (b) is more appropriate as the reference quoted here mentions the glucocorticoid potential of dexamethasone to be 30 as compared to arbitrarily assigned a value of 1 for hydrocortisone.

13. **Ans. (a) Myopathy and bruising**
    [Williams 13th ed pg 509]
    Myopathy and bruising are two of the most discriminatory features of Cushing's syndrome.

14. **Ans. (c) Exposed areas and new scar**
    [Williams 13th ed pg 528]
    Pigmentation in Addison's disease is seen in sun-exposed areas, recent scars, axillae, nipples, palmar creases, pressure points, and mucous membranes (buccal, vaginal, vulval, anal).

15. **Ans. (c) >90% due to de novo mutation**
    [Williams 13th ed pg 493, 494, 533, 536; Greenspan's 9th ed]

Biochemical Pathways Involved in Adrenal Steroidogenesis

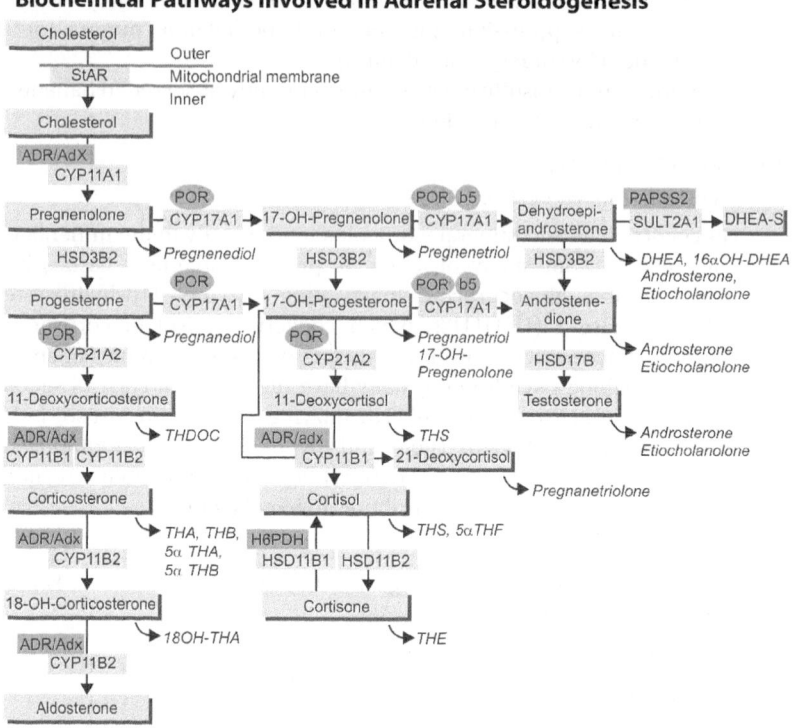

- Steroidogenesis involves action of several enzymes, including a series of cytochrome P450 enzymes
- Cytochrome P450 enzymes are classified into two types according to their subcellular localization and their specific electron shuttle system.
  a. Mitochondrial (type I) cytochrome P450 enzymes
     i. CYP11A1, P450 side-chain cleavage enzyme (P450scc),
     ii. 11β-hydroxylase (CYP11B1, or P450c11b1),
     iii. Aldosterone synthase (CYP11B2, or P450aldo)
  These enzymes rely on electron transfer facilitated by adrenodoxin and adrenodoxin reductase.
  b. Micrososomal (type II) cytochrome P450 enzymes (localized to the endoplasmic reticulum)
     i. 17α-hydroxylase (CYP17A1, or P450c17),
     ii. 21-hydroxylase (CYP21A2, or P450c21),
     iii. P450 aromatase (CYP19A1, or P450aro).
  These enzymes crucially depend on P450 oxidoreductase (POR), which provides electrons.

Congenital Adrenal Hyperplasia due to 21 Hydroxylase Deficiency
- Congenital adrenal hyperplasia is a group of disorders caused by deficient adrenal corticosteroid biosynthesis resulting from defects in one of the steroidogenic enzymes.
- Between 90% and 95% of cases of CAH are caused by 21-hydroxylase deficiency.
- The *CYP21A2* gene and its highly homologous pseudogene (*CYP21A1P*) are located on the short arm of chromosome 6 (6p21.3).
- Most of the mutations causing 21-hydroxylase deficiency are generated by gene conversion events.
- 21-Hydroxylase deficiency is inherited as an autosomal recessive trait.
- Approximately 65% to 75% of patients with 21-hydroxylase deficiency are compound heterozygotes (i.e. they have a different genetic mutation on each of their P450c21B allelic genes) having inherited a mutant gene from each of their parents. A spontaneous mutation in the 21-hydroxylase gene occurs in 1% to 2% of patients.

16. **Ans. (a) StAR deficiency**
    [Williams 13th ed pg 534]
    - DSD associated with various enzyme defects causing congenital adrenal hyperplasia
        - 46, XX DSD
            * 21-Hydroxylase deficiency
            * 11β-Hydroxylase deficiency
            * P450 Oxidoreductase deficiency
        - 46, XY DSD
            * 17α-Hydroxylase deficiency
            * 3β-Hydroxysteroid dehydrogenase deficiency type 2 deficiency
            * P450 Oxidoreductase deficiency
            * *StAR deficiency:* Congenital lipoid adrenal hyperplasia
            * P450 Side-chain cleavage deficiency
    - While both StAR deficiency and P450 Oxidoreductase deficiency are known to cause 46, XY DSD, P450 Oxidoreductase deficiency usually produces ambiguous genitalia, while StAR deficiency is usually known to result in female-typical genitalia.

17. **Ans. (b) Iatrogenic**
    [Williams 13th ed pg 514]
    See discussion of Chapter 9, Question 27.

18. **Ans. (b) Increased secretion of glucocorticoid and androgen**
    [Williams 13th ed pg 546]
    Eighty percent of primary adrenal carcinomas are functional, most commonly secreting glucocorticoids alone (45%), glucocorticoids and androgens (45%), or androgens alone (10%). Fewer than 1% of all tumors secrete aldosterone. Patients usually present with features of the hormone excess state (glucocorticoid, androgen, or both).

19. **Ans. (c) Hydrocortisone**
    [Harrison's Endocrinology 2nd ed pg 131, De Groot 7th ed pg 1743]
    See discussion of Chapter 9, Question 7.

20. **Ans. (b) Dexamethasone**
    [De Groot 7th ed pg 1742; National Center for Biotechnology Information. PubChem Compound Database; CID=31307, https://pubchem.ncbi.nlm.nih.gov/compound/31307 (accessed Fe Ans. (b) 14, 2018)]
    See discussion of Chapter 9, Question 7.
    T½ of triamcinolone is 1-2 hours.

21. **Ans. (d) Ca^+ restriction**

22. **Ans. (e) Thick skin**
    [Williams 13th ed pg 507-510; Professional Guide to Diseases 9th ed pg 631; Case Rep Dermatol. 2017 Jan-Apr; 9(1): 45-50]

23. **Ans. (d) None has very high caloric value**
    Cholesterol is the precursor of a large number of steroids
    Examples of steroids: cholesterol, bile acids, adrenocortical hormones, sex hormones, D vitamins, cardiac glycosides, sitosterols of the plant kingdom, and some alkaloids.
    All steroids have a similar cyclic nucleus resembling phenanthrene (rings A, B, and C) to which a cyclopentane ring (D) is attached.
    The hexagonal rings denote completely saturated six-carbon ring with all valences satisfied by hydrogen bonds.

    - Steroids are hydrophobic
    - Because of their hydrophobicity, they must be complexed with a plasma protein.

24. **Ans. (a) 24 hr UFC**
    [Journal of Clinical Endocrinology & Metabolism, May 2008, 93(5):1536]

25. **Ans. (d) Fluconazole**
    [J Clin Endocrinol Metab, August 2015, 100(8):2820-2822; Endocrine Reviews, August 2015, 36(4):427-458]
    See discussion of Chapter 9, Question 8.

26. **Ans. (d) Lipoid CAH (StAR deficiency)**
   See discussion of Chapter 9, Question 16.

   Both options (c) and (d) are correct.

   Although POR deficiency can be associated with underandrogenization of 46, XY males, mutations in StAR typically cause a marked deficiency in testosterone synthesis by fetal Leydig cells so that female-typical genitalia are seen.

   Thus, option (d) is a better choice than option (c).

27. **Ans. (c) Low dose dexamethasone test cannot differentiate from true Cushing's syndrome**
   [Williams 13th ed pg 514]

   - A pseudo-Cushing's state is defined as the presence of some clinical features of Cushing's syndrome with biochemical evidence of hypercortisolism that has arisen from some other causes.
   - The most commonly associated conditions are alcoholism, depression, and obesity.
   - It is hypothesized that these stressful conditions increase the activity of the CRH neuron, resulting in excessive ACTH secretion, adrenal hyperplasia, and increased cortisol production.
   - Utility of various tests in distinguishing between pseudo-Cushing's states and true Cushing's syndrome
     – *Urinary free cortisol:* Pseudo-Cushing's states may produce false positive elevations of urinary free cortisol (up to four fold normal)
     – Late-night salivary cortisol: The circadian rhythm is blunted in many patients with depressive illness and obese subjects
     – Longer low dose dexamethasone suppression test (2 mg/d for 48 h): Optimal test
     – 1 mg overnight dexamethasone suppression test: Specificity is lower compared with the 2-day test, with potential misclassification in patients with pseudo-Cushing's states
     – Other tests that have been used to distinguish Cushing's syndrome from pseudo-Cushing's states
       ♦ Dexamethasone-CRH test
       ♦ Insulin tolerance test.

28. **Ans. (a) Represent free cortisol**
   [J Clin Endocrinol Metab, May 2008, 93(5):1533]

   - Free cortisol in the blood is in equilibrium with cortisol in the saliva. Good correlation exists between salivary and simultaneous serum cortisol values
     – The concentration of salivary cortisol is not affected by the rate of saliva production.
     – Saliva sample is collected on two separate evenings between 2300 and 2400 h.

- Saliva is collected either by passive drooling into a plastic tube or by placing a cotton pledget (salivette) in the mouth and chewing for 1-2 min. Samples collected using the salivette device had lower cortisol concentrations than those collected from passive drooling, but they correlated better with total and free serum cortisol levels.
- Normal values: <145 ng/dL (4 nmol/liter).
- Conditions which may affect the result:
  - Shift workers/those with variable bedtimes/those with bedtimes consistently long after midnight
  - Individuals crossing widely different time zones
  - Depression
  - Stress
  - Critical illness
  - Licorice or chewing tobacco/smoking
  - Contamination with blood/steroid-containing lotion or oral gels
  - Age ≥60 yr
  - Diabetes
  - Hypertension
  - Obesity.

29. **Ans. (d) All of the above**
    [De Groot 7th ed pg 2680]

    Corticotropin-releasing Hormone Stimulation Test
    - *Indication:*
      - Suspected pituitary adrenocorticotropic hormone (ACTH) deficiency
      - Suspected pituitary Cushing's; rule out ectopic disease.
    - *Medication*: 1.0 μg/kg (100 μg/1.73 m^2; maximum dose 100 μg) synthetic sheep or human CRH administered as IV bolus throughout 30 s. Patient fasting 4 h.
    - *Sampling*: Blood measurements of cortisol and ACTH at -5 and -1 minute before CRH and at 15, 30, 45, and 60 minutes after CRH.
    - *Interpretation*: Baseline ACTH increases 20% to 40% in 95% of normal subjects. Peak values (usually in the 20 to 100 pg/mL range) are observed at 30 to 60 minutes. Serum cortisol peaks at 30 to 60 min in the 20 to 25 μg/dL range.
    - *Comments:*
      - Patients with pituitary ACTH deficiency have subnormal responses; those with hypothalamic disease tend to exhibit augmented and prolonged ACTH responses with reduced cortisol response. Patients with primary adrenal insufficiency have high baseline ACTH, an augmented response to CRH, and low cortisol levels before and after CRH.
      - Patients with Cushing's disease (pituitary Cushing's) usually show a >20% rise in cortisol and a >50% increase in ACTH. Patients with adrenal causes of Cushing's syndrome or ectopic ACTH syndrome

do not respond to CRH. Rarely, bronchial carcinoids producing ACTH may respond to CRH.

CRH Stimulation Test, Petrosal Venous Sinus Sampling
- *Indication:* Differentiation between ectopic and pituitary causes of Cushing's disease.
- *Medication:* Ovine CRH (1 µg/kg body weight) administered as IV bolus.
- *Sampling:* Catheters are inserted via the jugular or femoral veins into both inferior petrosal veins. Blood is obtained from a peripheral vein via a third catheter or from a port in the iliac vein. Blood samples are drawn simultaneously from both inferior petrosal sinuses and the peripheral vein for plasma ACTH. At least 4 sets of 3 samples each are obtained: 2 sets are drawn immediately before injection of CRH as a baseline, and 2 more are drawn between 2 and 3 and between 5 and 6 minutes after peripheral intravenous injection of CRH.
- *Interpretation:* A central-to-peripheral plasma ACTH gradient of 2.0 before CRH administration, or 3.0 after CRH, is diagnostic of a pituitary source of ACTH.

30. **Ans. (c) Clinical**
    [J Clin Endocrinol Metab, February 2016, 101(2):365]

31. **Ans. (a) Hypoaldosteronemia**
    [De Groot 7th ed pg 2678, 2680]

32. **Ans. (a) ACTH stimulation test**
    [Textbook of Diabetes 4th ed pg 923]

    Several endocrine disorders are associated with T1DM because of a common etiology and similar pathology (e.g. autoimmune adrenalitis [Addison's disease] or autoimmune thyroid disease). Attention is warranted to look for the onset of these disorders.

33. **Ans. (a) Dexamethasone**
    [Williams 13th ed pg 506]

34. **Ans. (b) Petrosal venous sinus sampling will lateralize the pituitary adenoma**
    [De Groot 7th ed pg 2681]

    The lateralization of the adenoma in pituitary Cushing's through this procedure is of dubious value, because it is only 70% accurate.

35. **Ans. (b) Ketoconazole**
    [J Clin Endocrinol Metab, August 2015, 100(8):2820-2822; Endocrine Reviews, August 2015, 36(4):427-458]

    See discussion of Chapter 9, Question 8.

36. **Ans. (b) Overnight dexamethasone suppression used to differentiate from true Cushing's**
    [Williams 13th ed pg 514; Endocrine Reviews, Volume 19, Issue 5, 1 October 1998, pg 663, 664]

See discussion of Chapter 9, Question 27.

The use of the opiate agonist loperamide has also been suggested for the purpose of discriminating between Cushing's syndrome and pseudo-Cushing's states.

37. **Ans. (c) Cushingoid stigmata**
    [Williams 13th ed pg 498, 524, 582, 1198; De Groot 7th ed pg 1890]
    See discussion of Chapter 10, Question 36.

38. **Ans. (d) Dexamethasone**
    [Harrison's Endocrinology 2nd ed pg 131, De Groot 7th ed pg 1742, 1743]
    See discussion of Chapter 9, Question 7.

39. **Ans. (c) Anti-21 hydroxylase antibody**
    [Williams 13th ed pg 525]

40. **Ans. (b) 5 mg**
    [Harrison's Endocrinology 2nd ed pg 131; De Groot 7th ed pg 1742, 1743]
    See discussion of Chapter 9, Question 7.

41. **Ans. (a) 11βhydroxylase**
    [Williams 13th ed pg 534]

CHAPTER

10

Endocrine Hypertension

QUESTIONS

1. Best test to diagnose hyperaldosteronism is:
   a. Aldosterone: PRA > 20
   b. Aldosterone: PRA < 20
   c. Decrease PRA
   d. Increased PRA

2. Cost effective investigation for diagnosis of pheochromocytoma difficult to locate:
   a. I 131 MIBG
   b. I 123 MIBG
   c. Whole body MRI
   d. Octreoscan

3. Mineralocorticoid receptor is found in all except:
   a. Liver
   b. Distal colon
   c. Hippocampus
   d. Kidney

4. Preoperative management of pheochromocytoma, true is:
   a. α-blocker before β-blocker
   b. β-blocker before α-blocker
   c. α-blocker is never used
   d. β-blocker is never used

5. Malignant pheochromocytoma commonly secretes:
   a. VMA
   b. Metanephrines
   c. Epinephrine
   d. Dopamine

6. Pheochromocytoma not associated with:
   a. VHL syndrome
   b. von Recklinghausen's disease
   c. McCune-Albright syndrome
   d. Sipple syndrome

7. Decreased renin action seen in all except:
   a. GRA
   b. Bartter's syndrome
   c. Liddle's syndrome
   d. Cushing's syndrome

8. All of the following are true about primary hyperaldosteronism except:
   a. HTN
   b. Renin/aldosterone ratio is used for screening
   c. Aldosterone suppression tests are used for confirmation
   d. Decreased PRA activity

9. Not done in case of adrenal adenoma:
   a. Urine metanephrines
   b. PRA, aldosterone
   c. FNAC
   d. Contrast CT

10. Aldosterone synthase causes following action:
    a. 18-hydroxylation of corticosterone
    b. 11-beta hydroxylation
    c. 17-alfa hydroxylation
    d. 18-oxidation

11. Aldosterone is stimulated by:
    a. K^+
    b. Na^+
    c. RAA
    d. ACTH

12. All of the following are correct about GRA except:
    a. AD
    b. PRA↑
    c. HTN in childhood
    d. Family H/O present

13. Hyperkalemia is seen in all except:
    a. Tubulointerstitial disease
    b. Mineralocorticoid deficiency
    c. Mineralocorticoid resistance
    d. Glomerulonephritis

14. All of the following statements are true about pheochromocytoma in MEN-II except:
    a. 50% bilateral
    b. Recurrence on other side common
    c. Less capsular invasion
    d. Mostly malignant

15. MIBG is imported into the storage vesicles in the adrenal medulla by:
    a. NIS
    b. Na-Pi transporter
    c. Vesicular monoamine transporter
    d. Na-K ATPase

16. In patients with CAH, fertility is least in:
    a. Atypical CAH
    b. Adult onset CAH
    c. Virilizing CAH
    d. Salt wasting CAH

17. Rate limiting step in catecholamine metabolism:
    a. Tyrosine hydroxylase
    b. Dopa decarboxylase
    c. PNMT
    d. Dopamine beta hydroxylase

18. Which of the following is true about GRA?
    a. X-linked/AR
    b. Hypertension is due to decreased 17αhydroxylase and 11βhydroxylase
    c. Hypertension and increased K^+ respond to dexamethasone
    d. Elevated urinary excretion of 18-hydroxycortisol and 18-oxycortisol

19. Gene for 21-hydroxylase is located on chromosome number:
    a. 12
    b. 20
    c. 8
    d. 6

20. Glucocorticoid responsive hypertension:
    a. Glucocorticoid resistance syndrome
    b. FHA 1
    c. FHA 2
    d. 11βHSD deficiency
    e. 3βHSD deficiency

21. Syndrome of apparent mineralocorticoid excess:
    a. High renin
    b. Macrosomia
    c. Childhood HTN
    d. Hypokalemia
    e. 11βHSD-1 defect

22. Difference between 1° and 2°, hyperaldosteronism:
    a. High ACTH
    b. High PRA
    c. Hypovolemia
    d. HTN
    e. Hypokalemia

23. Aldosterone synthesis is stimulated by all except:
    a. ACTH
    b. Cortisol
    c. Renin
    d. Potassium

24. ↓ renin levels:
    a. CAH
    b. GRA
    c. Liddle's syndrome
    d. Bartter's syndrome

25. Pheochromocytoma rule out and confirm:
    a. Urine fractionated metanephrines
    b. Plasma free metanephrines
    c. Urine total metanephrines
    d. Plasma catecholamines

26. Pheochromocytoma:
    a. Adrenal is more commonly malignant than extra adrenal
    b. Neuroectodermal in origin
    c. Extra adrenal more common
    d. 40% are familial

27. Not true about CAH:
    a. 21-hydroxylase deficiency is seen exclusively in females
    b. Ambiguous genitalia are not seen in StAR deficiency
    c. All are inherited in autosomal recessive manner
    d. HTN is seen in 17-hydroxylase and 11-hydroxylase deficiency

28. Features that differentiate primary from secondary aldosteronism:
    a. Hypokalemia
    b. Hypertension
    c. PRA
    d. Hypovolemia
    e. High ACTH

29. Triad of pheochromocytoma include all except:
   a. Tremor
   b. Sweating
   c. Headache
   d. Palpitations

30. Pheochromocytoma—tests with high precision:
   a. Fractionated metanephrines
   b. Chromogranin A
   c. VMA
   d. Free metanephrines
   e. Dopa PET

31. A 26-year-old woman presents with episodes of dizziness mainly on standing. Her biochemical profile shows hyperkalemic acidosis. Which underlying condition is she most likely to have?
   a. Cushing's syndrome
   b. Addison's disease
   c. Conn's syndrome
   d. Type 1 renal tubular acidosis
   e. Bulimia nervosa

32. A 36-year-old male presents with lethargy. He takes no medication and has generally been otherwise well. Examination reveals that he is obese with a BMI of 36.4 kg/m² and a blood pressure of 120/72. There are no abnormalities of the cardiovascular, respiratory or abdominal systems. Investigations reveal a sodium of 141 mmol/L, a potassium of 2.8 mmol/L, a urea of 5.6 mmol/L and a creatinine of 76 μmol/L. What is the most likely diagnosis?
   a. Conn's syndrome
   b. Apparent mineralocorticoid excess
   c. Cushing's syndrome
   d. Hypokalemic periodic paralysis
   e. Bartter's syndrome

33. A 29-year-old female presents with headaches. She is noted to be hypertensive with a blood pressure of 180/100 mm Hg and initial investigations reveal a hypokalemia of 2.9 mmol/L. On closer questioning she is found to consume a large quantity of liquorice. Inhibition of which enzyme is responsible for the pseudohyperaldosteronism associated with liquorice.
   a. 5-alpha-reductase
   b. 21-hydroxylase
   c. 11-beta hydroxysteroid dehydrogenase (11-β HSD)
   d. 17-alpha hydroxylase (17-α OH)
   e. 11-beta hydroxylase (11-β OH)

34. 17 OHP measurement—all except:
   a. High in first 48 hours
   b. High in premature, sick infant
   c. Measured after 72 hours
   d. ELISA in gold standard

35. Which is the best drug treatment of hypertension in pheochromocytoma?
   a. Atenolol
   b. Phentolamine
   c. Phenoxybenzamine
   d. Enalapril
   e. Nifedipine

36. Manifestation of glucocorticoid resistance include all except:
    a. Hypokalemia
    b. Hypertension
    c. Virilization
    d. Adrenal insufficiency

37. All of the following may be associated with hypokalemia except:
    a. Hyperaldosteronism
    b. Cushing's syndrome
    c. Renal tubular acidosis
    d. Lactic acidosis
    e. Ureterosigmoidostomy

38. CAH due to CYP 21 deficiency in a female is associated with all except:
    a. Labioscrotal fusion
    b. Hyperkalemia
    c. Suppressed plasma renin activity
    d. Increased androstenedione

39. Hypertension in endogenous hypercortisolism is mainly due to oversaturation of:
    a. 11-beta HSD 1
    b. 11-beta HSD 2
    c. 11-beta hydroxylase
    d. 17-beta HSD 3

40. 17-hydroxy progesterone may be elevated in all except:
    a. 3-beta HSD 2 deficiency
    b. POR deficiency
    c. 17-beta HSD 3 deficiency
    d. CYP 21 deficiency

41. False about MIBG scintigraphy for pheochromocytoma:
    a. I 123 MIBG is superior than I 131 MIBG
    b. MIBG is less sensitive than MRI
    c. Indicated for less than 10 cm adrenal mass on CT
    d. Indicated for suspected paraganglioma

42. Which of the following statement is wrong regarding primary hyperaldosteronism?
    a. Bilateral idiopathic hyperaldosteronism (IHA) is more common than aldosterone producing adenoma (APA)
    b. Hypokalemia is more common in APA than IHA
    c. APA have higher aldosterone concentration than IHA
    d. Hypertension is cured by bilateral adrenalectomy in IHA

43. All of the following inhibit the synthesis of aldosterone, except:
    a. Dopamine
    b. Potassium ion
    c. ANP
    d. Ouabain-like factor

44. Which of the following regimens is best for the preoperative management of a patient with a known pheochromocytoma?
    a. Propranolol alone
    b. Propranolol followed by phenoxybenzamine
    c. Phenoxybenzamine followed by propranolol
    d. Prazosin alone
    e. Propranolol followed by prazosin

45. Which of the following statements concerning the diagnosis of pheochromocytoma is correct?
    a. Measurement of plasma catecholamines is the preferred initial screening test.
    b. Random urine samples are equivalent in diagnostic accuracy to the measurement of catecholamines or catecholamine metabolites in a 24-h urine collection.
    c. After collection, the urine should be treated with dilute sodium hydroxide and refrigerated.
    d. The ideal time to collect urine is during a period of clinical stability.

46. The most common cause of primary aldosteronism is:
    a. Aldosterone producing carcinoma
    b. Unilateral adrenal hyperplasia
    c. Bilateral idiopathic hyperplasia
    d. Aldosterone producing adenoma

47. The cut off value for cortisol corrected aldosterone ratio to indicate unilateral disease in primary aldosteronism during bilateral AVS is:
    a. 1.5
    b. 2.5
    c. 4.0
    d. 8.5

48. Following are true about imaging in pheochromocytoma on CT except:
    a. Smooth margins
    b. Absence of calcification
    c. Marked enhancement
    d. Growth of 1 cm/year

Endocrine Hypertension | **131**

ANSWERS

1. **Ans. (a) Aldosterone: PRA > 20**
   [Williams 13th ed pg 576, 577]

2. **Ans. (b) I 123 MIBG**
   [Williams 13th ed pg 568]

3. **Ans. (a) Liver**
   [Williams 13th ed pg 574]

4. **Ans. (a) α-blocker before β-blocker**
   [Williams 13th ed pg 570]
   Combined α- and β-adrenergic blockade is one approach to control blood pressure and prevent intraoperative hypertensive crises.
   - α-adrenergic blockade should be started 7–10 days preoperatively
   - After adequate α-adrenergic blockade has been achieved, β-adrenergic blockade is initiated, typically 2–3 days preoperatively.

5. **Ans. (d) Dopamine**
   [Greenspan's 9th ed]
   Metastases usually secrete norepinephrine and normetanephrine. Some metastases secrete predominantly dopamine. Metastases rarely secrete epinephrine or metanephrine, with the exception of some metastases from epinephrine-secreting adrenal pheochromocytomas. About 20% of primary paragangliomas and their metastases do not secrete catecholamines or metanephrines, but most continue to secrete CgA.

6. **Ans. (c) McCune-Albright syndrome**
   [Williams 13th ed pg 562, 563]

7. **Ans. (b) Bartter's syndrome**
   [Williams 13th ed pg 575, 582; Brenner & Rector's The Kidney 9th ed pg 658]

   Adrenocortical Causes of Hypertension
   Low Renin and High Aldosterone
   - Primary aldosteronism
     - Aldosterone-producing adenoma (APA)—30% of cases
     - Bilateral idiopathic hyperplasia (IHA)—60% of cases
     - Primary (unilateral) adrenal hyperplasia—2% of cases
     - Aldosterone-producing adrenocortical carcinoma—<1% of cases
     - Familial hyperaldosteronism (FH)
       - Glucocorticoid-remediable aldosteronism (FH type 1)—<1% of cases
       - FH type 2 (APA or IHA)—<6% of cases
       - FH type 3 (germline KCNJ5 mutations)—<1% of cases
     - Ectopic aldosterone-producing adenoma or carcinoma—<0.1% of cases

Low Renin and Low Aldosterone
- Hyperdeoxycorticosteronism
  - Congenital adrenal hyperplasia
    - 11β-Hydroxylase deficiency
    - 17α-Hydroxylase deficiency
  - Deoxycorticosterone-producing tumor
  - Primary cortisol resistance
  - Apparent mineralocorticoid excess (AME)/11β-HSD deficiency
    - Genetic
      - Type 1 AME
    - Acquired
      - Licorice or carbenoxolone ingestion (type 1 AME)
      - Cushing syndrome (type 2 AME)
- Cushing's syndrome
  - Exogenous glucocorticoid administration—most common cause
  - Endogenous
    - ACTH-dependent—85% of cases
      - Pituitary
      - Ectopic
    - ACTH-independent—15% of cases
      - Unilateral adrenal disease (adenoma or carcinoma)
      - Bilateral adrenal disease
        - Massive macronodular hyperplasia (rare)
        - Primary pigmented nodular adrenal disease (rare)

Liddle Syndrome
- Renal disorder with a presentation similar to primary aldosteronism.
- Inheritance: Autosomal dominant
- Caused by mutations in the β- or γ-subunit of the amiloride sensitive epithelial sodium channel. This mutation results in enhanced activity of the epithelial sodium channel, and increased renal sodium reabsorption, potassium wasting.
- Affected individuals usually present as children or young adults with hypertension, hypokalemia and low levels of aldosterone and renin.
- *Diagnosis*:
  - Exclusion of other causes
  - Treatment trial with amiloride or triamterene.
  - Genetic testing.
- Liddle syndrome can be distinguished from apparent mineralocorticoid excess based on the good clinical response to amiloride or triamterene combined with a sodium restricted diet, lack of efficacy of spironolactone and dexamethasone, and normal 24-hour urine cortisone/cortisol ratio.

Bartter's Syndrome
- Bartter's syndrome is characterized by marked elevations in plasma angiotensin II, plasma aldosterone and plasma rennin levels

Endocrine Hypertension | **133**

8. **Ans. (b) Renin/aldosterone ratio is used for screening**
   [Williams 13th ed pg 576, 577]

9. **Ans. (c) FNAC**
   [Williams 13th ed pg 545; De Groot 7th ed pg 1806; Endocr Pract. 2009; 15(Suppl 1) pg 16]

10. **Ans. (a) 18-hydroxylation of corticosterone**
    [Williams 13th ed pg 494, 495]

    See discussion of Chapter 9, Question 15.
    CYP11B2 (aldosterone synthase) can carry out
    - 11β-hydroxylation (conversion DOC to corticosterone)
    - 18-hydroxylation (conversion of corticosterone to 18-OH corticosterone)
    - 18-methyloxidation (conversion of 18-OH corticosterone to aldosterone).

11. **Ans. (a) K^+, (c) RAA and (d) ACTH**
    [De Groot 7th ed pg 1757, 1758]

    Factors Regulating Renin Release

Stimulatory	Inhibitory
Decreased perfusion pressure	Increased chloride delivery at the macula densa
PGI2	Angiotensin II
ACTH	Atrial natriuretic factor
B-Adrenergic stimulation	Vasopressin
	α-Adrenergic stimulation
	Dopamine

    Factors Regulating Aldosterone Secretion

Factor	Stimulatory	Inhibitory
Peptides	Angiotensin II	Atrial natriuretic peptide
	Angiotensin III	Somatostatin
	ACTH	
	Vasopressin	
	Endothelin	
Ions	Plasma potassium	
Other	Serotonin	Dopamine
		Ouabain

12. **Ans. (b) PRA↑**
    [Williams 13th ed pg 579, 580; De Groot 7th ed pg 1887]

13. **Ans. (d) Glomerulonephritis**
    [Harrison's Principles of Internal Medicine 19th edition pg 309]

Causes of Hyperkalemia
- Pseudohyperkalemia
  - Cellular efflux; thrombocytosis, erythrocytosis, leukocytosis, *in vitro* hemolysis
  - Hereditary defects in red cell membrane transport
- Intra- to extracellular shift
  - Acidosis
  - Hyperosmolality; radiocontrast, hypertonic dextrose, mannitol
  - B_2-Adrenergic antagonists (noncardioselective agents)
  - Digoxin and related glycosides (yellow oleander, foxglove, bufadienolide)
  - Hyperkalemic periodic paralysis
  - Lysine, arginine, and E-aminocaproic acid (structurally similar, positively charged)
  - Succinylcholine; thermal trauma, neuromuscular injury, disuse atrophy, mucositis, or prolonged immobilization
  - Rapid tumor lysis
- Inadequate excretion
  - Inhibition of the renin-angiotensin-aldosterone axis:
    * Angiotensin-converting enzyme (ACE) inhibitors
    * Renin inhibitors; aliskiren
    * Angiotensin receptor blockers (ARBs)
    * Blockade of the mineralocorticoid receptor: spironolactone, eplerenone, drospirenone
    * Blockade of the epithelial sodium channel (ENaC): amiloride, triamterene, trimethoprim, pentamidine, nafamostat
  - Decreased distal delivery
    * Congestive heart failure
    * Volume depletion
  - Hyporeninemic hypoaldosteronism
    * Tubulointerstitial diseases: systemic lupus erythematosus (SLE), sickle cell anemia, obstructive uropathy
    * Diabetes, diabetic nephropathy
    * Drugs: nonsteroidal anti-inflammatory drugs (NSAIDs), cyclooxygenase 2 (COX2) inhibitors, β-blockers, cyclosporine, tacrolimus
    * Chronic kidney disease, advanced age
    * Pseudohypoaldosteronism type II: defects in WNK1 or WNK4 kinases, Kelch-like 3 (KLHL3), or Cullin 3 (CUL3)
  - Renal resistance to mineralocorticoid
    * *Tubulointerstitial diseases:* SLE, amyloidosis, sickle cell anemia, obstructive uropathy, postacute tubular necrosis
    * *Hereditary:* Pseudohypoaldosteronism type I; defects in the mineralocorticoid receptor or the epithelial sodium channel (ENaC)

- Advanced renal insufficiency
  - Chronic kidney disease
  - End-stage renal disease
  - Acute oliguric kidney injury
- Primary adrenal insufficiency
  - *Autoimmune:* Addison's disease, polyglandular endocrinopathy
  - *Infectious:* HIV, cytomegalovirus, tuberculosis, disseminated fungal infection
  - *Infiltrative:* Amyloidosis, malignancy, metastatic cancer
  - *Drug-associated:* Heparin, low-molecular-weight heparin
  - *Hereditary:* Adrenal hypoplasia congenita, congenital lipoid adrenal hyperplasia, aldosterone synthase deficiency
  - Adrenal hemorrhage or infarction, including antiphospholipid syndrome

14. **Ans. (d) Mostly malignant**
    [De Groot 7th ed pg 1911, 1912]
    - MEN 2-associated pheochromocytomas
      - Pheochromocytomas develop in ~50% of patients
      - Secrete epinephrine
      - Almost always intra-adrenal; often multifocal and bilateral (~30% at diagnosis, ~70% lifetime risk)
      - Almost exclusively benign (<5% are malignant).
    - In children with MEN 2B-associated pheochromocytomas, a higher risk of malignancy compared with MEN 2A or sporadic disease is found.

15. **Ans. (c) Vesicular monoamine transporter**
    [Williams 13th ed pg 558]

16. **Ans. (d) Salt wasting CAH**
    [Journal of Clinical Endocrinology & Metabolism, September 2010; 95(9):4149]

17. **Ans. (a) Tyrosine hydroxylase and (b) Dopa decarboxylase**
    [Williams 13th ed pg 557]

    Biosynthetic Pathway for Catecholamines

    Tyrosine →(TH)→ Dopa →(AADC)→ Dopamine →(DBH)→ Norepinephrine →(PNMT)→ Epinephrine

    Tyrosine hydroxylase (TH); Aromatic L-amino acid decarboxylase (AADC); dopamine β-hydroxylase (DBH); phenylethanolamine N-methyltransferase (PNMT).

Tyrosine is converted to 3,4-dihydroxyphenylalanine (dopa) by tyrosine hydroxylase (TH); this is the rate-limiting step.

18. **Ans. (d) Elevated urinary excretion of 18-hydroxycortisol and 18-oxycortisol**
    [Williams 13th ed pg 579, 580; De Groot 7th ed pg 1887]

    Glucocorticoid-remediable Aldosteronism:
    Familial Hyperaldosteronism Type I [GRA (FH type I)]
    - Autosomal-dominant disorder.
    - GRA results from CYP11B1/CYP11B2 chimeric gene that combines the regulatory sequences of the 11β-hydroxylase gene with the coding region of the aldosterone synthase gene. This results in the expression of aldosterone synthase in the zona fasciculata. Mineralocorticoid production is regulated by ACTH instead of angiotensin II (therefore, hypersecretion of aldosterone can be reversed with physiologic doses of glucocorticoid).
    - This mutation results in overproduction of aldosterone and the hybrid steroids 18-hydroxycortisol and 18-oxycortisol.
    - PRA is suppressed.
    - Characterized by early-onset severe hypertension; hypokalemia may be present.
    - Genetic testing for GRA should be considered for patients with primary aldosteronism who have
      - Family history of primary aldosteronism
      - Onset of primary aldosteronism at a young age (<20 years)
      - Family history of strokes at a young age.

19. **Ans. (d) 6**
    [Williams 13th ed pg 536]

20. **Ans. (b) FHA 1**
    [Williams 13th ed pg 579, 580; De Groot 7th ed pg 1887, 1888]

21. **Ans. (c) Childhood HTN and (d) Hypokalemia**
    [Williams 13th ed pg 582]

    Option (d) is more appropriate than option (c).

    Apparent Mineralocorticoid Excess Syndrome
    - Result of impaired activity of the enzyme HSD11B2, which normally inactivates cortisol in the kidney by converting it to inactive cortisone.
    - High levels of cortisol accumulate in the kidney and can act as a potent mineralocorticoid.
    - Decreased HSD11B2 activity may be
      - Congenital (Hereditary)
      - Acquired: Secondary to inhibition of enzyme activity by glycyrrhizic acid, the active principle of licorice root (Glycyrrhiza glabra).
    - In addition, HSD11B2 may be overwhelmed by massive cortisol hypersecretion associated with Cushing's syndrome due to ectopic ACTH syndrome.

- Congenital apparent mineralocorticoid excess
  - Autosomal recessive
  - Presents in childhood with hypertension, hypokalemia, low birth weight, failure to thrive, hypertension, polyuria and polydipsia, and poor growth.
- The clinical phenotype of patients with apparent mineralocorticoid excess includes hypertension, hypokalemia, metabolic alkalosis, low renin, low aldosterone, and normal plasma cortisol levels.
- Diagnosis of apparent mineralocorticoid excess is confirmed by an abnormal (high) ratio of cortisol to cortisone in a 24-hour urine collection (typically increased 10-fold above the normal value).

22. **Ans. (b) High PRA**
[Mosby's Manual of Diagnostic and Laboratory Tests 5th ed pg 448]

Patients with primary hyperaldosteronism will have increased aldosterone production associated with decreased renin activity.

Patients with secondary hyperaldosteronism will have increased levels of aldosterone and plasma renin.

23. **Ans. (b) Cortisol**
[De Groot 7th ed pg 1757, 1758]

See discussion of Chapter 10, Question 11.

24. **Ans. (d) Bartter's syndrome**
[Williams 13th ed pg 575, 582; Brenner & Rector's The Kidney 9th ed pg 658]

See discussion of Chapter 10, Question 7.

25. **Ans. (b) Plasma free metanephrines**
[De Groot 7th ed pg 1915]

26. **Ans. (d) 40% are familial**
[Williams 13th ed pg 559, 567; De Groot 7th ed pg 1902; Greenspan's 9th ed]

- Approximately 85% of these pheochromocytomas are found in the adrenal glands, and 95% are found in the abdomen and pelvis.
- Pheochromocytomas and paragangliomas are neuroendocrine tumors.
- Metastases occur in about 10% of pheochromocytomas and 30% of non-head-neck sympathetic paragangliomas.

27. **Ans. (a) 21 hydroxylase deficiency is seen exclusively in females and (b) Ambiguous genitalia are not seen in StAR deficiency**
[Williams 13th ed pg 533-536]

28. **Ans. (c) PRA**
[Mosby's Manual of Diagnostic and Laboratory Tests 5th ed pg 448]

See discussion of Chapter 10, Question 22.

29. **Ans. (a) Tremor**
[De Groot 7th ed pg 1907, Harrison's Endocrinology 3rd ed pg 127]

The triad of headache, sweating, and palpitations constitutes the most common symptoms in patients with a pheochromocytoma, and their presence in patients with hypertension should arouse immediate suspicion for a pheochromocytoma.

30. **Ans. (d) Free metanephrines**
 [De Groot 7th ed pg 1915]

31. **Ans. (b) Addison's disease**
 [Williams 13th ed pg 528]
 See discussion of Chapter 9, Question 3.

32. **Ans. (d) Hypokalemic periodic paralysis**

33. **Ans. (c) 11-beta hydroxysteroid dehydrogenase (11-β HSD)**
 [Williams 13th ed pg 582]
 See discussion of Chapter 10, Question 21.

34. **Ans. (d) ELISA in gold standard**
 [J Clin Endocrinol Metab, September 2010;95(9):4135]
 - First-tier screens for CAH employ immunoassays to measure 17-OHP. Both RIAs and ELISAs have been almost completely supplanted by automated time-resolved dissociation-enhanced lanthanide fluoro-immunoassay (DELFIA).
 - In interpreting these tests, it must be remembered that 17-OHP levels are normally high at birth and decrease rapidly during the first few postnatal days. In contrast, 17-OHP levels increase with time in infants affected with CAH. Thus, diagnostic accuracy is poor in the first 2 days. Additionally, premature, sick, or stressed infants typically have higher levels of 17-OHP than term infants and generate many false positives.

35. **Ans. (c) Phenoxybenzamine**
 [Williams 13th ed pg 570]

36. **Ans. (d) Adrenal insufficiency**
 [Williams 13th ed pg 498, 524, 582, 1198; De Groot 7th ed pg 1890]

 Glucocorticoid Resistance (Primary Cortisol Resistance)
 - Caused by genetic defects in the glucocorticoid receptor and the steroid-receptor complex.
 - Feedback inhibition is principally mediated via the glucocorticoid receptor (GR). Patients with glucocorticoid resistance have ACTH and cortisol hypersecretion due to perceived lack of negative feedback. Elevated ACTH levels lead to increased adrenal production of androgens and DOC.
 - *Presentation:* There may be features of androgen excess (acne, hirsutism, male-type baldness, menstrual irregularities, oligoanovulation and infertility) or mineralocorticoid excess (hypokalemic alkalosis, hypertension), or both.
 - Because of the compensatory increases in ACTH and cortisol secretion, patients do not usually experience symptoms of adrenal insufficiency.

- *Diagnosis:*
  - ↑ blood levels of cortisol, DOC, 11-deoxycortisol, androstenedione, testosterone, and DHEAS
  - ↑ 24-hour urinary cortisol excretion, serum ACTH is not suppressed.
  - Confirmatory test: germline mutation testing.
- These patients are resistant to suppression of cortisol with low-dose dexamethasone but respond to high doses.
- Treatment with dexamethasone (usually >3 mg/day) adequate to suppress ACTH results in a fall in adrenal androgens, decreases virilization and often returns plasma potassium and blood pressure to normal levels.
- *Differentiation from Cushing's syndrome:*
  - No stigmata of Cushing's syndrome
  - Bone mineral density is preserved (or even increased in females because of the androgen excess)
  - Circadian rhythm for ACTH and cortisol is preserved.

37. **Ans. (d) Lactic acidosis**
    [Campbell-Walsh Urology 11th ed pg 391; Harrison's Principles of Internal Medicine 19th edition pg 309]

38. **Ans. (c) Suppressed plasma renin activity**
    [De Groot 7th ed pg 1814, 1816; Williams 13th ed pg 940, 941]

39. **Ans. (b) 11-beta HSD 2**
    [Williams 13th ed pg 582]
    See discussion of Chapter 10, Question 21.

40. **Ans. (c) 17-beta HSD-3 deficiency**
    [Williams 13th ed pg 534, 542; J Clin Endocrinol Metab, September 2010;95(9):4136]

    17-Hydroxy progesterone may be elevated in
    - 21-Hydroxylase deficiency
    - 11β-Hydroxylase deficiency
    - P450 Oxidoreductase deficiency
    - 3β-Hydroxysteroid dehydrogenase deficiency

41. **Ans. (c) Indicated for less than 10 cm adrenal mass on CT**
    [Williams 13th ed pg 568]

    ### Indications for ^{123}I MIBG Scintigraphy
    - Negative abdominal imaging
    - Abdominal pheochromocytoma >10 cm
    - Paraganglioma identified on CT/MRI

42. **Ans. (d) Hypertension is cured by bilateral adrenalectomy in IHA**
    [Williams 13th ed pg 575, 578, 580, 581]
    - Compared with those who have IHA, patients with APAs have
      - More severe hypertension

- More frequent hypokalemia
- Higher levels of plasma aldosterone
- Younger age (< 50 years)

Also see discussion of Chapter 10, Question 7.
- Principles of treatment:
  - *APA and unilateral hyperplasia:* Unilateral laproscopic adrenalectomy
  - *IHA and GRA:* Medical treatment.

43. **Ans. (b) Potassium ion**
    [De Groot 7th ed pg 1757, 1758]
    See discussion of Chapter 10, Question 11.

44. **Ans. (c) Phenoxybenzamine followed by propranolol**
    [Williams 13th ed pg 570]
    See discussion of Chapter 10, Question 4.

45. **Ans. (d) The ideal time to collect urine is during a period of clinical stability**
    [Williams 13th ed pg 565, 1916, 1919; J Clin Endocrinol Metab, June 2014, 99(6):1920; https://www.mayomedicallaboratories.com/test-catalog/Specimen/83006]
    - Measurements of plasma free or urinary fractionated metanephrines are superior to other tests for diagnosis of PPGLs. Initial biochemical testing for PPGLs should include measurements of plasma free metanephrines or urinary fractionated metanephrines.
    - There is no evidence to suggest that a spot urine sample should replace the standardized 24-hour urine collection method.
    - Urine preservatives used: 50% acetic acid, Boric acid
    - Catecholamine secretion may be increased in situations of physical stress or illness (e.g. stroke, myocardial infarction, congestive heart failure, obstructive sleep apnea). There are no reliable references ranges for fractionated metanephrines or catecholamines in patients requiring intensive care unit hospitalization.

46. **Ans. (c) Bilateral idiopathic hyperplasia**
    [Williams 13th ed pg 575]
    See discussion of Chapter 10, Question 7.

47. **Ans. (c) 4.0**
    [Williams 13th ed pg 579]
    Cortisol corrected aldosterone ratio (i.e. the ratio of PAC/cortisol from the APA side to that from the normal side):
    - >4.0:1 indicates unilateral aldosterone excess
    - < 3.0:1 suggests bilateral aldosterone hypersecretion
    Ratios > 3.0 but <4.0 represent a zone of overlap.

48. **Ans. (b) Absence of calcification**
    [Williams 13th ed pg 566]

Typical Imaging Phenotypes of Adrenal Masses

Tumor type	Size (cm)	Shape	Texture	Laterality	Contrast enhancement	CT[1]	MRI[2]	Necrosis, hemorrhage or calcifications	Growth
Cortical adenoma	≤3	Round to oval with smooth margins	Homogeneous	Usually unilateral	Limited	<10 HU; >50% washout	Isointense (both T1 & T2)	Rare	Slow
Cortical carcinoma	>4	Irregular with unclear margins	Inhomogeneous	Usually unilateral	Marked	>10 HU; <50% washout	Hyperintense	Common	Rapid
Pheochromocytoma	>3	Round to oval with smooth margins	Inhomogeneous with areas of cystic degeneration	Usually solitary and unilateral	Marked	>10 HU; <50% washout	Hyperintense	Common	1 cm/year
Metastasis	Variable	Oval to irregular with unclear margins	Inhomogeneous	Often bilateral	Marked	>10 HU; <50% washout	Hyperintense	Common	Variable

[1] Precontrast radiodensity (HU) and percentage of contrast medium washout at 10 min;
[2] Relative intensity compared with liver on T2-weighted images.

CHAPTER 11

Female Reproductive Axis

QUESTIONS

1. Least common cause of virilization in a female:
   a. Adrenal tumor
   b. CAH
   c. PCOS
   d. Arrhenoblastoma

2. Testosterone secretion in female:
   a. 33.3% peripheral conversion of androstenedione to testosterone, 33.3% adrenals, 33.3% ovaries
   b. 50% peripheral conversion of A to T, 25% adrenals, 25% ovaries
   c. 100% peripheral conversion of A to T, 0% adrenals, 0% ovaries
   d. 80% peripheral conversion of A to T, 10% adrenals, 25% ovaries

3. A 22-year-old lady with hirsutism, diagnosed with PCOD recently, going to get married after 2 months, best treatment to initiate:
   a. Cyproterone acetate
   b. Finasteride
   c. Aldosterone
   d. Manual epilation

4. PCOD on aldosterone antagonist c/o intermittent bleeding, all can be done to remedy this except:
   a. Increase dose of aldosterone antagonist
   b. Decrease dose of aldosterone antagonist
   c. Add DC pills
   d. Give a drug free period from aldosterone antagonist at end of the month

5. Most common side effect of spironolactone:
   a. Irregular bleeding
   b. Hyperkalemia
   c. Hypernatremia
   d. Skin rashes

6. Early menopause is associated with:
   a. Obesity
   b. Smoking
   c. Alcohol
   d. Multiparity

7. Most effective treatment for affective disorders of post menopause:
   a. Danazol
   b. OCP
   c. Anti-depressant

8. A 21-year-old female with sec. amenorrhea after an abortion 1 year back. Her TFT and LH, FSH were normal, she had no menstruation after 10 days of progesterone and 21 days OCP therapy the next approach will be:
   a. Karyotyping
   b. Hystoscopy
   c. USG abdomen
   d. CT brain

9. Primary ovarian failure:
   a. 46 X O
   b. Radiotherapy
   c. Chemotherapy
   d. Hypogonadotropic hypogonadism
   e. MRKH syndrome

10. Estradiol in ovulatory cycles:
    a. Single peak
    b. Double peak
    c. High in early phase followed by decline
    d. Low in early phase followed by rise

11. All of the following statements are correct about PCOD except:
    a. Can be a manifestation of hypothyroidism
    b. Diagnostic criteria are specific/sensitive
    c. Present in patients with a family history of DM
    d. Associated with increased risk of pregnancy complications

12. Amenorrhea and infertility is associated with all except:
    a. PCOS
    b. Hyperthyroidism
    c. Hypothyroidism
    d. Prolactinoma

13. All are correct about HRT except:
    a. ↑Venous thromboembolism
    b. ↓IHD
    c. ↓ endometrial Ca
    d. ↑ breast Ca

14. Raloxifene is associated with:
    a. Endometrial hyperplasia
    b. Decreased hot flashes
    c. Thromboembolism
    d. Dyslipidemia

15. A 20-year-old lady with primary amenorrhea without clitoromegaly with no bleed on progesterone withdrawal:
    a. Mayer-Rokitansky-Küster-Hauser syndrome
    b. Ashermann syndrome
    c. Denys-Drash syndrome
    d. Reifenstein syndrome

16. Progesterone is given in PCOS to prevent endometrial hyperplasia for:
    a. 5 days
    b. 7 days
    c. 14 days
    d. 28 days

17. Waist/hip ratio suggestive of android obesity in PCOS is:
    a. > 0.35
    b. > 0.45
    c. > 0.65
    d. > 0.85

18. A 23-year-old female presents with weight gain and a 4 month history of amenorrhea. Examination reveals a BMI of 33 and mild hirsuitism. Relevant investigations reveal an estradiol concentration of 1200 pmol/L (NR 130–800 pmol/L), a testosterone concentration of 2.8 nmol/L (NR less than 3 nmol/L), a prolactin concentration of 1500 mU/L (NR 50–450 mU/L), an LH of 1.2 u/L (NR 1.2–8 u/L) and a FSH of 1.5 u/L (NR 1. 5–8 u/L). What is the most likely diagnosis:
    a. Polycystic ovarian syndrome
    b. Prolactinoma
    c. Pregnancy
    d. Ovarian tumor
    e. Cushing's syndrome

19. All of the following statements about PCOS are correct except:
    a. ↑FSH/LH ratio
    b. Starts at puberty
    c. ↑ risk of genitourinary Ca
    d. ↑ testosterone

20. The drug most likely to reduce the effect of oral contraceptives:
    a. Sodium valproate
    b. Phenytoin
    c. Warfarin

21. All of the following are produced by the corpus leuteum except:
    a. Estrogen
    b. Progesterone
    c. Relaxin
    d. FSH

22. AMH (Anti-Müllerian Hormone) is secreted by:
    a. Leydig cell
    b. Sertoli cell
    c. Germ cell
    d. Peg cells

23. Chiari Frommel Syndrome is associated with all except:
    a. Postpartum galactorrhea in a non-nursing mother
    b. Amenorrhea
    c. Utero ovarian atrophy
    d. Future infertility occurs as a rule even with medical therapy

24. Which one of the following is a C-18 steroid?
    a. Hydrocortisone
    b. Progesterone
    c. Estradiol
    d. Testosterone

25. Best evidence to diagnosis amenorrhea due perimenopausal transition is:
    a. Random FSH > 25 IU/L
    b. Low to undetectable estradiol
    c. Inhibin B
    d. AMH (anti-Müllerian hormone)

26. For development of primary follicle from primordial follicle, which factor is required:
    a. FSH
    b. GDF9
    c. IGF-1
    d. AMH

27. Increased gonadal production of estrogen is characteristic of:
    a. Testicular feminization
    b. Polycystic ovarian disease
    c. Congenital adrenal hyperplasia
    d. Third trimester of pregnancy
    e. Arrhenoblastoma

28. Anovulatory cycles are characterized by which of the following?
    a. Elevated levels of plasma progesterone
    b. Dysmenorrhea
    c. A shortened luteal phase
    d. Lack of a normal LH and FSH surge
    e. The absence of any uterine bleeding

29. A 27-year-old Italian woman presents for evaluation of hirsutism and a 2-year history of irregular heavy menses. Menarche was at age 13, and her periods were always irregular, except when she was on OCPs (ages 18–24 years). Thelarche and adrenarche were normal. She noted the onset of significant acne at the age of 17 years, for which she was treated with antibiotics and isotretinoin (Accutane). Accutane had to be discontinued because of severe hypertriglyceridemia. At about the same time, she noted the development of hirsutism, which has slowly progressed. She had been trying to become pregnant for the past 3 years.

    On examination, her weight is 170 pounds; height is 5 feet, 3 inches. She has hyperpigmentation of the neck and axillary folds; a small goiter; and hirsutism on the chin, upper lip, and side of her face as well as periareolar and periumbilical coarse, dark terminal hair. Her blood pressure is 120/82 mm Hg. Waist-to-hip ratio is 0.95 and no striae. Liver edge is palpable 1 cm below the costal margin. The differential diagnosis in this case would include:
    a. Genetic hirsutism
    b. Adult-onset congenital adrenal hyperplasia
    c. Polycystic ovarian disease
    d. Cushing's syndrome
    e. a, b, and c
    f. a and c
    g. All of the above

30. In this same case, the appropriate laboratory tests include:
    a. Serum DHEAS, testosterone, free testosterone
    b. Serum TSH, prolactin
    c. Serum 17-hydroxyprogesterone
    d. Gonadotropins and E2
    e. a, b, and c
    f. All of the above laboratory tests

31. A 51-year-old woman seeks attention because she has not had a menstrual period for 4 months. She is not pregnant, and her follicle stimulating hormone level returns to 112 uIU/dL (normal <14). She is menopausal and is deficient in estrogen and:
   a. Activin
   b. Inhibin
   c. GnRH
   d. Corticosterone

32. Hot flushes occurring in postmenopausal ladies is due to:
   a. Increased circulating gonadotropin levels
   b. Beta endorphin
   c. Decreased estrogen and progestin
   d. All of the above

33. A 31-year-old lady with 2 healthy kids presents with 6 months amenorrhea, increased LH and FSH levels with low estradiol, likely cause can be:
   a. Turners
   b. Ovarian failure
   c. CAH
   d. PCOS

34. Following are true for hormone replacement therapy with estrogen and progesterone except:
   a. Increase in dementia
   b. Increase gall bladder disease
   c. Decrease in incidence of hip fractures
   d. Increase in colon cancers

ANSWERS

1. **Ans. (d) Adrenal tumor**
   [Williams 13th ed pg 623, 624, 629, 633, 1198]
   - Common cause of androgen excess disorders
     - PCOS—72.1%
     - Idiopathic hyperandrogenism—15.8%
     - Idiopathic hirsutism—7.6%
     - 21-hydroxylase-deficient nonclassic adrenal hyperplasia—4.3%
     - Androgen-secreting tumors (ovarian/adrenal)—0.2%
   - Virilizing ovarian tumors (e.g. Sertoli-Leydig cell tumors, hilus cell tumors, lipoid cell tumors, and infrequently, granulosa-theca tumors) are encountered much more frequently than those of adrenal origin. Arrhenoblastoma, also called Sertoli tumor of the ovary, is the most common virilizing ovarian tumor
   - While Idiopathic hirsuitism is not associated with virilization, virilization is unusual in PCOS. Ovarian hyperthecosis is a severe variant of PCOS in which virilization is common

2. **Ans. (a) 33.3% peripheral conversion of androstenedione to testosterone, 33.3% adrenals, 33.3% ovaries**
   [Williams 13th ed pg 622; Greenspan's 9th ed]
   During the reproductive years, the ovaries are directly responsible for one-third of the testosterone production. The remaining two-thirds come from the periphery and is derived from ovarian and adrenal gland precursors—notably androstenedione, which is produced in equal proportions by the adrenal gland and the ovary. Thus, option (a) is most appropriate.

3. **Ans. (d) Manual epilation**
   [Williams 13th ed pg 626, 627; The Journal of Clinical Endocrinology & Metabolism, Vol. 93, issue 4, pg 1114, 1115]

   Treatment of Hirsuitism
   Treatment of Cause
   Lifestyle Modification
   - Moderate lifestyle modification (i.e., diet with a 500-kcal/day deficit and 30 minute/day of exercise) should be a part of hirsutism management in obese patients.

   Drugs
   I. Oral contraceptives
      - Reduce circulating testosterone and androgen precursors by suppression of LH and stimulation of SHBG levels.
      - An oral contraceptive containing 30 or 35 µg of ethinyl estradiol should be used.

II. Spironolactone
- Most commonly used androgen blocker for the treatment of hirsutism.
- Aldosterone antagonist structurally related to progestins. Apart from inhibiting steroidogenesis and acting as an androgen antagonist, spironolactone has a significant effect in inhibiting 5α-reductase activity.
- LH levels have occasionally been reported to decrease.
- Dose: 100 to 200 mg/day
- *Side effects:*
  - Gastritis
  - Dry skin
  - Anovulation
  - Menstrual irregularity (most frequent side effect; remedied by a downward dose adjustment or the addition of an oral contraceptive)
  - Diuretic effect (transient- noticed initially)
  - Hyperkalemia (rare)
  - Hypotension (rare)
  - In utero feminizing effect on the genitalia of a 46,XY fetus (effective contraception should always be provided in women taking spironolactone)

III. Cyproterone acetate
- 17-hydroxyprogesterone acetate derivative
- Acts as an antiandrogen by competing with DHT and testosterone for binding to the androgen receptor has strong progestagenic properties. There is also some evidence of effect in inhibiting 5α-reductase activity in skin.
- The drug usually is administered in doses of 50 to 100 mg on days 5 through 15 of the treatment cycle.
- When ethinyl estradiol is added, it is usually administered in 50-μg doses on days 5 through 26.
- This regimen is referred to as the *reverse sequential regimen.*
- Cyproterone acetate 2 mg in daily combination with 50 or 35 μg of ethinyl estradiol has been administered as an oral contraceptive. This regimen is primarily suited for individuals with mild hyperandrogenism.

IV. Finasteride
- Inhibits 5α-reductase type 2. Because hirsutism results from the combined effects of type 1 and type 2, this agent is only partially effective.
- Dose: 5 mg/day.
- Finasteride may cause congenital genital ambiguity in a 46, XY fetus (effective contraception should be provided during its use).

V. Others
   a. Flutamide
      - Potent antiandrogen
      - Occasional severe hepatotoxicity makes this drug unsuitable for the indication of hirsutism.
   b. Metformin and thiazolidinediones
      - Have been used in PCOS
      - Mitigate insulin resistance
      - Metformin (1500 to 2700 mg/day)
      - Rosiglitazone (4 mg/day)
      - Pioglitazone (30 mg/day)

Direct Hair Removal Methods
I. Temporary methods of hair removal
   a. Epilation (extract hairs to above the bulb): e.g. Plucking, Waxing
   b. Depilation (removal of the hair shaft from the skin surface): e.g. Shaving, Chemical depilartory agent
II. Permanent methods of hair reduction
   a. Electrolysis
   b. Photoepilation
III. Topical treatment
   a. Eflornithine (Ornithine decarboxylase)
   b. Bleaching

A Comprehensive Treatment Strategy for Hirsutism
- Patients with PCOS, nonclassic adrenal hyperplasia, or idiopathic hirsutism are often initially treated with a combination of two agents, one that suppresses the ovary (e.g. an oral contraceptive) and another that suppresses the extraovarian (peripheral) action of androgens (e.g. spironolactone).
  An oral contraceptive containing 30 to 35 µg of ethinyl estradiol combined with spironolactone (100 mg/day) is the initial treatment of choice.
- For women with only minor hirsutism, an oral contraceptive alone may be an appropriate first approach.
- Because the growth phase of body hairs lasts 3 to 6 months, a response should not be expected before 6 months after onset of treatment.
- Suppression of androgen production and action inhibits only new hair growth. Existing coarse hair should be removed mechanically. Electrolysis is the method of choice.

As discussed above, drugs take about 6 months for response to be apparent. Therefore, in the above patient, who is going to get married after 2 months, mechanical hair removal is the best possible option. Also the aldosterone antagonist spironolactone and finasteride have feminizing effect on the genitalia of a 46, XY fetus and should not be prescribed in the absence of effective contraception.

4. **Ans. (a) Increase dose of aldosterone antagonist**
   [Williams 13th ed pg 626]
   See discussion of Chapter 11, Question 3.

5. **Ans. (a) Irregular bleeding**
   [De Groot 7th ed pg 2294]
   See discussion of Chapter 11, Question 3.

6. **Ans. (b) Smoking**
   [De Groot 7th ed pg 2312-2313]

   Etiologic Factors in Early Menopause
   - Race/ethnicity
   - Parity (nulliparous women have earlier menopause than parous women—there is a trend of increasing age at menopause with increasing number of live births)
   - Prior oral contraceptive use status (associated with later age at menopause)
   - Socioeconomic status
     - Lower educational attainment
     - Marital status (earlier menopause in separated, divorced, or widowed women)
     - Stress
   - Familial/genetic factors
     - Blepharophimosis gene
     - POF1/POF2 gene
     - Fragile X syndrome
     - Pvu II polymorphic allele
   - Environmental toxins
     - Smoking
     - Chemotherapy
     - Irradiation
     - Galactose consumption
   - Body mass index (BMI) (those with higher weight have later menopause)
   - Depression.

7. **Ans. (c) Anti-depressant**
   [Menopause: The Journal of The North American Menopause Society Vol. 21, No. 2, pg. 198-206]

8. **Ans. (b) Hysteroscopy**
   [Greenspan's 9th ed; Fertility and Sterility April 2008, Volume 89, Issue 4, pg 759, 765, 776]

Assessment of patients with amenorrhea
Absent breast development; uterus present

• Gonadal failure
  – Gonadal agenesis
  – Gonadal dysgenesis
    - 45, X (Turner syndrome)
    - 46, X abnormal X (e.g. short- or long-arm deletion)
    - Mosaicism (e.g. X/XX, X/XX/XXX)
    - 46, XX or 46, XY (Swyer syndrome) gonadal dysgenesis

• Defects in estrogen biosynthesis (46, XX)
  – 17,20-Lyase deficiency
  – CYP17α deficiency

• Hypothalamic failure secondary to inadequate GnRH release
  – Insufficient GnRH secretion
    - FHA
    - Anorexia nervosa and bulimia
    - CNS neoplasm (craniopharyngioma, gliomas)
    - Excessive exercise
    - Constitutional delay
  – Inadequate GnRH synthesis (Kallmann syndrome)
  – Developmental anatomic abnormalities in central nervous system

• Pituitary failure
  – Isolated gonadotropin insufficiency
  – GnRH resistance
  – Pituitary tumors (hyperprolactinemia)
  – Pituitary insufficiency
    - Infections (mumps, encephalitis)
    - Newborn kernicterus
  – Prepubertal hypothyroidism

Breast development; uterus absent
• Androgen resistance (androgen insensitivity syndrome)
• Congenital absence of uterus (utero-vaginal agenesis)
Absent breast development; uterus absent

• Defects in testosterone biosynthesis (46, XY)
  – 17,20-Lyase deficiency
  – CYP17α deficiency
  – 17β-Hydroxysteroid dehydrogenase deficiency

• Testicular regression syndrome (46, XY)
Breast development; uterus present
• Pregnancy

• Hypothalamic etiology
  – FHA
  – Anorexia nervosa and bulimia
  – Psychogenic (depression)
  – CNS neoplasm
  – Chronic disease

Contd...

Contd...

Breast development; uterus present
• Pituitary etiology 　– Pituitary tumors (hyperprolactinemia) 　– Pituitary insufficiency 　　- Hypotensive event (Sheehan syndrome) 　　- Infections 　　- Autoimmune destruction 　　- Iatrogenic (surgery, radiation)
• Ovarian etiology 　– POF 　　- Mosaicism (46, XX/XO, XX/XY) 　　- Autoimmune destruction 　　- Iatrogenic (radiation, chemotherapy) 　　- Fragile X syndrome 　　- Infections 　– Resistant ovarian syndrome (Savage syndrome)
• Chronic estrogenized anovulation 　– Hyperandrogenic 　　- PCOS 　　- Nonclassical congenital adrenal hyperplasia 　　- Cushing's syndrome 　　- Androgen secreting tumors 　– Other 　　- Adrenal insufficiency 　　- Thyroid disorders
• Outflow tract 　– Congenital abnormalities 　　- Transvaginal septum 　　- Imperforate hymen 　– Asherman syndrome

Female Reproductive Axis

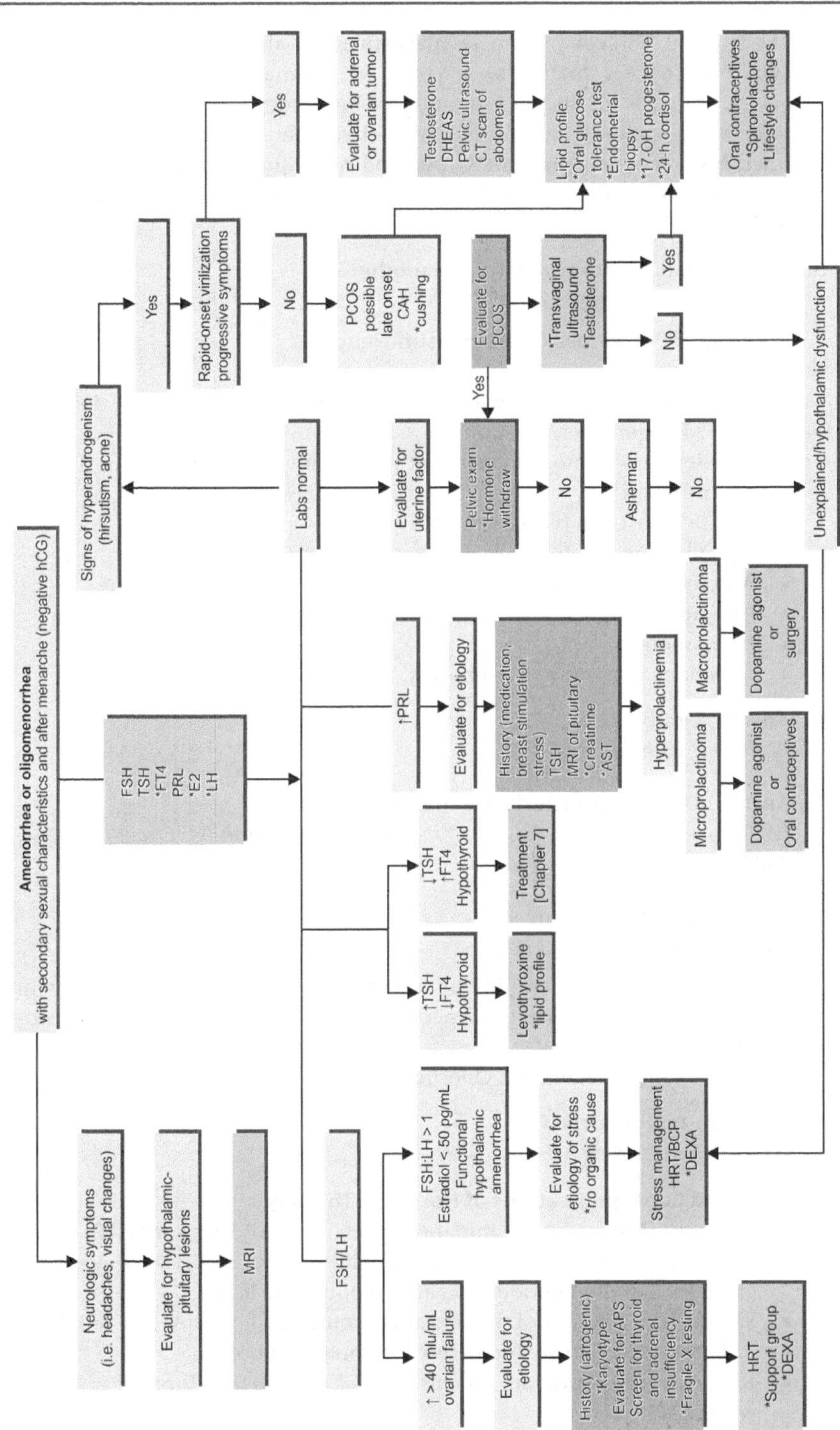

The current clinical picture is suggestive of Asherman syndrome. This syndrome occurs mainly as a result of trauma to the gravid uterine cavity, which leads to the formation of intrauterine and/or intracervical adhesions. Patients can present with hypomenorrhea or amenorrhea, infertility, recurrent pregnancy loss, and other pregnancy complications. Hysteroscopy is the method of choice for the investigation and treatment of this condition.

9. **Ans. (b) Radiotherapy and (c) Chemotherapy**
   [Williams 13th ed pg 637]
   Etiology of Premature Ovarian Insufficiency
   - Genetic
     - Gonadal dysgenesis with primarily mosaic X-chromosome defects
     - FMR1 gene permutation
     - Blepharophimosis-ptosis-epicanthus inversus syndrome [FOXL2 mutation]
     - Galactosemia (GALT mutation)
     - Other gene defects, e.g. FSHR, CYP17A1, CYP19A1
   - Autoimmune (including autoimmune polyendocrine syndrome)
   - Chemotherapy
   - Irradiation
   - Infections, e.g. mumps oophoritis.

10. **Ans. (b) Double peak**
    [Williams 13th ed pg 610]

11. **Ans. (b) Diagnostic criteria are specific/sensitive**
    [Williams 13th ed pg 628, 630; J Clin Endocrinol Metab 98: Dec 2013; 4566, 4567]

12. **Ans. (c) Hypothyroidism**
    [Williams 13th ed pg 373, 422]

    Although all of the conditions mentioned may be associated with amenorrhoea and infertility, hyperthyroidism appears to be most appropriate answer.
    See discussion of Section 11, Question 8.

13. **Ans. (c) ↓ endometrial Ca**
    [Williams 13th ed pg 649, 651, 652]

    Risks and Contraindications of Hormone Therapy
    - *Coronary heart disease:* Initiation of HT (HT-EP but not HT-E) many years after menopause is associated with excess CHD risk, whereas HT given for a limited period soon after menopause is not.
    - *Stroke:* Increased risk of stroke among women assigned to HT-E or HT-EP.
    - *Pulmonary embolism:* Increased pulmonary embolism
    - *Breast cancer:* Moderate increase in risk with HT-E. The risk is higher with HT-EP

Female Reproductive Axis

- *Ovarian cancer:* HT-E, particularly when taken for 10 or more years, significantly increases the risk of ovarian cancer.
- *Dementia:* HT significantly increase probable dementia risk.
- *Hyperlipidemia:* Hyperlipidemia is a rare side effect of oral estrogen regimen observed in patients with severe familial hypertriglyceridemia.
- *gallbladder disease:* Both (HT-E and HT-EP) show higher risk for cholecystitis and cholelithiasis.

Indications for Hormone Therapy
- *Hot flashes:* HT-E or HT-EP reliably treats hot flashes in most women. Hot flashes constitute the most common indication for a short course of HT (<5 years).
- *Fractures:* HT-EP or HT-E significantly decreased the incidence of hip, vertebral, and other osteoporotic fractures.
- *Colon cancer:* Colon cancer was significantly less common with HT-EP but not with HT-E. It is possible that progestin is the protective hormone in this case.

Postmenopausal women who have undergone a hysterectomy ordinarily receive HT with estrogen only (HT-E). A progestin is added to estrogen (HT-EP) in the postmenopausal woman with a uterus to prevent endometrial hyperplasia and cancer. Although both options (b) and (c) are correct, option (c) is a better choice as a number of observational studies had suggested benefits of HT for CVD including coronary heart disease (CHD).

14. **Ans. (c) Thromboembolism**
    [Williams 13th ed pg 655, 1355]
    - Raloxifene has
        - Estrogen-like actions on bone, lipids, and the coagulation system
        - Estrogen antagonist effects on the breast
        - No detectable action in the endometrium (unlike Tamoxifene which has estrogen agonistic properties on the uterus)
    - Inhibit bone resorption- approved by the FDA for the prevention and treatment of osteoporosis.
    - Reduces new cases of breast cancer- Approved by FDA for reducing the risk of invasive breast cancer in postmenopausal women.
    - Raloxifene use is not associated with endometrial cancer
    - Low-density lipoprotein cholesterol levels are reduced.
    - Adverse effects:
        - Hot flashes
        - Leg cramps
        - Deep venous thrombosis.

15. **Ans. (a) Mayer-Rokitansky-Küster-Hauser syndrome**
    [Greenspan's 9th ed.; De Groot 7th ed pg 2057, 2090; Williams 13th ed pg 759, 951]
    See discussion of Chapter 11, Question 8.

Mayer-Rokitansky-Küster-Hauser (MRKH) syndrome is a heterogeneous disorder characterized by uterovaginal atresia in 46, XX females. Abnormalities of the genital tract may range from upper vaginal atresia to total Müllerian agenesis associated with urinary tract abnormalities, and even cervicothoracic somite dysplasia (MURCS association). Presents with primary amenorrhea in a girl who has developed in puberty.

Denys-Drash syndrome and Reifenstein syndrome are associated with genital ambiguity.

16. Ans. (c) 14 days
    [De Groot 7th ed pg 2294]

17. Ans. (d) >0.85
    [Clinical Gynecologic Endocrinology and Infertility 7th ed pg 479]

18. Ans. (a) Polycystic ovarian syndrome
    [De Groot 7th ed pg 110; Williams 13th ed pg 617, 629]
    - Menstrual disturbances are prevalent in patients with polycystic ovary syndrome and in patients with prolactinomas, and sometimes the distinction between the two conditions may be difficult.
    - Polycystic ovary syndrome also may be associated with hyperprolactinemia.
    - The presence of mild hyperprolactinemia, negative pituitary imaging, high luteinizing hormone/follicle stimulating hormone ratio, and clinical features suggestive of polycystic ovary syndrome can help in the differential diagnosis.
    - In this case, the following findings support the diagnosis of polycystic ovary syndrome:
        - The hyperprolactinemia is mild
        - Weight gain
        - Features of hyperandrogenism (mild hirsuitism and elevated testosterone concentration)
        - Raised estradiol concentration (prolactinoma patients are estrogen deficient).

19. Ans. (a) ↑ FSH/LH ratio
    [Williams 13th ed pg 623, 628, 629]
    - PCOS is associated with
        - Ovulatory dysfunction (i.e. amenorrhea, oligomenorrhea, or other forms of irregular uterine bleeding)
        - Infertility
        - Increased pregnancy loss
        - Increased risk for endometrial cancer
        - Hyperandrogenism: hirsutism (seborrhea, acne, and alopecia are other clinical signs of androgen excess) and/or hyperandrogenemia
        - Increased metabolic and cardiovascular risk factors

- *Multifactorial:* May be inherited in polygenic fashion
- Usually pubertal onset—history of cyclic predictable menses of menarchal onset makes the diagnosis of PCOS unlikely; however acquired insulin resistance associated with significant weight gain or an unknown cause may induce PCOS in a woman with a history of previously normal ovulatory function.
- LH/FSH ratio is elevated in PCOS.

20. **Ans. (b) Phenytoin**
    [Williams 13th ed pg 670]
    The following drug may reduce the efficacy of oral contraceptives:
    - Anticonvulsants (phenytoin, carbamazepine, barbiturates, primidone, topiramate, and oxcarbazepine) that
    - Antibiotic (rifampicin/rifabutin)
    - Antiretrovirals
        - Nonnucleoside reverse transcriptase inhibitors (efavirenz and nevirapine)
        - Ritonavir-boosted (/r) protease inhibitors (darunavir/r, fosamprenavir/r, lopinavir/r, saquinavir/r, and tipranavir/r).

21. **Ans. (d) FSH**
    [Williams 13th ed pg 590, 835]
    Hormones secreted by corpus luteum—estradiol, progesterone, inhibin A, relaxin.

22. **Ans. (b) Sertoli Cell**
    [Williams 13th ed pg 601, 868, 903, 912, 1103, 1237]
    In the male fetus, anti-Müllerian hormone (AMH) is first secreted from about 7–8 weeks after conception. It is produced by testicular Sertoli cells and reaches the müllerian ducts largely by diffusion. AMH causes regression of müllerian ducts (prevents the development of müllerian structures e.g. fallopian tubes, uterus, upper two thirds of the vagina) by its paracrine action on the AMH type 2 receptor (AMHR2). Müllerian structures appear to be maximally sensitive to AMH between 9 and 12 weeks' gestation, a time when the developing testis is producing peak concentrations of AMH but before the onset of significant AMH production by the developing ovary (in a female fetus). AMH also has autocrine and paracrine effects on testicular steroidogenic function during fetal life. AMH biosynthesis continues throughout gestation. Concentrations of AMH rise from birth to relatively high levels during the first year of life in males, decrease by age 10 years, and decrease further during puberty.

    In the female fetus, AMH is produced later in gestation by granulosa cells of the fetal ovary. Newborn females have low or nondetectable serum levels of AMH, which rise only slightly thereafter; serum AMH concentrations are virtually nondetectable in most girls just before puberty. After an initial increase until early adulthood, AMH concentrations slowly decrease with increasing age until becoming undetectable approximately

5 years before menopause when the stock of primordial follicles is exhausted. Serum AMH may be a useful marker of ovarian reserve and predictor of ovarian insufficiency. Antral follicle number is positively correlated with AMH levels. AMH has been proposed as a marker to predict age at natural menopause.

23. **Ans. (d) Future infertility occurs as a rule even with medical therapy**
    [Williams 13th ed pg 187]

    The Chiari-Frommel syndrome comprises postpartum galactorrhea, amenorrhea, and "utero-ovarian atrophy" in patients not nursing. This disorder is usually self-limiting, and fertility eventually returns after normalization of PRL levels.

24. **Ans. (c) Estradiol**
    [Williams 13th ed pg 492]

    Estrogens have 18 carbon atoms (C18 steroids) and androgens have 19 carbon atoms (C19), whereas glucocorticoids and progestogens are C21-steroid derivatives.

25. **Ans. (a) Random FSH > 25 IU/L**
    [De Groot 7th ed pg 2311]

    Staging system for reproductive aging in women.

Stage	−5	−4	−3b	−3a	−2	−1	+1a	+1b	+1c	+2
Terminology	Reproductive				Menopausal transition		Postmenopause			
	Early	Peak	Late		Early	Late	Early			Late
						Perimenopause				
Duration	Variable				Variable	1–3 years	2 years	(1+1)	3–6 years	Remaining lifespan
Principal criteria										
Menstrual cycle	Variable to regular	Regular	Regular	Subtle changes in flow/length	Variable length persistent ≥7-day difference in length of consecutive cycles	Interval of amenorrhea of ≥60 days				
Supportive criteria										
Endocrine FSH AMH inhibin B			Low Low	Variable* Low Low	↑Variable* Low Low	↑>25 IU/L** Low Low	↑Variable Low Low	Stabilizes Very low Very low		
Antral follicle count			Low	Low	Low	Low	Very low	Very low		
Descriptive characteristics										
Symptoms						Vasomotor symptoms Likely	Vasomotor symptoms Most likely			Increasing symptoms of urogenital atrophy

26. **Ans. (b) GDF 9**
    [De Groot 7th ed pg 2180, 2181]

    Developmental Stages of the Ovarian Follicle
    - Primordial follicle
    - Primary follicle

- Secondary follicle
- Tertiary follicle
- Graafian follicle

Primordial Follicle
- The primordial follicles comprise a pool of nongrowing follicles from which all preovulatory follicles are ultimately derived.
- A primordial follicle consists of a small oocyte arrested in the dictyotene stage of meiosis, a single layer of squamous granulosa cells, and a thin basal lamina that encloses both cell types.
- The primordial follicles are formed in the fetal ovaries between the 6th and 9th months of gestation.
- Notch and Wnt signaling are critical for the formation/maintenance of the primordial follicle.
- Once the primordial follicles are formed, some are recruited to grow. As a woman ages, the process of recruitment continues on a regular basis until the total primordial follicle compartment is exhausted. This event, the menopause, occurs in most women at about 51 years of age. The loss of primordial follicles or ovary reserve (OR) is not constant during aging. An accelerated decrease in OR occurs at about 37 years of age in most women.
- Primordial-to-primary follicle transition is regulated by negative and positive growth factors.
  - Follicle maturation is inhibited by
    - Epidermal growth factor
    - Anti-Müllerian hormone (AMH)
  - Follicle development is stimulated by
    - Kit ligand
    - Insulin
    - Testosterone
    - Bone morphogenetic protein (BMP)-7 and BMP-15
    - Growth and differentiation factor (GDF)-9
    - Restricted food intake
- The PI3K/AKT pathway is involved in activation of follicles.

27. **Ans. (b) Polycystic ovarian disease**
    [Williams 13th ed pg 631]

28. **Ans. (d) Lack of a normal LH and FSH surge**
    [Women's Health-Menstrual Disorders by ACP pg 10, 11]

Anovulatory Cycles
- GnRH pulsations from hypothalamus cause pulsatile release of FSH from pituitary gland, which acts on follicles in ovary resulting in estrogen production
- FSH and LH midcycle surges are not produced, and follicular maturation and ovulation do not occur.

- In the absence of ovulation, corpus luteum formation and progesterone production do not occur
- Estrogen levels remain high and progesterone levels remain relatively low
- Endometrial lining displays intense vascularity, back-to-back granularity, and little stromal matrix. This tissue is relatively fragile and sheds sporadically and unevenly, resulting in variable intervals between bleeding episodes and variation in amount of blood flow
- Moliminal symptoms (premenstrual symptoms, including cramping, bloating, moodiness and breast tenderness) typically associated with ovulatory cyclea are typically absent with anovulatory bleeding.

29. **Ans. (e) a, b, and c**
    [Williams 13th ed pg 623-626, 628, 629]
    - Causes of androgen excess in women of reproductive age
        - *Ovarian:*
            * Polycystic ovary syndrome (PCOS)
            * Hyperthecosis (a severe PCOS variant)
            * Ovarian tumor (e.g. Sertoli-Leydig cell tumor)
        - *Adrenal:*
            * Nonclassic adrenal hyperplasia
            * Cushing's syndrome
            * Glucocorticoid resistance
            * Adrenal tumor (e.g. adenoma, carcinoma)
        - *Specific conditions of pregnancy:*
            * Luteoma of pregnancy
            * Hyperreactio luteinalis
            * Aromatase deficiency in fetus
        - *Other causes:*
            * Hyperprolactinemia, hypothyroidism
            * Medications (danazol, testosterone, anabolizing agents)
            * Idiopathic hirsutism (normal serum testosterone in an ovulatory woman)
            * Idiopathic hyperandrogenism (patients who do not fall into any of the other categories listed)
    - Common cause of androgen excess disorders
        - PCOS- 72.1%
        - Idiopathic hyperandrogenism- 15.8%
        - Idiopathic hirsutism- 7.6%
        - 21-hydroxylase-deficient nonclassic adrenal hyperplasia- 4.3%
        - Androgen-secreting tumors (ovarian/adrenal)- 0.2%
    - Polycystic ovary syndrome (PCOS)
        - The most common cause of androgen excess.
        - *Characterized by:*
            * Ovulatory dysfunction (i.e. amenorrhea, oligomenorrhea, or other forms of irregular uterine bleeding)

- Infertility
- Increased pregnancy loss
- Increased risk for endometrial cancer
- *Hyperandrogenism:* Hirsutism (seborrhea, acne, and alopecia are other clinical signs of androgen excess) and/or hyperandrogenemia
- Increased metabolic and cardiovascular risk factors.
- It is usually pubertal onset—history of cyclic predictable menses of menarchal onset makes the diagnosis of PCOS unlikely; however acquired insulin resistance associated with significant weight gain or an unknown cause may induce PCOS in a woman with a history of previously normal ovulatory function.
- *Diagnosis:* After exclusion of related disorders
- Idiopathic (constitutional) hirsutism
  - *Characterized by:*
    - Hirsutism in conjunction
    - Regular menstrual cycles
    - Absence of signs of virilization
    - Normal levels of serum testosterone.
  - It occurs more frequently in certain ethnic populations, particularly in women of Mediterranean ancestry.
- Androgen-secreting tumors of the ovary and adrenal
  - *Characterized by:*
    - Rapidly progressing symptoms of androgen excess—progressive hirsutism and virilization.
    - Defeminizing signs, such as loss of female body contour, increased muscle mass, and decreased breast size.
  - Ovarian tumors are associated with elevated serum testosterone levels.
  - Virilizing adrenal tumors commonly secrete large quantities of DHEAS, DHEA, and androstenedione, and testosterone is usually produced by extraovarian conversion of these precursors.
  - Testosterone levels three times the upper-normal range (i.e. >2 ng/mL) and DHEAS levels higher than 8 μg/mL have been used traditionally as guidelines to investigate further for neoplasms of the ovary or adrenal.
- Nonclassic adrenal hyperplasia
  - The clinical presentation is almost identical to that of PCOS.
  - The characteristic presentation consists of anovulatory uterine bleeding and progressive hirsutism of pubertal onset.
  - These individuals are born with normal genitalia, do not exhibit salt wasting, and are symptom-free until puberty.
  - High prevalence seen in Ashkenazi Jews, Hispanics, and patients of central European ancestry.

- A screening 8 AM serum level of 17-hydroxyprogesterone (on any day in an anovulatory patient during the follicular phase in an ovulatory patient) should be obtained for patients with
  - High-risk ethnic group
  - Premature pubarche
  - Androgen excess of early pubertal onset
  - Progressive hirsutism or virilisation
  - Strong family histories of severe androgen excess.
- Laboratory tests for the differential diagnosis of androgen excess
  - Initial testing
    - Total testosterone
    - Prolactin
    - Thyroid-stimulating hormone
  - Further testing based on clinical presentation
    - 17-hydroxyprogesterone (8 AM)
    - 17-hydroxyprogesterone 60 minutes after intravenous ACTH
    - Cortisol (8 AM) after 1 mg dexamethasone at midnight
    - DHEAS
    - Androstenedione
    - Imaging of ovaries (transvaginal ultrasonography)
    - Imaging of adrenal glands (abdominal ultrasonography, CT, MRI)
    - Nuclear imaging after intravenous administration of radio-labeled cholesterol.
- In the given patient the most likely diagnosis is PCOS. However, as PCOS is a diagnosis of exclusion, other related disorders (including non-classic adrenal hyperplasia) should be ruled out. There are no features suggestive of Cushing's syndrome in the patient.

30. **Ans. (e) a, b, and c**
    [Williams 13th ed pg 623-626, 628, 629]
    See discussion of Chapter 11, Question 29.

31. **Ans. (b) Inhibin**
    [De Groot 7th ed pg 2313, 2314]
    - Hormonal changes in the hypothalamic-pituitary-ovarian axis during menopause
      - ↑ FSH
      - ↓ Inhibin B
      - ↓ Estradiol
      - ↓ Progesterone
      - ↓ AMH

32. **Ans. (d) All of the above**
    [Nature Reviews Endocrinology volume14, pg 207 (2018)]

After menopause, the ovaries are depleted of follicles, estradiol (E2) and inhibin B production falls. The loss of ovarian sensitivity to follicle-stimulating hormone (FSH) and luteinizing hormone (LH) and the loss of negative feedback of E2 and inhibin B on the hypothalamic–pituitary unit result in increased production and release of gonadotropin release hormone (GnRH), FSH and LH. Modifications of gonadotropins, E2, alterations in the function of noradrenergic and serotoninergic pathways, and opioid tone in the hypothalamus (↑ Noradrenaline, ↓ Dopamine, ↓ Serotonin, ↑ Neurokinin B, ↑ Kisspeptin, ↑ Dynorphin, and ↑ Cortisol) cause the vasomotor symptoms. Thermoregulatory dysfunction might be a result of a maladaptation of the brain to kisspeptin, neurokinin B and dynorphin (KNDy) neuron hypertrophy, which project to the preoptic thermoregulatory area.

33. **Ans. (b) Ovarian failure**
    [Greenspan's 9th ed.]
    See discussion of Chapter 11, Question 8.

34. **Ans. (d) Increase in colon cancers**
    [Williams 13th ed pg 649, 651, 652]
    See discussion of Chapter 11, Question 13.

CHAPTER 12

Testicular Disorders

QUESTIONS

1. A 25-year-old male patient is on testosterone replacement therapy. Monitoring required:
   a. Hematocrit
   b. PSA
   c. Lipid profile
   d. Platelet count

2. True about androgen receptors are all except:
   a. Intracellular
   b. Testosterone has highest affinity
   c. DHT more stable and less dissociation
   d. Similar to GR, MR and progesterone receptor

3. In hepatic dysfunction, which oral testosterone causes least hepatoxicity:
   a. Fluoxymesterone
   b. Methyl testosterone
   c. Testosterone undecanoate
   d. Testosterone succinate

4. Testosterone synthesis not inhibited by:
   a. Nitrofurantoin
   b. Ketoconazole
   c. Spironolactone
   d. Finasteride

5. Androgen replacement all are CI except:
   a. Prostate cancer
   b. Severe CHF
   c. Severe urinary obstruction
   d. HCT < 52%

6. Low testosterone levels in males are seen in all except:
   a. Klinfelter
   b. Uncorrected cryptoorchidism
   c. Testicular feminization syndrome
   d. Hyperprolactinemia

7. Feature of hypogonadism in adult male are all except:
   a. Normal voice pitch
   b. Decreased beard growth
   c. Small prostate
   d. Decreased lipids

Testicular Disorders

8. **Klinfelter in childhood can be suspected by:**
   a. Limb disproportion
   b. Gynecomastia
   c. Small testis
   d. Ambiguous genetalia

9. **Decreased free testosterone levels with ageing due to:**
   a. Increased SHBG
   b. Decreased synthesis
   c. Increases degradation
   d. Decreased aromatase

10. **Gynecomastia is associated with all except:**
    a. Tamoxifen
    b. Marijuana
    c. Omeprazole
    d. Spironolactone

11. **All of the following are true about cryptorchidism except:**
    a. 1/3rd of premature crypto-orchid at birth
    b. 12% of term crypto-orchid at birth
    c. At 9 months 1% crypto-orchid
    d. Increased malignancy

12. **All of the following are contraindications of androgen replacement except:**
    a. Lung Ca
    b. Prostatism
    c. PSA>4
    d. Urinary tract obstruction

13. **Gynecomastia is seen in all except:**
    a. Rifampicin
    b. Refenstein syndrome
    c. KFS
    d. Testicular feminization syndrome

14. **46, XX male syndrome all except:**
    a. Variant of KFS
    b. Testes small, firm
    c. Short height
    d. Hypogonadotropic hypogonadism

15. **Conversion of T to DHT is:**
    a. 17,20 lyase
    b. 3βHSD-2
    c. 5α-reductase
    d. Aromatase

16. **C/I of testosterone treatment include all except:**
    a. Aplastic anemia
    b. NYHA grade 2 CHF
    c. Breast Ca
    d. Unexplained PSA elevation
    e. LUTS

17. **Pathological gynecomastia:**
    a. >3 cm size
    b. Tenderness
    c. Hormone duct syndrome
    d. Hypogonadotropic hypogonadism

18. **Testicular descent is caused by:**
    a. FSH
    b. LH
    c. DHEAS
    d. DHT

19. **Which of the following supports the diagnosis of AIS?**
    a. Hiatal hernia
    b. Femoral hernia
    c. Umbilical hernia
    d. Inguinal hernia

20. **AIS; inheritance:**
    a. From mother
    b. From father
    c. From either
    d. De novo

21. A 64-year-old male presents with difficulty in micturition. He is diagnosed with benign prostatic hyperplasia and elects to receive finasteride. Production of which of the following hormones would be selectively inhibited?
    a. Testosterone
    b. Dihydroepiandrostenedione sulphate (DHEAS)
    c. Androstenedione
    d. Dihydrotestosterone (DHT)
    e. IGF-1

22. **Testosterone:**
    a. Is a steroid hormone
    b. Acts via cell surface receptors
    c. Acts via g-protein second messengers
    d. Is manufactured through the breakdown of estradiol
    e. In the circulation is mostly bound to albumin

23. **Nitric oxide:**
    a. Is synthesized by the vascular smooth muscle
    b. Acts via cAMP as the second messenger
    c. Is manufactured from Glycine
    d. Is inactivated by superoxide dismutase
    e. Inhibits platelet aggregation

24. Which of the following is most likely to be associated with the development of gynecomastia?
    a. Congenital adrenal hyperplasia
    b. Prolactinoma
    c. Hypopituitarism
    d. Hypothyroidism
    e. Seminoma

25. **Testes decent all except:**
    a. Mechanical
    b. Androgen
    c. InSL3
    d. LGR8

26. **Refenstein syndrome gynecomastia due to:**
    a. ↑ aromatase
    b. Adrenal sources
    c. INSL3
    d. Liver conversion

27. A man with reduced libido and failure of erection is given parenteral testosterone. What is the least-likely side effect?
    a. Gynecomastia
    b. Worsens sleep apnea
    c. ↑ symptoms due to prostatic enlargement
    d. Reduced HDL cholesterol
    e. ↑ risk of hepatocellular carcinoma

28. **Cryptorchidism means:**
    a. Descent of testis
    b. Hypogonadism
    c. Hyperfunction of the testis
    d. Undescended testis

29. **Androgen binding protein is produced by:**
    a. Adrenals
    b. Hypothalamus
    c. Sertoli cells
    d. Leydig cells

30. **The testis is kept at a temperature of 2-3°C below core temperature due to:**
    a. Contraction of cremasteric muscle
    b. Contraction of dartos muscle
    c. Contraction of internal oblique muscle
    d. Relaxation of cremasteric muscle and due to position of the testis outside the pelvic cavity

ANSWERS

1. **Ans. (a) Hematocrit**
   [Williams 13th ed pg 770]

2. **Ans. (b) Testosterone has highest affinity**
   [Williams 13th ed pg 712]

3. **Ans. (c) Testosterone undecanoate**
   [Williams 13th ed pg 761, 762, 768, 769]

4. **Ans. (a) Nitrofurantoin**
   [De Groot 7th ed pg 2413, 2414]

5. **Ans. (d) HCT < 52 %**
   [Williams 13th ed pg 769-771; Journal of Clinical Endocrinology & Metabolism, June 2010, Vol. 95(6):2537-8]

   Contraindications of Testosterone Treatment
   - Prostate cancer (testosterone therapy should not be started without further urological evaluation in patients with palpable prostate nodule or induration or PSA > 4 ng/ml or PSA > 3 ng/ml in men at high risk of prostate cancer, such as men with first-degree relatives with prostate cancer)
   - Breast cancer.
   - Untreated obstructive sleep apnea
   - Baseline hematocrit > 50
   - Severe edematous conditions (e.g. uncontrolled or poorly controlled CHF)
   - Severe lower urinary tract symptoms (LUTS) due to BPH, such as in men with IPSS greater than 19
   - Those desiring fertility.

6. **Ans. (c) Testicular feminization syndrome**
   [Williams 13th ed pg 735, 759]

   Causes of Primary Hypogonadism
   Androgen Deficiency and Impairment of Sperm Production
   - Congenital or developmental disorders
     Common causes
     – Klinefelter syndrome (XXY) and variants
     Uncommon causes
     – Myotonic dystrophy
     – Uncorrected cryptorchidism
     – Noonan syndrome
     – Bilateral congenital anorchia
     – Polyglandular autoimmune syndrome
     – Testosterone biosynthetic enzyme defects

- CAH (testicular adrenal rest tumors)
- Complex genetic syndromes
- Down syndrome
- LH receptor mutation
- Acquired disorders
  Common causes
  - Bilateral surgical castration or trauma
  - Drugs (spironolactone, ketoconazole, abiraterone, enzalutamide, alcohol, chemotherapy agents)
  - Ionizing radiation

  Uncommon causes
  - Orchitis
- Systemic disorders
  Common causes
  - Chronic liver disease (hepatic cirrhosis)*
  - Chronic kidney disease*
  - Aging*

  Uncommon causes
  - Malignancy (lymphoma, testicular cancer)
  - Sickle cell disease*
  - Spinal cord injury
  - Vasculitis (polyarteritis)
  - Infiltrative disease (amyloidosis, leukemia)

Isolated Impairment of Sperm Production or Function

- Congenital or developmental disorders
  Common causes
  - Cryptorchidism
  - Varicocele
  - Y-chromosome microdeletions

  Uncommon causes
  - Myotonic dystrophy
  - Sertoli cell–only syndrome
  - Primary ciliary dyskinesia
  - Down syndrome
  - FSH receptor mutation
- Acquired disorders
  Common causes
  - Orchitis
  - Ionizing radiation
  - Chemotherapy agents
  - Thermal trauma

  Uncommon causes
  - Environmental toxins
- Systemic disorders
  Common causes
  - Acute febrile illness

- Malignancy (testicular cancer, Hodgkin disease)*
- Idiopathic azoospermia or oligozoospermia

Uncommon causes
- Spinal cord injury

Causes of Secondary Hypogonadism
Androgen Deficiency and Impairment of Sperm Production
- Congenital or developmental disorders

  Common causes
  - Constitutional delayed puberty
  - Hemochromatosis

  Uncommon causes
  - IHH and variants
    - IHH
    - Kallmann syndrome
    - Congenital adrenal hypoplasia
    - Isolated LH deficiency, LHβ mutations
  - Complex genetic syndromes
- Acquired disorders

  Common causes
  - Hyperprolactinemia
  - Opioids
  - Androgenic anabolic steroids, progestins, estrogen excess
  - GnRH agonist or antagonist

  Uncommon causes
  - Hypopituitarism
    - Pituitary or hypothalamic tumor
    - Surgical hypophysectomy, pituitary or cranial irradiation
    - Vascular compromise, traumatic brain injury
    - Granulomatous or infiltrative disease
    - Infection
    - Pituitary stalk disease
  - Lymphocytic or autoimmune hypophysitis
- Systemic disorders

  Common causes
  - Glucocorticoid excess (Cushing's syndrome)*
  - Chronic organ failure*
  - Chronic liver disease (hepatic cirrhosis), chronic kidney disease, chronic lung disease, chronic heart failure
  - Chronic systemic illness*
  - Type 2 diabetes mellitus
  - Malignancy
  - Rheumatic disease (rheumatoid arthritis)
  - HIV disease
  - Starvation,* malnutrition,* eating disorders, endurance exercise
  - Morbid obesity, obstructive sleep apnea

Testicular Disorders | **171**

- Acute and critical illness
- Aging*

Uncommon causes
- Chronic systemic illness*
- Spinal cord injury
- Transfusion-related iron overload (β-thalassemia)
- Sickle cell disease
- Cystic fibrosis

Isolated Impairment of Sperm Production or Function
- Congenital or developmental disorders
  Uncommon causes
  - Congenital adrenal hyperplasia (21-hydroxylase deficiency, 11β-hydroxylase deficiency)
  - Isolated FSH deficiency, FSHβmutations
- Acquired disorders
  Common causes
  - Testosterone, androgenic anabolic steroids
  - Malignancy (Hodgkin disease, testicular cancer)*
  Uncommon causes
  - Androgen- or hCG-secreting tumors
  - Hyperprolactinemia

Also see discussion of Chapter 16, Question 5.

7. **Ans. (d) Decreased lipids**
   [Williams 13th ed pg 714, 715]

   Some of the masculinizing changes induced by testosterone during puberty are permanent.
   Testosterone is not necessary for maintenance of
   - Penis size,
   - Scrotal development,
   - Linear growth,
   - Laryngeal size,
   - Vocal cord thickness, or voice pitch.

8. **Ans. (a) Limb disproportion**
   [Williams 13th ed pg 1147]

   Prepubertally, patients can be detected by
   - Disproportionate length of the extremities: decreased U/L body ratio without an increase in arm span
   - Behavior problems.

9. **Ans. (a) Increased SHBG and (b) Decreased synthesis**
   [Williams 13th ed pg 744]

10. **Ans. (a) Tamoxifen**
    [Williams 13th ed pg 724]

Causes of Gynecomastia
- Physiologic causes
  - Maternal estrogen exposure: Neonatal gynecomastia
  - Transient increase in estrogen to androgen concentrations: Pubertal gynecomastia
- Estrogen excess
  - *Estrogens or estrogen receptor agonists:* e.g. Estrogens, marijuana smoke, digitoxin, testosterone or other aromatizable androgens
  - *Increased peripheral aromatase activity:* Obesity, aging, familial
  - *Estrogen-secreting tumors:* Adrenal carcinoma, Leydig or Sertoli cell tumor
  - *hCG-secreting tumors:* Germ cell, lung, hepatic carcinoma
  - hCG treatment
- Androgen deficiency or resistance
  - Androgen deficiency
    - Primary or secondary hypogonadism
    - Hyperprolactinemia causing androgen deficiency
  - Androgen resistance disorders
    - Congenital and acquired androgen resistance
    - *Drugs that interfere with androgen action:* e.g. Spironolactone, androgen receptor antagonists, marijuana, 5α-reductase inhibitors, histamine 2 receptor antagonists
- Systemic disorders
  - *Organ failure:* Hepatic cirrhosis, chronic kidney disease
  - *Endocrine disorders:* Hyperthyroidism, acromegaly, growth hormone treatment, Cushing's syndrome
  - *Nutritional disorders:* Refeeding, recovery from chronic illness (hemodialysis, insulin, isoniazid, antituberculous medications, HAART)
- Idiopathic causes
  - *Drugs:* e.g. HAART, calcium channel antagonists, amiodarone, antidepressants (SSRIs, tricyclic antidepressants), alcohol, amphetamines, penicillamine, sulindac, phenytoin, omeprazole, theophylline
  - Adult-onset idiopathic gynecomastia
  - Persistent prepubertal macromastia

11. **Ans. (b) 12% of term crypto-orchid at birth**
    [Williams 13th ed pg 740; Greenspan's 9th ed]
    - Cryptorchidism is unilateral or bilateral absence of the testes from the scrotum because of failure of normal testicular descent from the genital ridge through the external inguinal ring.
    - 2–4% of full-term and 20% to 25% of premature male infants have cryptorchidism.
    - In most cases, spontaneous testicular descent occurs during the first year of life, reducing the incidence to 0.2% to 0.8% by 1 year of age.

- Approximately 0.75% of adult males are crypto-orchid.
- Unilateral cryptorchidism is 5 to 10 times more common than bilateral cryptorchidism.
- The risk of testicular cancer in an undescended testis is 2.5- to 8-fold greater than in a scrotal testis.

12. **Ans. (a) Lung Ca**
    [Williams 13th ed pg 769-771; Journal of Clinical Endocrinology & Metabolism, June 2010, Vol. 95(6):2537-8]
    See discussion of Chapter 12, Question 5.

13. **Ans. (a) Rifampicin**
    [Williams 13th ed pg 724, 738, 759, 933, 934]
    Reifenstein syndrome is a form of partial androgen sensitivity syndrome. See discussions of Chapter 12, Question 10 and Chapter 16, Questions 4 and 5.

14. **Ans. (d) Hypogonadotropic hypogonadism**
    [De Groot 7th ed pg 2096, 2097]

    46, XX Males
    - Previously called XX sex reversal
    - Characterized by testicular development and complete virilization of the internal and external genitalia in subjects who have two X chromosomes and lack a Y chromosome.
    - Most cases are sporadic.
    - A form of X-Y paternal interchange is suggested when part of the short arm of the Y chromosome carrying SRY is transferred to one of the two X chromosomes. ~10% of XX males lack SRY sequences. Some SRY(-) XX males have overexpression of *SOX3*, *SOX9*, or *SOX10* resulting from gene duplication.
    - Before puberty, testicular endocrine function does not seem to be affected in XX males.
    - The condition is often diagnosed at puberty or adulthood owing to
        - Small testes
        - Gynecomastia
        - Sterility
        - Some degree of testosterone deficiency and elevated gonadotropins.
    - Similarities to Klinefelter's syndrome include small testis size and azoospermia. However, XX males show shorter stature than Klinefelter patients.

15. **Ans. (c) 5α-reductase**
    [Williams 13th ed pg 711]

16. **Ans. (a) Aplastic anemia**
    [Williams 13th ed pg 769-771; Journal of Clinical Endocrinology & Metabolism, June 2010, Vol. 95(6):2537-8]
    See discussion of Chapter 12, Question 5.

17. **Ans. (b) Tenderness**
    Pathologic gynecomastia is defined as
    - "Tender, palpable breast tissue" or
    - "Nontender breast tissue >4 cm."
    - Documentation of growth of breast tissue over time (even when the diameter is < 4 cm).

18. **Ans. (d) DHT**
    [Greenspan's 9th ed; Williams 13th ed pg 699, 700]

    Testis Descent
    The developing testis is attached to the diaphragm by the cranial suspensory ligament and anchored to the inguinal region by a caudal ligament known as the *gubernaculum*.

    Descent of the testis occurs in two phases.
    - *Transabdominal phase*
        - Testis descends within the abdomen to the inguinal region
        - Occurs between 10 and 23 weeks of gestation
        - Depends on two processes:
            ◆ Regression of the cranial suspensory ligament which frees the testes to descend: induced by testosterone
            ◆ Thickening of the gubernaculums: controlled by INSL3 (produced by leydig cells and acts through relaxin family peptide receptor 2 (RXFP2, also known as leucine-rich repeat–containing G protein–coupled receptor 8 [LGR8] or G protein–coupled receptor affecting testis descent [GREAT]).
    - *Inguinoscrotal phase*
        - Begins at 26 to 28 weeks of gestation. Testes descent is usually complete by 7 months of gestation to birth.
        - The testis descends into the scrotum
        - Depends on gubernacular shortening and contractions: controlled by testosterone

    The effects of testosterone may be mediated in part by the neurotransmitter, calcitonin gene-related peptide (CGRP), which is released by the genitofemoral nerve. DHT is also required for normal testicular descent.

19. **Ans. (d) Inguinal hernia**
    [Williams 13th ed pg 933]

    See discussion of Chapter 16, Question 5.

20. **Ans. (a) From mother**
    [De Groot 7th ed pg 2107]

    AIS is an X-linked recessive disorder, inheritance usually occurs from mother.
    About 30% of mutations occur de novo.
    Thus, option (a) is a better choice than option (d).

Testicular Disorders | **175**

21. **Ans. (d) Dihydrotestosterone (DHT)**
    [Williams 13th ed pg 711]
    Testosterone is converted to dihydrotestosterone (DHT) by SRD5A1 and SRD5A2 (isoenzymes of 5α-reductase). Inhibitors of SRD5A2 (finasteride) or of both SRD5A1 and SRD5A2 (dutasteride) are used to treat lower urinary tract symptoms, improve urinary flow, and prevent complications related to BPH.

22. **Ans. (a) Is a steroid hormone**
    [Williams 13th ed pg 709, 710, 712; De Groot 7th ed pg]
    Testosterone is a steroid hormone and can be converted to estradiol. It binds to intracellular receptors.
    Under physiologic conditions,
    - 60% of circulating testosterone is bound to sex hormone–binding globulin (SHBG), a high affinity, low capacity binding protein.
    - 38% is weakly bound to albumin, a lower affinity, high-capacity binding protein.
    - 1% to 2% is nonprotein bound (free testosterone).

    Also see discussions of Chapter 1, Questions 1, 2 and 37.

23. **Ans. (e) Inhibits platelet aggregation**
    [Robbins & Cotran Pathologic Basis of Disease, 8th ed]
    - Nitric oxide (NO) is produced by endothelial cells, macrophages and some neurons in the brain.
    - NO is synthesized from L-arginine by the enzyme nitric oxide synthase (NOS). There are three different types of NOS: endothelial (eNOS), neuronal (nNOS), and inducible (iNOS). eNOS and nNOS are constitutively expressed at low levels and can be activated rapidly by an increase in cytoplasmic Ca^{2+}. iNOS, in contrast, is induced when macrophages and other cells are activated by cytokines (e.g. TNF, IFN-γ) or microbial products.
    - It acts in a paracrine manner through induction of cyclic guanosine monophosphate
    - NO relaxes vascular smooth muscle and promotes vasodilation, reduces platelet aggregation and adhesion, inhibits several features of mast cell-induced inflammation and inhibits leukocyte recruitment. Because of these inhibitory actions, production of NO is thought to be an endogenous mechanism for controlling inflammatory responses. NO and its derivatives are microbicidal, and thus NO is a mediator of host defense against infection.

24. **Ans. (c) Hypopituitarism**
    [Williams 13th ed pg 724-725]

25. **Ans. (a) Mechanical**
    [Greenspan's 9th ed; Williams 13th ed pg 699,700]
    See discussion of Chapter 12, Question 18.
    Although none of the options is correct, option (a) appears to be the single best answer.

26. Ans. (c) Testicular secretion
    [Williams 13th ed pg 724, 1202]
    See discussions of Chapter 12, Question 10.

27. Ans. (e) ↑ risk of hepatocellular carcinoma
    [Williams 13th ed pg 771-3]

28. Ans. (d) Undescended testis
    [Williams 13th ed pg 740]

29. Ans. (c) Sertoli cells
    [Williams 13th ed pg 706]

30. Ans. (d) Relaxation of cremasteric muscle and due to position of the testis outside the pelvic cavity
    [Williams 13th ed pg 695]

CHAPTER 13

Multiple Endocrine Neoplasia

QUESTIONS

1. MEN 2 is characterized by all except:
   a. Parathyroid adenoma
   b. Islet hyperplasia
   c. MTC
   d. Pheochromocytoma

2. MEN 1 all are true except:
   a. Parathyroid hyperplasia
   b. Parathyroid adenoma
   c. Pituitary adenoma
   d. Pheochromocytoma

3. MEN 2A is associated with all except:
   a. MTC
   b. Pheochromocytoma
   c. Mucosal neuromas
   d. Hyperparathyroidism

4. In MEN 1, most common tumor is:
   a. Insulinoma
   b. Gastrinoma
   c. Somatostatinoma
   d. Glucagonoma

ANSWERS

1. **Ans. (b) Islet hyperplasia**
   [Harrison's Endocrinology 3rd ed pg 363]

MEN 1	MEN 2

• Parathyroid hyperplasia or adenoma
• Islet cell hyperplasia, adenoma, or carcinoma
• Pituitary hyperplasia or adenoma
• Other less common manifestations:
  – Foregut carcinoid
  – Pheochromocytoma
  – Subcutaneous or visceral lipomas
	MEN 2A
	• MTC
	• Pheochromocytoma
	• Parathyroid hyperplasia or adenoma
	MEN 2A with cutaneous lichen amyloidosis
	MEN 2A with Hirschsprung disease
	Familial MTC
	MEN 2B
	• MTC
	• Phaeochromocytoma
	• Mucosal and gastrointestinal neuromas
	• Marfanoid features

2. **Ans. (d) Pheochromocytoma**
   [Harrison's Endocrinology 3rd ed pg 363; Williams 13th ed pg 1726]

   See discussion of Chapter 13, Question 1.
   Pheochromocytoma is a less common manifestation of MEN 1 with a penetrance of <1%.

3. **Ans. (c) Mucosal neuromas**
   [Harrison's Endocrinology 3rd ed pg 363]

   See discussion of Chapter 13, Question 1.

4. **Ans. (b) Gastrinoma**
   [Williams 13th ed pg 1726]

   Features of Multiple Endocrine Neoplasia Type 1 in Adults

Tumor type	Penetrance

Endocrine features
• Parathyroid
  – Adenoma
• Pancreaticoduodenal
  – Gastrinoma
  – Insulinoma
  – Nonfunctioning—including pancreatic polypeptidoma
  – Other: glucagonoma, VIPoma, etc.
• Foregut Carcinoid
  – Thymic carcinoid nonfunctioning
  – Bronchial carcinoid nonfunctioning
  – Gastric enterochromaffin-like tumor nonfunctioning
	
	95%
	
	40%
	10%
	20%
	each <1%
	
	2%
	4%
	10%

   Contd...

Contd...

Tumor type	Penetrance
• Anterior Pituitary	
– Prolactinoma	25%
– Other	
- Nonfunctioning	10%
- Growth hormone + prolactin	
- Growth hormone	5%
- ACTH	2%
- Thyrotropin	5%
• Adrenal	
– Cortex	
- Nonfunctioning	30%
- Functioning or cancer	2%
– Medulla: pheochromocytoma	<1%
Nonendocrine features	
• Angiofibroma	85%
• Collagenoma	70%
• Lipoma	30%
• Leiomyoma	5%
• Meningioma	5%

CHAPTER
14

Endocrine Changes in Pregnancy

QUESTIONS

1. **HPA axis in pregnancy all except:**
   a. Cortisol 2-4 times ↑
   b. Stress response is impaired
   c. More resistant to suppression
   d. ACTH is secreted by placenta

2. **GDM; cut off sugar values after 100 gram GTT is:**
   a. Fasting 95, 1 hr 180, 2 hr 155, 3 hr 140
   b. Fasting 85, 1 hr 190, 2 hr 150, 3 hr 145
   c. Fasting 90, 1 hr 185, 2 hr 150, 3 hr 145
   d. Fasting 95, 1 hr 190, 2 hr 155, 3 hr 140

3. **FT4 highest in:**
   a. 1st trimester
   b. 2nd trimester
   c. 3rd trimester
   d. All equal

4. **Secondary amenorrhea can most commonly be caused in the following conditions except:**
   a. Age above 60 years
   b. Stress
   c. Pregnancy
   d. Competitive athletes

5. **In the first 20 weeks of pregnancy, placental function is best assessed by urinary:**
   a. Pregnanediol
   b. Pregnanetriol
   c. Chorionic gonadotropin
   d. Estriol

6. **Best method for diagnosing fetal lung maturity is:**
   a. Clinical examination
   b. Ultrasonography
   c. Amniocentesis
   d. Fetal kick counts

7. **Full lung maturity is indicated by L/S ratio:**
   a. 2:1
   b. 3:1
   c. 4:1
   d. 5:1
8. **The best method to diagnose Rh-sensitization in the mother is:**
   a. Direct coombs test
   b. Indirect coombs test
   c. "c" antigen
   d. "a" antigen
9. **Inhibin is secreted by all except:**
   a. Graafian follicle
   b. Corpus luteum
   c. Endometrium
   d. Placenta

ANSWERS

1. **Ans. (b) Stress response is impaired**
   [Williams 13th ed pg 836, 838, 843, 844; Journal of Clinical Endocrinology & Metabolism, May 2008, 93(5):1536]
   - As a result of the hyperestrogenemia, hepatic production of cortisol-binding globulin is increased. The increased cortisol-binding globulin, result in decreased metabolic clearance of cortisol and a three-fold rise in total plasma cortisol by week 26, when the levels reach a plateau until they rise at the onset of labor.
   - The rate of cortisol production is increased, and the plasma free cortisol concentrations are also increased. The enhanced cortisol production is due to an increase in the maternal plasma ACTH concentrations and hyperresponsiveness of the adrenal cortex to ACTH stimulation during pregnancy.
   - The syncytiotrophoblast synthesizes an ACTH-like peptide, human chorionic corticotropin (hCC). The elevation of free cortisol levels during pregnancy may be related in part to both placental hCC and pituitary ACTH production
   - The circadian rhythm and the ability to respond to stress are maintained throughout pregnancy
   - Suppression of serum cortisol by dexamethasone is blunted in pregnancy. Thus, dexamethasone testing has an increased potential for false-positive results in pregnancy.

2. **Ans. (a) Fasting 95, 1 hr 180, 2 hr 155, 3 hr 140**
   [Diabetes Care Volume 41, Supplement 1, January 2018 pg S22]
   See discussion of Chapter 21, Question 61.

3. **Ans. (a) 1st trimester**
   [De Groot 7th ed pg 1482]

   FT4 and FT3 levels may be slightly increased in the first trimester at between 6 and 12 weeks and may fall progressively throughout gestation, often to levels below the nonpregnant assay-specific reference ranges; TBG saturation is reduced.

   Summary of Effects of Pregnancy on Thyroid Physiology

Physiologic change	Thyroid-related consequences
↑ Serum thyroxine-binding globulin	↑ Total T4 and T3; ↑ T4 production
↑ Plasma volume	↑ T4 and T3 pool size; ↑ T4 production; ↑ cardiac output
Type 3 iodothyronine deiodinase (D3) expression in placenta and uterus	↑ T4 production

   Contd...

Contd...

Physiologic change	Thyroid-related consequences
First trimester ↑ in hCG	↑Free T4; ↓ basal thyrotropin; ↑ T4 production
↑ Renal iodide(I⁻) clearance	↑ Iodine requirements
↑ T4 production; fetal T4 synthesis during second and third trimesters	
↑ Oxygen consumption by fetoplacental unit, gravid uterus, and mother	↑ Basal metabolic rate; ↑ cardiac Output

4. **Ans. (a) Age above 60 years**
   [Williams 13th ed pg 616-620, 646]
   The median age at menopause is approximately 51 years.

5. **Ans. (d) Estriol**
   [Obstetrics and Gynaecology: An Evidence-based Text for MRCOG 3rd ed pg 275; Williams 13th ed pg 840; De Groot 7th ed pg 2496; Clinical Gynecologic Endocrinology and Infertility 8th ed pg 270, 271, 276]
   - *Biochemical tests of placental function:* Include measurement of estriol (E3), human placental lactogen (hPL), human chorionic gonadotropin (hCG) and placental growth factor (PGF) in maternal plasma, serum or urine.
   - hCG is first detected in maternal serum 6 to 9 days after conception. The levels rise in a logarithmic fashion, peaking 8 to 10 weeks after the last menstrual period, followed by a decline to a nadir at 18 weeks, with subsequent levels remaining constant until delivery.
   - A rise in estrone begins at 6–10 weeks. As pregnancy advances, the production of estriol, increases rapidly.
   - Pregnanediol and pregnanetriol are metabolites of progesterone. Until approximately the seventh week, progesterone is produced by the corpus luteum. After a transition period of shared function between the seventh week and tenth week, during which there is a slight decline in circulating maternal progesterone levels, the placenta emerges as the major source of progesterone synthesis, and maternal circulating levels progressively increase.
   - For years, measurement of estrogen in a 24-hour urine collection was a standard method of assessing fetal well-being. This was replaced by immunoassay of unconjugated estriol in the plasma. However, assessment of maternal estriol levels has been superseded by various biophysical fetal monitoring techniques such as nonstress testing, stress testing, and measurement of fetal breathing and activity.

6. **Ans. (c) Amniocentesis**
   [Clinical Gynecologic Endocrinology and Infertility 8th ed pg 325, 326]

7. **Ans. (a) 2:1**
   [Clinical Gynecologic Endocrinology and Infertility 8th ed pg 326]

8. **Ans. (b) Indirect coombs test**
   [Williams Obstetrics 24th ed pg 307]

9. **Ans. (c) Endometrium**
   [Williams 13th ed pg 609, 610]

   Inhibin
   - Synthesized in ovary (granulosa cells), adrenal, pituitary, and placenta.
   - *Two isoforms:*
     1. Inhibin A-heterodimer ($\alpha\beta A$) i.e. contains an identical α-subunit but distinct β-subunit (βA); LH-induced; levels are low during the first half of the follicular phase but increase gradually during the midfollicular phase and peak during the luteal phase.
     2. Inhibin B-heterodimer ($\alpha\beta_B$) i.e. contains an identical α-subunit but distinct β-subunit (β_B); influenced by FSH; secreted mainly during the early follicular phase, with levels decreasing in midfollicular phase and becoming undetectable after the LH surge.
   - All three subunits are detected in small antral follicles; the α- and β_A-subunits are found in the dominant follicle and in the corpus luteum.
   - Suppresses FSH production in the pituitary.

   Activin
   - Synthesized in ovary (granulosa cells), adrenal, pituitary (gonadotrophs), and placenta.
   - *Three isoforms:*
     1. Activin A-contains two β-subunits ($\beta_A\beta_A$)
     2. Activin B-contains two β-subunits ($\beta_B\beta_B$)
     3. Activin AB-contains two β-subunits ($\beta_A\beta_B$)
   - In the pituitary, activin stimulates the release of FSH. In the ovarian follicle, activin enhances FSH action.
   - Unlike inhibin, locally synthesized activin in the pituitary, rather than the ovarian-derived activin, is responsible for regulating FSH.

   Follistatin
   - Single-unit peptide
   - Produced in several human tissues, including pituitary and ovary
   - Binds and neutralizes the biologic functions of activin-inhibits pituitary FSH secretion.

CHAPTER 15

Endocrinology of Fetal Development

QUESTIONS

1. Fetal growth during intra-uterine phase is dependent on:
   a. Maternal insulin
   b. Placental GH
   c. Fetal GH
   d. Fetal thyroxine

2. Steroid hormone in fetal life:
   a. Testosterone
   b. Aldosterone
   c. Cortisol
   d. DHEA

3. All of the following are true about aromatase deficiency in adults except:
   a. Small testis
   b. Large testis
   c. Lack of gynecomastia
   d. Increased FSH

4. Aromatase is present in all tissues except:
   a. Brain
   b. Adipose tissue
   c. Heart
   d. Ovary

5. Can't cross the placenta:
   a. TSH
   b. TRH
   c. Vit-D
   d. GnRH

6. All of the following statements about hPL are true except:
   a. 191-amino acid polypeptide with 2 disulfide bridges
   b. 85% homology to GH and 13% to Prl
   c. A major regulator of IGF-2 production
   d. Synthesized from syncytiotrophoblast

ANSWERS

1. **Ans. (b) Placental GH**
   [Williams 13th ed pg 877-880; Endocrine Reviews, April 2006, 27(2):146]

   Factors Important for Fetal Growth
   - Insulin like Growth factors—IGF-1, IGF-2
   - Insulin
   - *Growth factors:*
     - Epidermal growth factor/transforming growth factor system (EGF/TGF-α system)
     - Nerve Growth Factor (NGF)
     - Others
       - Hematopoietic growth factors, e.g. Erythropoietin
       - Platelet-derived growth factors (PDGFs)
       - Fibroblast growth factors (FGFs)
       - Vascular endothelial growth factor (VEGF)
       - TGF-β superfamily

   The hormones most important for postnatal growth, including T4, GH, and gonadal steroids, have a limited role in fetal growth. Placental hormones including the human GH variant and hPLs play a limited role.

   The levels of insulin in maternal serum or amniotic fluid were not correlated with birth weight.

2. **Ans. (d) DHEA**
   [Williams 13th ed pg 858]

3. **Ans. (a) Small testis**
   [Nat Rev Endocrinol. 2009 Oct;5(10):560; Williams 13th ed pg 711]

   Aromatase Deficiency
   Caused by inactivating mutations of the aromatase gene (*CYP19A1*)

   Clinical Presentation
   - Lack of signs and symptoms during infancy and early adolescence
   - *Onset of signs and symptoms:* Late adolescence
   - Clinical features in adult men
     - Signs and symptoms that are highly likely to be present
       - Tall stature
       - Widespread bone pain
       - Continuing and progressive linear growth during adulthood
       - Delayed bone maturation
       - Unfused epiphyses
       - Eunuchoid proportions of the skeleton
       - Progressive genu valgum
       - Osteopenia or osteoporosis
     - Signs and symptoms that are often present
       - Abdominal adiposity

Endocrinology of Fetal Development | 187

- ♦ Acanthosis nigricans
- ♦ Early-onset metabolic syndrome
- ♦ Nonalcoholic fatty liver disease
- ♦ Dyslipidemia
- Signs and symptoms that are occasionally present
  - ♦ Oligozoospermia
  - ♦ Abnormalities in spermatogenesis
  - ♦ Cryptorchidism
  - ♦ Increased volume of the testes
  - ♦ Scoliosis

Laboratory Findings
- Impairments in glucose and lipid metabolism (insulin resistance, ↑ triglyceride, ↓HDL),
- Abnormal liver enzymes, fatty liver,
- Low sperm counts, infertility,
- Undetectable estradiol levels with normal to elevated serum testosterone and gonadotropin levels.

4. **Ans. (c) Heart**
   [Williams 13th ed pg 608, 710]

   Aromatase is present in:
   - Adipose tissue
   - Brain
   - Bone
   - Breast
   - Liver
   - Blood vessels
   - Ovaries (granulosa cells and granulosa lutein cells)
   - Testes (Sertoli cells and Leydig cells).

5. **Ans. (a) TSH**
   [Williams 13th ed pg 849, 850; Comprehensive Human Physiology: From Cellular Mechanisms to Integration pg 2339; Endocrinol Metab Clin North Am. 2010 Jun;39(2):308; The onset of labor: cellular and integrative mechanisms: a National Institute of Child Health & Human Development Research Planning Workshop, November 29-December 1, 1987 pg 220]
   - The placenta is impermeable to most peptide hormones.
   - Hormones larger than 0.7 to 1.2 kDa have little or no access to the fetal compartment.
   - Hormones that do not cross the placenta include the hypothalamic releasing factors (except for TRH and somatostatin), anterior and posterior pituitary hormones, insulin, glucagon, parathyroid hormone (PTH), calcitonin and renin.
   - Steroid, thyroid hormones and catecholamines do cross the placenta, but several of them are metabolized en route, including cortisol, estradiol, thyroxine (T4), triiodothyronine (T3), and catecholamines.

- Placental 11β-hydroxysteroid dehydrogenase type 2 (11β-HSD2) catalyzes the conversion of most of the maternal cortisol to inactive cortisone.
- Placental 17β-HSD prevent passage of excessive estrogens to the fetus by catalyzing inactivation of estradiol to estrone.
- Placental iodothyronine inner-ring monodeiodinase deiodinates most of the T4 to inactive reverse triiodothyronine (rT3) and converts 3,5,3-T3 to inactive diiodothyronine (T2).
  Thus, there is limited permeability to thyroid hormones.
- Placental tissue monoamine oxidase and catechol O-methyltransferase converts catecholamines to metabolites like metanephrine and dihydroxymandelic acid.

25-OHD readily crosses the placenta. Vitamin D and $1,25(OH)_2D$ do not cross the placenta into the fetus in appreciable amounts.

6. **Ans. (c) A major regulator of IGF-2 production**
   [Williams 13th ed pg 842, 843]

   Human Placental Lactogen (hPL, also called chorionic somatomammotropin)
   - Single chain polypeptide composed of 191 amino acid residues and two disulfide bridges
   - Closely related to GH (85% amino acid homology) and prolactin (13% amino acid homology)
   - Gene is located on the long arm of chromosome 17
   - Synthesized and secreted by the syncytiotrophoblast
   - Detected in maternal serum between 20 and 40 days of gestation; the maternal serum levels rise rapidly and peak at 34 weeks, followed by a plateau
   - *Actions:*
     - Can bind to both hGH and prolactin receptors—biologic activities are similar to those of hGH and prolactin.
     - Major regulator of IGF-1 production.
     - *Affects the metabolism of maternal nutrients:* Stimulates pancreatic islet insulin secretion; promotes insulin resistance (diabetogenic); enhances lipolysis, leading to a rise in free fatty acids, which may in part be responsible for the insulin resistance.
     - Appears to play a role in providing the fetus with a constant supply of glucose and amino acids: lipolysis allows the mother to utilize free fatty acids for energy during fasting, allowing glucose, amino acids, and ketone bodies to be used by the fetus.
     - *Actions in the fetus:* Promoting amino acid uptake by muscle and stimulating protein production, IGF-1 production, and glycogen synthesis.
   - However, its absence (related to gene defects) does not appear to impair pregnancy.

CHAPTER 16

Pediatric Disorders of Sexual Development

QUESTIONS

1. XY sex reversal can occur due to duplication of:
   a. SRY
   b. DAX-1
   c. WT-1
   d. SF-1

2. 15 yr/F, primary amenorrhea, normal breast development, 46 XX, FSH/LH normal, E2 normal, Müllerian structures absent, ovaries normal. Diagnosis is:
   a. MRKH
   b. AIS
   c. Pure gonadal dysgenesis
   d. 5α-reductase deficiency

3. Turner stigmata include all except:
   a. Nail hypoplasia
   b. Café au lait spots
   c. Low posterior hairline
   d. Cubitus valgus

4. Klinefelter syndrome is characterized by all except:
   a. Tall children
   b. Small firm testes
   c. Hyposmia
   d. Taurodontism

5. In AIS, which of the following does not help in diagnosis:
   a. Penile response to testosterone is decreased
   b. Normal to high testosterone response to LH
   c. Increased SHBG levels
   d. Increased serum estradiol levels

6. Virilization in karyotype female (XX) is seen in all except:
   a. 21-hydroxylase deficiency
   b. 3 beta HSD deficiency
   c. Testicular feminization
   d. True hermaphrodite

7. Undervirilization of XY (male) karyotype seen in all except:
   a. True hermaphrodite (XY)
   b. Gonoadal dysgenesis
   c. LH receptor defect
   d. FSH receptor defect

8. **Short height in Turner syndrome is linked to:**
   a. DAX
   b. SHOX
   c. SF-1
   d. SOX9

9. **Scrotum develops from:**
   a. Genital ridge
   b. Genital swelling
   c. Genital tubercle
   d. Urogenital fold

10. **Ambiguous genitalia not seen in male:**
    a. 21-hydroxylase
    b. 17α-hydroxylase
    c. 3β-HSD
    d. Chol. side chain cleavage

11. **False about 5α reductase deficiency:**
    a. Autosomal dominant
    b. Virilization at puberty
    c. Absent Mullerian duct derivatives
    d. Small phallus with urogenital sinus and a blind vaginal pouch

12. **47xxx syndrome is associated with all except:**
    a. Extra X-chromosome is maternal in origin
    b. Ovarian failure is a must
    c. Behavioral disturbances may be seen
    d. Growth rate and height normal

13. **True about Klinefelter's syndrome are all except:**
    a. Osteoporosis
    b. Leg ulcers
    c. Pituitary hypoplasia
    d. Dysgenesis

14. **SF-1:**
    a. Orphan receptor
    b. Synergize WT1 and antagonize DAX1
    c. Mutation not identified in human
    d. Chromosome 10q

15. **All of the following are true about DAX 1 except:**
    a. Located on the X chromosome
    b. Duplication → 46, XY sex reversal
    c. Deletion → 46, XY sex reversal
    d. Hypogonadotropic hypogonadism

16. **Syndrome associated with ambiguous genitalia:**
    a. Robinow syndrome
    b. Carney complex
    c. Extrophy of bladder
    d. McCune-Albright syndrome
    e. Fraser syndrome

17. **Kallmann syndrome:**
    a. Nystagmus
    b. Anosmia
    c. Ambiguous genitalia
    d. Microcephaly

18. **17α-hydroxylase deficiency is characterized by all except:**
    a. Female unambiguity
    b. Primary amenorrhea
    c. Hypervirilization in male
    d. Hypertension

19. **Not true about Klinefelter's syndrome:**
    a. Advanced maternal age is risk factor
    b. Meiotic nondisjunction is MC cause
    c. Peritubular elastin deposition is MC histopath finding
    d. Gynecomastia is seen

20. **Androgen insensitivity syndrome can be differentiated from Mayer Rokitansy Kuster Hauser syndrome by:**
    a. Absence of pubic hair
    b. Blind vagina
    c. Short stature
    d. Well developed breasts

21. **Androgen insensitivity syndrome can be differentiated from Swyer syndrome by:**
    a. Female phenotype
    b. Palpable Mullerian structures
    c. 46 XY
    d. Developed breasts

22. **All are associated with brachydactyly except:**
    a. Turner's
    b. Klinefelter's
    c. PHP
    d. Achondroplasia

23. **Labia majora are developed by:**
    a. Genital tubercle
    b. Genital folds
    c. Genital swellings
    d. Genital ridge

24. **Cause of cubitus valgus in Turner's syndrome is:**
    a. Defect in medial epicondyle
    b. Defect in head of radius
    c. Defect in olecranon process
    d. Defect in trochlea of ulna

25. **Chondrodysplasia is characterized by all except:**
    a. Disproportionate body segments
    b. Can be seen in Turner syndrome
    c. Can be seen in Klinefelter syndrome
    d. Is usually inherited

26. **Turner syndrome true is:**
    a. Deafness is common
    b. Short stature is due to hypothyroidism
    c. Hypogonadism is due to low LH
    d. Diabetes is due to decreased insulin secretion

27. **Gene acting only on genital ridge not on Bipotential gonads:**
    a. WT-1
    b. SF-1
    c. SOX-9
    d. DAX-1

ANSWERS

1. **Ans. (b) DAX-1**
   [Williams 13th ed pg 898, 899]
   Factors involved in sex determination and sex differentiation

   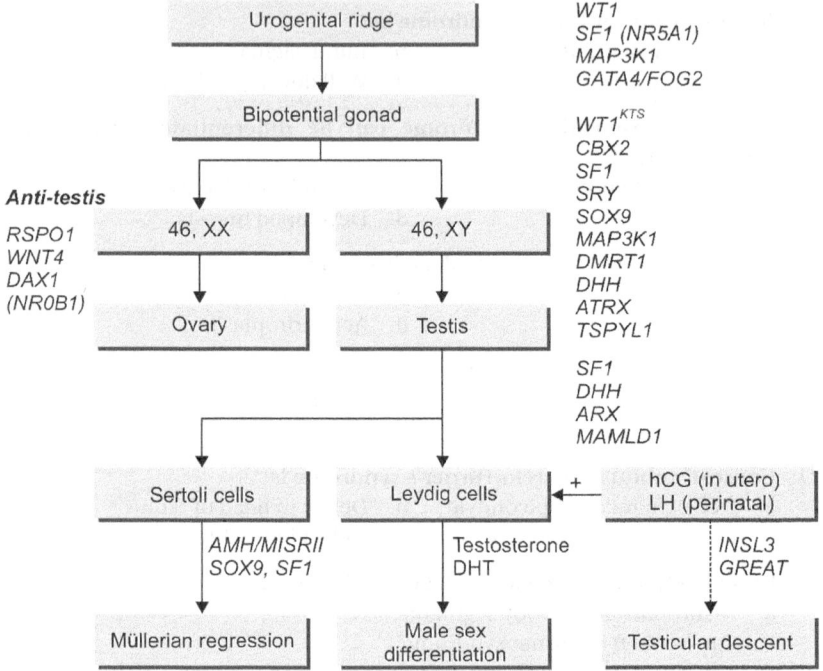

   Overexpression of DAX1 (NR0B1), WNT4 and RSPO1 have been implicated in 46, XY DSD.

2. **Ans. (a) MRKH**
   [Greenspan's 9th ed; De Groot 7th ed pg 2090; Williams 13th ed pg 951]
   See discussion of Chapter 11, Questions 8 and 15.

3. **Ans. (b) Café au lait spots**
   [Williams 13th ed pg 910]

   Features of Turner syndrome
   - *Childhood:* Lymphedema, shield chest, web neck, low hairline; cardiac defects and coarctation of the aorta; renal and urinary abnormalities; short stature, cubitus valgus, hypoplastic nails, scoliosis; otitis media and hearing loss; ptosis and amblyopia; nevi; autoimmune thyroid disease; visuospatial learning difficulties.

- *Adulthood:* Pubertal failure, primary amenorrhea; hypertension; aortic root dilatation and dissection; sensorineural hearing loss; increased risk of CVD, IBD, colon cancer, thyroid disease, glucose intolerance and diabetes mellitus, osteoporosis.
  Uterus is present, Gonads-streak gonad or immature ovary.

4. **Ans. (c) Hyposmia**
   [Williams 13th ed pg 737, 738, 1147, 1148]

   Klinefelter Syndrome
   - Most common form of male hypogonadism.
   - Risk increases with both maternal and paternal age
   - Characterized by presence of one or more extra X chromosomes due to maternal/paternal meiotic nondisjunction
   - Karyotype: 47,XXY (in 90%), mosaic (47,XXY/46,XY) (in 10%), others (rare): 48,XXXY, 49,XXXXY
   - Mosaicism occurs as a result of postfertilization mitotic nondisjunction.
   - *Clinical features:*
     - Male phenotype
     - Small, firm testes as an adult (< 3.5 cm long)
     - Impaired spermatogenesis
     - Gynecomastia
     - Tall stature
     - Long legs but not long arms (decreased U/L body ratio without an increase in arm span)
     - Muscle tone may be low
     - *Behavior problems:*
       - Neurobehavioral abnormalities, primarily in language, speech, learning, and frontal executive functions
       - Adjustment problems in adolescence
       - Crime rates for sexual abuse and arson are increased, whereas traffic offenses and drug-related crime are decreased
     - The global IQ is normal or near normal, but verbal IQ, is usually lower (e.g. 10 to 20 points) than performance IQ.
   - Conditions associated with Klinefelter syndrome
     - Aortic valvular disease
     - Mitral valve prolapse
     - Ruptured berry aneurysms
     - Breast carcinoma
     - Acute leukemia
     - Deep vein thrombosis, and pulmonary embolism
     - Non-Hodgkin Lymphoma
     - Germ cell tumors at any midline site
     - Systemic lupus erythematosus
     - Rheumatoid arthritis

- Sjögren syndrome
- Osteoporosis
- Diabetes mellitus
- Thyroid disease
- Fatigue
- Depression and schizophrenia
- Varicose veins, venous stasis ulcers
- Deep vein thrombosis, and pulmonary embolism
- Essential tremor.
- Taurodontism (enlarged molar teeth).
- *Gonadal function:*
  - There is a normal increase in testosterone, INSL3, and inhibin B before puberty
  - By midpuberty testosterone and INSL3 concentrations remain in the low-normal range
  - AMH levels decrease at an age later than in normal boys
  - Serum LH and FSH usually rise by midpuberty
  - Prepubertal testes show only subtle histologic changes, although the testes are small, and the germ cell content is reduced. Seminiferous tubules are normal
  - The testes degenerate in an accelerated manner at the onset of puberty
  - Hyalinization and fibrosis of the seminiferous tubules and pseudoadenomatous changes of the Leydig cells develop after puberty
  - Adult-type spermatogonia are found in peripubertal boys, but older boys had no germ cells
  - The plasma concentration of testosterone fails to rise to normal adult levels
  - The onset of puberty usually is not delayed, but impaired Leydig cell reserve and low testosterone levels may lead to slow progression or arrest of pubertal changes.
- Mortality is increased.

5. **Ans. (c) Increased SHBG levels**
[Williams 13th ed pg 759, 933, 934]
Complete Androgen Insensitivity Syndrome (previously known as testicular feminization syndrome)
- Karyotype: 46,XY
- Inheritance: X-linked recessive; mutations in AR gene
- Patients appear as normal females at birth.

- Typically presents in an adolescent female who has breast development with a pubertal growth spurt but who has not had her menarche (primary amenorrhea). Pubic and axillary hair is absent or scanty. The vagina is short and blind ending, and the uterus is absent as a result of normal AMH action, although there may be Müllerian remnants. The Wolffian ducts are stabilized in many patients, with well-developed vas deferens and epididymis. The testes are usually located in the inguinal canal or the labia majora.
- They may be diagnosed in infancy because of an inguinal hernia containing a palpable gonad that turns out to be a testis, or prenatally because of discordance between genotype and phenotype.

Partial Androgen Insensitivity Syndrome
- Karyotype: 46,XY
- Inheritance X-linked recessive; mutations in AR gene
- Characterized by incomplete masculinization resulting from a partial biologic response to androgens.
- The prototypic phenotype for PAIS comprises penoscrotal hypospadias, micropenis, and a bifid scrotum. The testes may be undescended; The most severe form of PAIS manifests as isolated clitoromegaly; The milder end of the spectrum includes isolated hypospadias.
- Wolffian duct derivatives: Often normal; Müllerian duct derivatives: Absent.
- Decreased to normal axillary and pubic hair, beard growth, and body hair; gynecomastia is common at puberty.

Minimal or Mild Androgen Insensitivity Syndrome
- Associated with normal male development but gynecomastia at puberty and infertility in adulthood.

Breast cancer risk is increased in MAIS and in those with PAIS raised male. In contrast, breast cancer has not been reported in women with CAIS.

Hormone Profiles in Androgen Insensitivity Syndromes
- Increased LH and testosterone levels
- Increased estradiol (for male reference range)
- FSH levels are often normal or slightly increased
- Complete or partial resistance to androgenic and metabolic effects of testosterone
- Concentrations of sex hormone–binding globulin (SHBG) are sexually dimorphic, with levels in patients with CAIS similar to those found in normal females.
- Serum AMH concentration is typically increased in CAIS.

6. **Ans. (c) Testicular feminization**
[Williams 13th ed pg 909]

DSD Classification System		
Sex Chromosome DSD	46,XY DSD	46,XX DSD

• 47,XXY (Klinefelter syndrome and variants)
• 45,X (Turner syndrome and variants)
• 45,X/46,XY (mixed gonadal dysgenesis)
• 46,XX/46,XY (chimerism)
	• Disorders of gonadal (testis) development
	  – Complete or partial gonadal dysgenesis (e.g. *SF1/NR5A1,WT1, GATA4, FOG2/ZFPM2, CBX2, SRY, SOX9, MAP3K1, DMRT1, TSPYL1, DHH, ARX, MAMLD1/CXorf6*)
	  – Ovotesticular DSD
	  – Testis regression
	• Disorders in androgen synthesis or action
	  – Disorders of androgen synthesis
	    - Luteinizing hormone (LH) receptor mutations
	    - Smith-Lemli-Opitz syndrome
	    - StAR protein mutations
	    - Cholesterol side-chain cleavage (CYP11A1)
	    - 3β-Hydroxysteroid dehydrogenase 2 (HSD3B2)
	    - 17α-Hydroxylase/17,20-lyase (CYP17)
	    - P450 oxidoreductase (POR)
	    - Cytochrome b5 (CYB5A)
	    - Aldo-keto reductase 1C2 (AKR1C2)
	    - 17β-Hydroxysteroid dehydrogenase (HSD17B3)
	    - 5α-Reductase 2 (SRD5A2)
	  – Disorders of androgen action
	    - Androgen insensitivity syndrome
	    - Drugs and environmental modulators
	• Other
	  – Syndromic associations of male genital development (e.g. cloacal anomalies, Robinow, Aarskog, hand-foot-genital, popliteal pterygium)
	  – Persistent Müllerian duct syndrome
	  – Vanishing testis syndrome
	  – Isolated hypospadias
	  – Congenital hypogonadotropic hypogonadism
	  – Cryptorchidism (INSL3, GREAT)
	  – Environmental influences
		• Disorders of gonadal (ovary) development
		  – Gonadal dysgenesis
		  – Ovotesticular DSD
		  – Testicular DSD (e.g. SRY+, dup SOX9, dup SOX3, RSPO1, WNT4)
		• Androgen excess
		  – Fetal
		    - 3β-Hydroxysteroid dehydrogenase 2 (HSD3B2)
		    - 21-Hydroxylase (CYP21A2)
		    - P450 oxidoreductase (POR)
		    - 11β-Hydroxylase (CYP11B1)
		    - Glucocorticoid receptor mutations
		  – Fetoplacental
		    - Aromatase (CYP19) deficiency
		    - Oxidoreductase (POR) deficiency
		  – Maternal
		    - Maternal virilizing tumors (e.g. luteomas)
		    - Androgenic drugs
		• Other
		  – Syndromic associations (e.g. cloacal anomalies)
		  – Müllerian agenesis/hypoplasia (e.g. MKRH)
		  – Uterine abnormalities (e.g. MODY5)
		  – Vaginal atresias (e.g. McKusick-Kaufman)
		  – Labial adhesions

NB: True hermaphrodite is currently called ovotesticular DSD; Testicular feminization syndrome is preferable called complete androgen insensitivity syndrome.

Pediatric Disorders of Sexual Development | **197**

7. **Ans. (d) FSH receptor defect**
   [Williams 13th ed pg 909]
   See discussion of Chapter 16, Question 6.

8. **Ans. (b) SHOX**
   [Williams 13th ed pg 1007]

9. **Ans. (b) Genital swelling**
   [Williams 13th ed pg 903; Langman's Embryology 11th ed pg 258]
   In the male:
   - Urogenital sinus develops into the prostate and prostatic urethra,
   - Genital tubercle develops into the glans penis,
   - Urogenital (urethral) folds fuse to form the shaft of the penis,
   - Urogenital (labioscrotal) swellings form the scrotum.

   In the female:
   - Genital tubercle forms the clitoris
   - Urethral folds develop into the labia minora
   - Genital swellings form the labia majora
   - The urogenital groove is open and forms the vestibule.

10. **Ans. (a) 21-hydroxylase deficiency**
    [Williams 13th ed pg 534, 909]
    See discussions of Chapter 9, Question 16 and Chapter 16, Question 6.

11. **Ans. (a) Autosomal dominant**
    [Williams 13th ed pg 930, 931]

    Steroid 5α-reductase Type 2 Deficiency
    - 5α-reductase type 2 deficiency is transmitted as an autosomal recessive trait.
    - Two microsomal 5α-reductase enzymes catalyze the conversion of testosterone to DHT.
      - The type 2 isoenzyme is expressed predominantly in the primordia of the prostate and external genitalia but not in the wolffian ducts until after their differentiation into the male internal genital ducts.
      - The type 1 isoenzyme is expressed in skin, including human genital skin fibroblasts. The action of type 1 isoenzyme may contribute to virilization at puberty.
    - At birth, there is typically a bifid scrotum, a urogenital sinus, a blind vaginal pouch, and a clitoris-like, hypospadiac phallus.
    - Testes differentiate normally and are located in the inguinal canal or in the labioscrotal folds.
    - Müllerian structures are absent.
    - The Wolffian ducts are stabilized so that the epididymides, vasa deferentia, and seminal vesicles are well differentiated.
    - The prostate is hypoplastic.
    - Up to a third of cases may present with isolated hypospadias.

- Individuals virilize to various degrees at puberty. The voice deepens, muscle mass increases, the phallus lengthens to 4 to 8 cm, the bifid scrotum becomes rugated and pigmented, and the testes enlarge and descend into the labioscrotal folds.
- Gender role changes occur frequently.
- Postpubertal affected males do not have acne, temporal hair recession, or enlargement of the prostate, and they do not develop gynecomastia.
- There is normal libido with penile erections.
- Infertility is common.
- Biochemical profile
    - Elevated testosterone-to-DHT ratio basally or after hCG stimulation (ratio > 10 : 1 had a sensitivity and specificity of 78% and 72%, respectively).
    - Serum LH and FSH levels may be normal or elevated after puberty.
    - Analysis of a urinary steroid profile by gas chromatography and mass spectrometry demonstrate a diminished ratio of urinary 5α- to 5β-reduced C19 and C21 steroids.

12. **Ans. (b) Ovarian failure is a must**
[De Groot 7th ed pg 2097; Clinical Laboratory Medicine 2nd ed pg 624]
- 47,XXX Females.
- Most cases are oligo- or asymptomatic.
- Gonadal development and function is normal in the majority of cases, except for a few XXX women who develop premature ovarian failure.
- Children are long-legged, with accelerated growth from infancy resulting in increased height at pubertal onset.
- Behavior disturbances may occur.

13. **Ans. (c) Pituitary hypoplasia**
[Williams 13th ed pg 738, 1147, 1148]
See discussion of Chapter 16, Question 4.

14. **Ans. (a) Orphan receptor**
[Williams 13th ed pg 899; De Groot 7th ed pg 2055]
Steroidogenic factor 1 (SF1):
- Orphan nuclear receptor transcription factor
- Also referred to as *nuclear receptor subfamily 5, group A, member 1* [NR5A1]
- Gene is located on chromosome 9q33
- Affects reproductive function at all three levels of the hypothalamic-pituitary gonadal axis and gonadal and adrenal development in males and females
- Plays a critical role in testis development and facilitates SRY regulation of SOX9 expression. SF1 is also an important regulator of ovarian integrity and function
- Mutations identified in the human SF1 gene account for approximately 20% of cases of 46,XY gonadal dysgenesis.

WT1 -KTS isoforms synergize with SF1 to promote AMH expression; WT1-KTS can also activate the DAX1 promoter. However, DAX1 antagonizes the synergy between SF1 and WT1, most likely through a direct protein-protein interaction with SF1, suggesting that WT1 and DAX1 functionally oppose each other in testis development by modulating SF1-mediated transactivation. Thus, the relative dosages of WT1 -KTS and DAX1 and the timing of their expression during embryogenesis are vital for gonadal development.

15. **Ans. (c) Deletion → 46,XY sex reversal**
    [Williams 13th ed pg 899]

    DAX1
    - DAX1 is an orphan nuclear receptor.
    - The gene (NROB1) coding for DAX1 is located on the short arm of the X chromosome.
    - DAX1/NROB1 is expressed throughout the HPG axis.
    - The DAX1 protein functions as a transcriptional repressor of many genes, including NR5A1.
    - Duplication of the DAX1/NROB1 locus is associated with male-to-female sex reversal. External genitalia ranges from female to ambiguous. Internal genitalia include the presence of Müllerian and Wolffian structures. Gonads are typically streaks.
    - Loss-of-function mutations are associated with X-linked adrenal hypoplasia congenita (AHC). Adrenal insufficiency generally manifests in infancy or early childhood.
    - At the age of expected puberty, hypogonadotropic hypogonadism due to hypothalamic and pituitary dysfunction may occur among affected males. Delayed puberty has been recognized in heterozygous females.

16. **Ans. (a) Robinow syndrome**
    [Williams 13th ed pg 909]
    See discussion of Chapter 16, Question 6.

17. **Ans. (b) Anosmia**
    [Williams 13th ed pg 1134-1138]
    See discussion of Chapter 18, Question 24.
    Option (b) is a more appropriate than option (a).

18. **Ans. (c) Hypervirilization in male**
    [Williams 13th ed pg 539, 541]

    17α-Hydroxylase Deficiency
    - Mutations within the *CYP17A1* gene result in failure to synthesize cortisol (17α-hydroxylase activity), adrenal androgens (17,20-lyase activity), and gonadal steroids.
    - Rare patients with isolated deficiency 17,20-lyase deficiency have been reported.

- Loss of negative feedback results in increased secretion of steroids proximal to the block, and mineralocorticoid synthesis is enhanced.
- Corticosterone has weak glucocorticoid activity, corticosterone excess generally prevents adrenal crises.
- Accumulation of corticosterone and DOC results in severe hypokalemic hypertension.
- Sex steroid deficiency results in hypergonadotropic hypogonadism. There is lack of pubertal development in both sexes. Female patients (XX) have primary amenorrhea with absent sexual characteristics, whereas 46,XY individuals present with 46,XY DSD with female external genitalia but absent uterus and fallopian tubes.
- The diagnosis is usually made at the time of puberty when patients present with hypertension, hypokalemia, and hypergonadotropic hypogonadism.
- The intra-abdominal testes should be removed, and such patients are usually reared as females.
- Glucocorticoid replacement lowers blood pressure. Sex steroid replacement is required from puberty onward.

19. Ans. (c) Peritubular elastin deposition is MC histopath finding
 [Williams 13th ed pg 737, 738, 1147, 1148]
 See discussion of Chapter 16, Question 4.

20. Ans. (a) Absence of pubic hair
 [Williams 13th ed pg 951]
 Both the conditions may present as primary amenorrhea in a girl who has developed in puberty.
 Differentiating feature:
 - Karyotype-In Mayer-Rokitansky-Küster-Hauser (MRKH) syndrome the karyotype is 46,XX. In complete androgen insensitivity syndrome (CAIS) the karyotype is 46,XY.
 - Girls with CAIS often have reduced pubic and axillary hair.

21. Ans. (d) Developed breasts
 [Williams 13th ed pg 914, 919, 933]
 - *Complete testicular dysgenesis* (Swyer syndrome) is associated with a complete lack of androgenization of the external genitalia and persistent Müllerian structures due to insufficient AMH production.
 - XY complete gonadal dysgenesis (Swyer syndrome) is distinguished from CAIS absence of pubertal development- poor breast development, taller stature, decreased ratio of upper to lower body segments, and a different hormone profile.

22. Ans. (b) Klinefelter's
 [De Groot 7th ed pg 494, 997, 1149, 1153; Williams 13th ed pg 749; Sparling-Pediatric Endocrinology 4th ed pg 124, 746, 828, 985; Pediatric Endocrine Disorders pg 79]

See discussion of Chapter 2, Question 1.
Klinefelter's syndrome is associated with arachnodactyly.

23. **Ans. (c) Genital swellings**
    [Williams 13th ed pg 903; Langman's Embryology 11th ed pg 258]
    See discussion of Chapter 16, Question 9.

24. **Ans. (d) Defect in trochlea of ulna**
    [Sparling-Pediatric Endocrinology 4th ed pg 673]
    - Cubitus valgus can be measured as the angle of intersection of the long axis of the upper arm with the long axis of the supinated forearm when the elbow is fully extended.
    - Normally, in adult women this angle is approximately 12 degrees—whereas in adult men it is approximately 6 degrees.
    - The major determinant of the angle is the depth of the inner lip of the trochlea of the ulna relative to the outer lip.
    - In many patients with Turner syndrome, the angle is between 15 and 30 degrees as a consequence of developmental abnormalities of the trochlear head.

25. **Ans. (c) Can be seen in Klinefelter syndrome**
    [De Groot 7th ed pg 400; Williams 13th ed pg 1007]

26. **Ans. (a) Deafness is common**
    [Sparling-Pediatric Endocrinology 4th ed pg 675, 680, 682]
    - Turner syndrome is commonly associated with conductive hearing loss (bilateral otitis media is common) and sensorineural hearing loss. Conductive hearing loss is most common and severe in children whereas sensorineural hearing loss is more common in adults.
    - Short stature in Turner syndrome has been attributed to SHOX haploinsufficiency.
    - Hypogonadism is due to ovarian insufficiency.
    - The etiology of glucose intolerance has remained unclear. Early studies described insulin deficiency and insulin resistance Most recent data generally suggest that glucose intolerance in Turner syndrome is due to insulin deficiency rather than insensitivity.
    - Thus, option (a) appears more appropriate than option (d).

27. **Ans. (a) WT-1**
    [Sparling-Pediatric Endocrinology 4th ed pg 112]

CHAPTER 17

Normal and Aberrant Growth

QUESTIONS

1. **CDGP:**
   a. Ht. age = bone age
   b. Ht. age = Chr. age
   c. Bone age = Chr. age
   d. Ht. age/bone age = Chr. age

2. **GH stimulation test include all except:**
   a. Standing/erect
   b. Clonidine 4 ug/day
   c. Overnight fasting
   d. GH ≥ 10 ug/dL

3. **IGF binding protein:**
   a. Related to insulin
   b. Increased by GH
   c. α and β chain
   d. Acts on insulin receptor

4. **Bone age compatible to Chr. age in:**
   a. GH deficiency
   b. Celiac disease
   c. Constitutional DP
   d. Familial

5. **Growth retardation is seen in all except:**
   a. Cushing disease
   b. Addison disease
   c. Pseudohypoparathyroidism
   d. Vit D resistant rickets

6. **Main growth promoting hormone in infancy:**
   a. Thyroxin
   b. GH
   c. Cortisol
   d. Nutrition

7. **Primary regulator of IGF-1 is:**
   a. GH
   b. Insulin
   c. Cortisol
   d. Thyroxine

8. **hGH has therapeutic role in all except:**
   a. GH deficiency
   b. CRF
   c. Turner syndrome
   d. Laron syndrome

9. GH action independent of IGF-1 include all except:
   a. Increase in bone mass
   b. Hepatic protein synthesis
   c. Lipolysis
   d. Nitrogen retention
10. A 3-year-old girl presents with short stature, h/o secondary hypothyroidism at birth, adrenal axis normal and now has GH deficiency, diagnosis is:
    a. Laron dwarfism
    b. Multiple pituitary hormone deficiency
    c. Turner syndrome
    d. None of the above
11. Increased in Prader-Willi syndrome:
    a. GH
    b. Ghrelin
    c. LH
    d. FSH
12. Least useful in evaluation of GH deficiency:
    a. Basal GH
    b. Insulin induced
    c. Exercise induced
    d. GHRH induced
13. All are stimuli for GH secretion except:
    a. Insulin
    b. Glucagon
    c. Arginine
    d. Bromocriptine
14. Bone age are delayed in all except:
    a. Constitutional
    b. Familial
    c. Hypothyroidism
    d. GH deficiency
15. The midparental height will be same for:
    a. True brother and sister
    b. Two true sister
    c. Cousin brother
    d. All grand daughter
16. A prepubertal boy of 12 years with a bone age of 10 with weight 10th percentile. Most likely diagnosis is:
    a. CDGD
    b. GHD
    c. Primary IGF-1 deficiency
    d. Multiple pituitary hormone deficiency
17. Following is GH-dependent IGF-1:
    a. IGFBP-1
    b. IGFBP-2
    c. IGFBP-3
    d. IGFBP-5
18. Side effect of hGH replacement include all except:
    a. Hypotension
    b. Arthralgia
    c. Carpal tunnel syndrome
    d. Melanocytic nevi
19. An 8-year-old boy with short stature, delayed bone age, no cushingoid features, normal TSH, ↓ FSH, ↓ LH. Next investigation is:
    a. GH stimulation test
    b. FT4
    c. Testosterone level to diagnose hypogonadism
    d. ACTH stimulation test

20. **Action of GH through IGF-1:**
    a. Lipolysis
    b. Amino acid transport
    c. Protein synthesis
    d. Promotes both osteoclast/osteoblast activity

21. **GH causes all except:**
    a. Increased IGFBP3
    b. Increased IGFBP1
    c. Decreased IGFBP2
    d. Increased IGF1

22. **Which of the following is not true?**
    a. Length at birth is 50 cm
    b. Increases by 25 cm in 1st year
    c. Increase of 6 cm in 2nd year
    d. Increase of 6 cm per year from 3rd to 10th year

23. **Height prediction is done by all except:**
    a. Radiological Atlas by Greulich and Pyle
    b. Bayley-Pinneau scale
    c. Midparental height ± 6.5 cm
    d. Specific charts have been prepared for Turner's syndrome and achondroplasia

24. **All are side effects of GH therapy in children except:**
    a. Hypoglycemia
    b. Scoliosis
    c. Raised ICT
    d. Edema of feet

25. **Which of the following causes of short stature does not have delayed bone age?**
    a. GH deficiency
    b. Hypothyroidism
    c. Familial short stature
    d. Constitutional delay of growth and puberty

26. **Drugs used to assess GH sufficiency include all except:**
    a. TRH
    b. GHRH
    c. Alpha methyldopa
    d. Propranolol

27. **Features of GH insufficiency; all except:**
    a. Levels >10 µg/L suggest normal response
    b. Increased HDL
    c. Increased waist hip ratio
    d. Decreased muscle mass
    e. Decreased IGF-1 and IGFBP-3

28. **Growth hormone deficiency is noted in:**
    a. Turner's syndrome
    b. Constitutional short stature
    c. Laron's syndrome
    d. Sheehan's syndrome
    e. Chronic renal failure

29. Side effects of recombinant human growth hormone therapy include all except:
   a. Proliferative retinopathy
   b. Aplastic anemia
   c. Leukemia
   d. Creutzfeldt-Jakob disease
   e. Benign intracranial hypertension

30. A 33-year-old female presents with tiredness and lethargy. Five years previously she had undergone a frontal surgery for a craniopharyngioma following presentation with amenorrhea and headache. Postoperatively she developed seizures and was treated with sodium valproate. She was demonstrated to be hypopituitary and receives hydrocortisone, thyroxine, estrogen replacement therapy and desmopressin. Which of the following investigations would you select to confirm a growth hormone deficiency?
   a. IGF-1 concentration
   b. Insulin tolerance test
   c. Clonidine test
   d. L-dopa test
   e. GHRH/Arginine test

31. GH therapy in adults is associated with all except:
   a. AF
   b. VT
   c. Carpal tunnel
   d. Benign ICT

32. All are correct about GH deficiency except:
   a. Glucagon-induced GH stimulation causes hypoglycemia
   b. Bone age < chronological age
   c. Priming with gonadal steroids improves specificity of GH provocative tests
   d. Growth failure usually manifests after 4 years of age

33. All of the following statements are correct about secretion of growth hormone except:
   a. Increases during REM sleep
   b. Increases during exercise
   c. Increases during starvation
   d. Increases during NREM sleep

ANSWERS

1. **Ans. (a) Ht. age = bone age**
   [Williams 13th ed pg 1022]

   Criteria for Presumptive Diagnosis of Constitutional Delay of Growth and Development
   - No history of systemic illness
   - Normal nutrition
   - Normal physical examination, including body proportions
   - Normal thyroid and growth hormone levels
   - Normal complete blood count, sedimentation rate, electrolytes, blood urea nitrogen
   - Height ≤3rd percentile but with annual growth rate >5th percentile for age
   - Delayed puberty
   - Delayed bone age
   - Normal predicted adult height.

2. **Ans. (a) Standing/erect and (b) Clonidine 4 ug/day**
   [Williams 13th ed pg 1019; Barts endocrine e-protocols pituitary function pg 11]

   Clonidine Test for Growth Hormone (GH) Reserve
   - *Precautions:* Systolic BP falls by 20–25 mm Hg in all subjects. Patient should lie down for 2 hours after the test or until blood pressure is satisfactory. The test can be highly sedative.
   - *Preparation:* Fast from midnight.
   - *Procedure:*
     - IV cannula at 8.30 AM and take basal GH at 8.30 AM.
     - Clonidine 0.15 mg/m^2 orally at 9 AM
     - Measure blood pressure every 30 minutes
     - Take further samples at 30, 45, 60, 90, 120 and 150 minutes for GH at all timepoints.
   - *Interpretation:* The test is more accurate in children. If the GH rises above 10 ng/mL, the GH reserve is probably normal.

3. **Ans. (b) Increased by GH**
   [Williams 13th ed pg 983-5; 1017]

4. **Ans. (d) Familial**
   [Williams 13th ed pg 1023]

   Genetic (Familial) Short Stature
   - Their height is appropriate for their genetic potential based on the parents' heights; i.e. their height standard deviation score (SDS) is within the target height SDS range.
   - Growth is at or below the 3rd percentile, but the velocity is usually normal.

- The onset and progression of puberty are normal.
- The skeletal age is concordant with chronologic age.
- By definition, the GH/IGF-1 system is normal (as are all other systems).
- Final height is below the 3rd percentile; however final heights are in the target height range for the family.

Distinguishing GSS from CDGD

Feature	CDGD	GSS
Midparental height	Lower	Normal
Puberty	Delayed	Normal
Bone age	Delayed	Concordant with chronologic age
Final height	< 3rd percentile	Normal

5. **Ans. (b) Addison disease**
   [Williams 13th ed pg 1004, 1005]

   Endocrine Causes of Growth Retardation
   - Hypothyroidism
   - Diabetes mellitus
   - Cushing's syndrome
   - Addison disease
   - Pseudohypoparathyroidism: Albright hereditary osteodystrophy
   - Rickets, hypophosphatemic rickets.

6. **Ans. (b) GH**

7. **Ans. (a) GH**
   [Williams 13th ed pg 978]
   - GH is the primary regulator of IGF-1 transcription
   - Another influential factor is estrogen. The sex-steroid effects on IGF-1 transcription play a role in the pubertal rise of IGF-1 levels in humans.

8. **Ans. (d) Laron syndrome**
   [Endocrine Secrets 6th ed pg 235, 236; De Groot 7th ed pg 328; Williams 13th ed pg 997, 1042]
   - Initially, rhGH was indicated for GH-deficient children.
   - rhGH is now indicated for growth promotion during childhood and adolescence in several conditions associated with growth impairment in the absence of GH deficiency.
   - US Food and Drug Administration (FDA)–approved indications of GH for the treatment of short stature:
     1. Chronic renal insufficiency before transplant
     2. Turner's syndrome (45 XO or mosaic variants)
     3. AIDS wasting syndrome
     4. Prader-Willi syndrome
     5. Short stature due to intrauterine growth retardation in the absence of "catch-up" growth

6. Idiopathic short stature in boys with predicted adult height less than 63 inches and girls with predicted height less than 59 inches (normal GH secretion)
7. Noonan's syndrome

Indications 2 through 6 do not require demonstration of GH deficiency.
- In addition, accepted medical uses in adults include treatment of GH deficiency and the wasting syndrome encountered with human immunodeficiency virus/acquired immunodeficiency syndrome (HIV/AIDS).
- Laron syndrome is characterized by GH insensitivity. Treatment consists of rhIGF-1.

9. **Ans. (b) Hepatic protein synthesis**
    [De Groot 7th ed pg 328; Williams 13th ed pg 977]

    IGF-independent Action of GH
    - Epiphysis—stimulation of epiphyseal growth (Note: GH and IGF-1 have distinct and overlapping functions in terms of growth)
    - Bone—stimulation of osteoclast differentiation and activity, stimulation of osteoblast activity, and increase in bone mass through endochondral bone formation
    - Adipose tissue—acute insulin-like effects, followed by increased lipolysis, inhibition of lipoprotein lipase, stimulation of hormone-sensitive lipase, decreased glucose transport, and decreased lipogenesis
    - Muscle—increased amino acid transport, increased nitrogen retention, increased lean tissue, and increased energy expenditure.

    NB: The "diabetogenic" actions of GH are contradictory to the glucose-lowering effects of IGFs.

10. **Ans. (b) Multiple pituitary hormone deficiency**

11. **Ans. (b) Ghrelin**
    [De Groot 7th ed pg 182]

12. **Ans. (a) Basal GH**
    [Williams 13th ed pg 1018, 1019]

    Provocative Tests for GH
    - Random GH levels cannot be used to diagnose GHD because GH secretion is pulsatile.
    - Evaluation of GH secretion requires that samples be obtained after an stimulation of GH secretion.
    - Physiologic stimuli include fasting, sleep, and exercise.
    - Pharmacologic stimuli include levodopa, clonidine, glucagon, propranolol, arginine, insulin and GHRH.
    - Failure to increase serum GH above a defined cutoff level (10 µg/L) indicate GHD.
    - The same cutoff level is applied without regard to the stimulus used with the exception of GHRH where the cutoff used is higher than that for other tests.

13. **Ans. (a) Insulin**
    [Williams 13th ed pg 1018, 1019; Greenspan's 9th ed]
    See discussions of Chapter 5, Question 20 and Chapter 17, Question 12.

14. **Ans. (b) Familial**
    [Williams 13th ed pg 1023]
    See discussion of Chapter 17, Question 4.

15. **Ans. (b) Two true sister**
    [Williams 13th ed pg 967]
    A boy's midparental height equals the average of his parents' heights plus 6.5 cm, and a girl's midparental height equals the average of her parents' heights minus 6.5 cm.

16. **Ans. (a) CDGD**

17. **Ans. (c) IGFBP-3**
    [Williams 13th ed pg 986]

18. **Ans. (a) Hypotension**
    [Williams 13th ed pg 198]
    See discussion of Chapter 17, Question 31.

19. **Ans. (a) GH stimulation test**
    [Williams 13th ed pg 1012]

20. **Ans. (c) Protein synthesis**
    [De Groot 7th ed pg 328; Williams 13th ed pg 977]
    See discussion of Chapter 17, Question 9.

21. **Ans. (b) Increased IGFBP1**
    [De Groot 7th ed pg 367-369]
    GH:↑IGF-1, ↑IGFBP-3, ↑IGFBP-5, ↓IGFBP-2

22. **Ans. (c) Increase of 6 cm in 2nd year**
    [Williams 13th ed pg 968; Nelson Essentials of Pediatrics 6th ed]
    Williams Textbook of Endocrinology states:
    Growth velocity averages about 15 cm per year during the first 2 years of life; it then slows to approximately 6 cm per year during middle childhood.
    Nelson Essentials of Pediatrics states:
    - Average length: 20 in at birth, 30 in at 1 year
    - At age 3 year, the average child is 3 ft tall
    - At age 4 year, the average child is 40 in tall (double birth length)
    - Average annual height increase: 2–3 in between age 4 year and puberty

    Option (c) appears most appropriate.

23. **Ans. (a) Radiological Atlas by Greulich and Pyle**
    [Williams 13th ed pg 967, 1014]
    See discussion of Chapter 17, Question 15.

24. **Ans. (a) Hypoglycemia**
    [Williams 13th ed pg 1040, 1041]

    Adverse Effects of Growth Hormone
    - Pituitary-derived human GH proved to be an agent for transmission Creutzfeldt-Jakob disease (CJD). Although pit-GH was removed from use. Recombinant DNA–derived GH does not carry this risk.
    - *Side effects of recombinant GH:*
        - Development of malignancies
            * Increased risk for post-transplant lymphoproliferative disease
        - Development of subsequent neoplasms in children who have survived cancer
            * Probable increased incidence in secondary malignances, predominantly CNS tumors (glioblastoma/glioma, astrocytoma, meningioma) and osteogenic sarcoma
        - Pseudotumor cerebri (idiopathic intracranial hypertension)
        - Slipped capital femoral epiphysis
        - Scoliosis
        - Diabetes mellitus
        - *Miscellaneous side effects:*
            * Prepubertal gynecomastia
            * Pancreatitis
            * Growth of nevi
            * Behavioral changes
            * Worsening of neurofibromatosis
            * Hypertrophy of tonsils and adenoids
            * Sleep apnea.

25. **Ans. (c) Familial short stature**
    [Williams 13th ed pg 1023]

    See discussion of Chapter 17, Question 4.

26. **Ans. (a) TRH**
    [Williams 13th ed pg 1018, 1019]

    See discussion of Chapter 17, Question 12.

27. **Ans. (b) Increased HDL**
    [Williams 13th ed pg 1018, 1019]

    See discussions of Chapter 5, Question 1.

28. **Ans. (d) Sheehan's syndrome**
    [Williams 13th ed pg 193]

29. **Ans. (b) Aplastic anemia**
    [Williams 13th ed pg 198, 1040, 1041; Oxford Textbook of Endocrinology and Diabetes 2nd ed pg 162]

    See discussions of Chapter 17, Questions 24 and 31.
    Retinopathy is an extremely unusual complication.

30. **Ans. (a) IGF-1 concentration**
    [Williams 13th ed pg 194, 195]
    Patients with three or more pituitary hormone deficiencies and an IGF-1 level below the reference range have a greater than 97% chance of being GH deficient and, therefore, do not require GH stimulation testing.

31. **Ans. (b) VT**
    [Williams 13th ed pg 198]
    Side Effects of Adult Growth Hormone Treatment
    - Edema
    - Arthralgias
    - Myalgias
    - Muscle stiffness
    - Paresthesias
    - Carpal tunnel syndrome
    - Atrial fibrillation
    - Headache
    - Benign intracranial hypertension
    - Increase in melanocytic nevi
    - Hyperglycemia
    - Sleep apnea
    - Iatrogenic acromegaly.

    Patients with active malignancies should not be treated with GH. The possibility that hGH might initiate new cancers or stimulate growth of preexisting benign tumors is an important theoretical issue.

32. **Ans. (d) Growth failure usually manifests after 4 years of age**
    [Williams 13th ed pg 1109, 1595; De Groot 7th ed pg 430]

33. **Ans. (a) Increases during REM sleep**
    [Greenspan's 9th ed]

    Factors Affecting GH Secretion

Increase	Decrease
Physiologic Sleep Exercise Stress (physical or psychologic) Postprandial • Hyperaminoacidemia • Hypoglycemia (relative)	Postprandial hyperglycemia Elevated free fatty acids

Contd...

Contd...

Increase	Decrease
Pharmacologic Hypoglycemia • *Absolute:* Insulin or 2-deoxyglucose • *Relative:* Postglucagon Hormones • GHRH • Ghrelin • Peptide (ACTH, α-MSH, vasopressin) • Estrogen Neurotransmitters, etc. • Alpha-adrenergic agonists (clonidine) • Beta-adrenergic antagonists (propranolol) • Serotonin precursors • Dopamine agonists (levodopa, apomorphine, bromocriptine) • GABA agonists (muscimol) • Potassium infusion • Pyrogens (Pseudomonas endotoxin)	Hormones • Somatostatin • Growth hormone • Progesterone • Glucocorticoids Neurotransmitters, etc. • Alpha-adrenergic antagonists (phentolamine) • Beta-adrenergic agonists (isoproterenol) • Serotonin agonists (methysergide) • Dopamine antagonists (phenothiazines)
Pathologic Protein depletion and starvation Anorexia nervosa Ectopic production of GHRH Chronic renal failure Acromegaly TRH GnRH	Obesity Acromegaly- dopamine agonists Hypothyroidism Hyperthyroidism

Peak levels occur 1–4 hours after the onset of sleep (during stages 3 and 4).

CHAPTER 18

Puberty

QUESTIONS

1. Central precocious puberty (CPP) true:
   a. Common in boys > girls
   b. CNS lesion is more common in boys
   c. CNS lesion is more common in girls
   d. Idiopathic is more common in boys

2. True about exaggerated thelarche is:
   a. Advanced bone age
   b. Elevated levels of LH and FSH with prepubertal response to GnRH stimulation
   c. Disproportionate breast enlargement
   d. Persistent breast growth

3. 5 yr 8 m/M, premature birth, birth wt. 1.8 kg, low PRA, low ACTH, increased FSH/LH, high testosterone, high DHEA:
   a. CAH
   b. CPP
   c. Adrenal adenoma
   d. Testotoxicosis

4. All are true regarding fibrous dysplasia except:
   a. Most common endocrine abnormality is precocious puberty
   b. Deactivating mutation in Gs-alpha
   c. Mono-ostotic or polyostotic
   d. Expansion of fibroblast and osteoblast

5. Premature thelarche, all are true except:
   a. Increased estradiol as compared to other girls
   b. Bone age > Chronological age
   c. GnRH in pre-pubertal range
   d. FSH in pubertal range

6. Carney's syndrome all except:
   a. ACTH independent Cushing's
   b. B/l pigmented nodule
   c. Medical therapy
   d. <30 yrs of age

7. Pseudoprecocious puberty not seen in:
   a. Ovarian tumor
   b. Adrenal tumor
   c. Organic brain disease
   d. McCune-Albright syndrome

8. Drug not given in testotoxicosis:
   a. Spironolactone
   b. Ketoconazole
   c. GnRH analogues
   d. Testolactone

9. True isosexual precocious puberty is found in all except:
   a. CAH
   b. Constitutional
   c. Hypothyroidism
   d. Hypothalamic

10. All are seen in McCune-Albright syndrome (MAC) except:
    a. Cardiac and skin myxoma
    b. Polyostotic fibrous dysplasia
    c. Precocious puberty
    d. Increased pigmentation

11. True about puberty:
    a. After 12 years in males → delayed
    b. Before 11 years in males → precocious
    c. Delayed puberty more common in males than females
    d. Precocious puberty more common in males than females

12. All of the following are used in treatment of precocious puberty except:
    a. Testolactone
    b. Medroxyprogesterone
    c. GnRH antagonist
    d. Leuprolide

13. True precocious puberty is due to:
    a. Organic brain disease
    b. Cranial tumors
    c. Adrenal tumors
    d. Gonadal tumors

14. Hypergonadotropic hypogonadism seen in all except:
    a. Kallmann's syndrome
    b. Klinefelter's syndrome
    c. Gonadal dysgenesis
    d. Premature ovarian insufficiency

15. Hypothalamic hamartoma is not associated with:
    a. Acromegaly
    b. Cushing
    c. Hypogonadism
    d. Seizure

16. Premature thelarche is characterized by all except:
    a. Infancy to 2 years
    b. Uterus and ovaries prepubertal
    c. Growth velocity increased
    d. Tanner Stage III

17. McCune-Albright syndrome:
    a. Only mono-ostotic fibrous dysplasia
    b. GPCR mutation
    c. GnRH dependent precocious puberty
    d. Ambiguous genitalia
    e. More common in female than male

18. All are true about precocious puberty except:
    a. Pubic hair < 7 yr
    b. Discordance between thelarche and menarche
    c. In female CPP-idiopathic more common
    d. Accelerated bone maturation
    e. Juvenile hypothyroidism

19. Hypogonadotropic hypogonadism is associated with mutations in all except:
    a. PROP 1
    b. HESX
    c. GPR52
    d. FGF8
    e. DAX1

20. All of the following statements about hypothalamic hamartoma are true except:
    a. Attached to posterior hypothalamus
    b. Transcranial surgery is the treatment of choice
    c. Precocious puberty
    d. Tuber cinereum

21. Delayed puberty is defined as:
    a. Age > 8 in girls and > 9 in boys
    b. Age > 13 in girls and > 14 in boys
    c. Age > 12 in girls and > 13 in boys
    d. Age > 14 in girls and > 15 in boys

22. CDGP is a/w all except:
    a. Bone age accelerated relative to height
    b. May or may not reach normal adult height
    c. Normal velocity
    d. Delayed adrenarche

23. Which is not a cause of precocious puberty in females?
    a. Peutz-Jeghers syndrome
    b. Ovarian cyst
    c. hCG secreting tumors in liver
    d. Hypothalamic hamartoma

24. Kallmann syndrome; not true is:
    a. Eunuchoid proportions
    b. Agenesis of olfactory lobe and sulci
    c. Gynecomastia absent in all
    d. Cleft palate, cerebellar ataxia

25. Kallmann syndrome is characterized by all except:
    a. Eunuchoid proportions
    b. Short stature
    c. Cerebellar ataxia
    d. Color blindness

26. SHBG binding decreased in all except:
    a. Hyperthyroidism
    b. Androgen
    c. Obesity
    d. Acromegaly

ANSWERS

1. **Ans. (b) CNS lesion is more common in boys**
   [Williams 13th ed pg 1164]
   - Precocious puberty is more prevalent (10-times) in girls compared with boys.
   - True precocious puberty (i.e. GnRH-dependent CPP) is more common (5-times) in girls than boys
   - Idiopathic CPP is more common (8-times) in girls than in boys
   - In boys CNS abnormalities occur at least as often as idiopathic CPP.
   - In girls neurologic lesions are one fifth as common as idiopathic CPP.

2. **Ans. (a) Advanced bone age**
   [Williams 13th ed pg 1199; De Groot 7th ed pg 2131]
   Premature Thelarche
   - *Clinical features*:
     - Unilateral or bilateral breast enlargement without other signs of sexual maturation (e.g. sexual hair, growth of the labia minora, growth of the uterus) is termed *premature thelarche*.
     - Usually, significant nipple and areola development is absent; usually does not exceed a Tanner stage III level of development.
     - Estrogen-induced thickening and dulling of the vaginal mucosa is uncommon.
     - Growth in stature is normal.
     - The disorder usually occurs by age 2 (>80% of cases) and rarely after age 4.
     - This is a benign, self-limited disorder that is compatible with normal pubertal development at an appropriate age.
     - About 10% of girls with premature thelarche progress to CPP.
   - Premature thelarche appears to result from the ovarian response to transient increases in FSH levels and possibly from variations in ovarian sensitivity to FSH.
   - *Laboratory findings*:
     - Measurement of the ellipsoid volume of the uterus is the most sensitive and specific discriminator between premature thelarche and early CPP. Usually, uterus volume is <1.8 mL, length is <36 mm.
     - The LH response to GnRH is prepubertal in all cases.
     - Plasma estradiol levels are prepubertal but slightly higher for age.
     - Plasma inhibin B and FSH levels are higher in girls with precocious thelarche than in control subjects, in a range similar to that observed in patients with precocious puberty. Nocturnal FSH pulsatility has been detected, and the rise in FSH elicited by administration of GnRH may be augmented for chronologic age, with an FSH/LH ratio higher in precocious thelarche than in normal individuals or in girls with CPP.

- Sonograms of the ovary often show one or several cysts larger than 0.5 cm that disappear and reappear, usually correlating with changes in the size of the breasts, but the volume of the ovary is prepubertal.

Exaggerated Thelarche
- Exaggerated thelarche is premature thelarche with the added findings of advanced bone age and increased growth rate, which are estrogen effects.
- The endocrine measurements in the basal state are in the normal prepubertal range, but after GnRH agonist stimulation, the level of FSH (but not of LH) rose higher than in control subjects or in patients with CPP.

3. **Ans. (c) Adrenal adenoma**
   [Williams 13th ed pg 1196, 1197]
   Presence of high DHEA is indicative of presence of adrenal tumor.

4. **Ans. (b) Deactivating mutation in Gs-alpha**
   [Williams 13th ed pg 1185, 1186, 1190]

   McCune-Albright Syndrome
   - It is characterized by the triad of
     - Café au lait spots
     - Polyostotic fibrous dysplasia
     - GISP

   At least two of the features must be present to consider the diagnosis.
   - *Clinical features:*
     - Café au lait spots: Irregularly edged (coast of Maine type); usually do not cross the midline; often located on the same side as the main bone lesions; have a segmented distribution.
     - Polyostotic fibrous dysplasia: The skeletal lesions often result in pathologic fractures and progressive deformities; If skull is involved, there may be entrapment and compression of optic or auditory nerve foramina, which can lead to blindness, deafness, facial asymmetry, and ptosis.
     - Autonomous endocrine hyperfunction:
       - Ovary (most common)
       - Thyroid gland (nodular hyperplasia with thyrotoxicosis or euthyroid status)
       - Adrenal gland (multiple hyperplastic nodules with Cushing's syndrome that may be followed by adrenal insufficiency)
       - Pituitary gland (adenoma or mammosomatotroph hyperplasia with gigantism, acromegaly, and hyperprolactinemia)
       - Parathyroid glands (adenoma or hyperplasia with hyperparathyroidism).
     - Hypophosphatemic vitamin D-resistant rickets or osteomalacia: occurs either because of overproduction of a phosphaturic factor, phosphatonin, by the bone lesions or because of an intrinsic renal

abnormality leading to decreased proximal tubule reabsorption of phosphate.
- Hepatocellular dysfunction, jaundice.
- Pancreatitis.
- Cardiac disease: patients carry the risk of cardiac arrhythmia and sudden death.
- Myxomas have been reported in extremities.
- *Sexual precocity:*
  - Girls
    - Sexual precocity often begins during the first 2 years of life and is frequently heralded by menstrual bleeding
    - The cause is autonomously functioning luteinized follicular cysts of the ovary
    - Serum estradiol is elevated
    - LH response to GnRH is prepubertal, and the pubertal pattern of nighttime LH pulses is absent during the initial years
    - An affected girl may progress from GnRH-independent puberty to GnRH-dependent puberty.
  - Boys
    - Sexual precocity is rare in boys; however, testicular disease occurs frequently.
    - Asymmetric enlargement of the testes.
    - The seminiferous tubules are enlarged and exhibit spermatogenesis, and Leydig cells may be hyperplastic.
- McCune-Albright syndrome occurs about twice as often in girls than in boys.
- It is sporadic.
- Caused by somatic activating mutations in the gene (GNAS1) encoding the α-subunit of the trimeric GTP-binding protein (Gsα).
- This leads to a constitutive activation of cellular function in a mosaic distribution, leading to a high variability of organ involvement and degree of severity.

5. **Ans. (b) Bone age > Chronological age**
   [Williams 13th ed pg 1199]
   See discussion of Chapter 18, Question 2.

6. **Ans. (c) Medical therapy**
   [Williams 13th ed pg 257, 512]

   Carney Complex
   - Autosomal dominant disorder
   - Results from inactivating mutations of type 1α regulatory subunit (R1α) of the cAMP-dependent protein kinase A (PRKAR1A) leading to abnormal PKA signaling.

- Clinical Features

Feature	Prevalence (%)

• Skin lesions
  – Pigmented lesions (spotty skin pigmentation)
  – Blue nevi
  – Cutaneous myxomas
	80

• Cardiac myxomas	72
• Pigmented nodular adrenal hyperplasia	45
• Breast lesions – Bilateral fibroadenomas	45 (females only)
• Testicular tumors	56 (males only)
• Pituitary lesions, usually growth hormone secreting	10
• Neural lesions (gastric schwannomas)	<5

• Miscellaneous
  – Thyroid cancers
  – Acoustic neuromas
  – Hepatomas
	
	Rare
	Rare
	Rare

Primary Pigmented Nodular Adrenal Hyperplasia and Carney Syndrome
- ACTH-independent Cushing's syndrome.
- Bilateral, small (2–4 mm), pigmented adrenal nodules.
- Adjacent adrenal tissue is atrophic.
- Presentation is with typical features of Cushing's syndrome in persons younger than 30 years of age.
- Bilateral adrenalectomy is curative.

7. **Ans. (c) Organic brain disease**
   [Williams 13th ed 1163-72]

   Classification of Sexual Precocity
   - True precocious puberty or complete isosexual precocity or central precocious puberty (GnRH-dependent sexual precocity or premature activation of the hypothalamic GnRH pulse generator)
     – Idiopathic true precocious puberty
     – CNS tumors
       ♦ Optic glioma associated with neurofibromatosis type 1
       ♦ Hypothalamic astrocytoma
     – Other CNS disorders
       ♦ Developmental abnormalities including hypothalamic hamartoma of the tuber cinereum
       ♦ Encephalitis
       ♦ Static encephalopathy
       ♦ Brain abscess
       ♦ Sarcoid or tubercular granuloma
       ♦ Head trauma
       ♦ Hydrocephalus
       ♦ Arachnoid cyst
       ♦ Myelomeningocele

- Vascular lesion
- Cranial irradiation
- Pineal cyst
- Cerebral atrophy/focal encephalomalacia
- Epilepsy
- Laughing seizures
- Developmental delay
- Septo-optic dysplasia
- Marfan syndrome
  - True precocious puberty after late treatment of congenital virilizing adrenal hyperplasia or other previous chronic exposure to sex steroids
  - True precocious puberty due to gain of function mutations:
    - In *KISS1R/GRP54* gene
    - In *KISS1* gene
  - True precocious puberty due to loss of function mutations:
    - In *MKRN3* gene
- Incomplete isosexual precocity or pseudoprecocious puberty or peripheral precocity or GnRH independent sexual precocity (Hypothalamic GnRH-Independent)
  - Males
    - Gonadotropin-secreting tumors
      - hCG-secreting CNS tumors (e.g. chorioepithelioma, germinoma, teratoma)
      - hCG-secreting tumors located outside the CNS (hepatoma, teratoma, choriocarcinoma)
    - Increased androgen secretion by adrenal or testis
      - Congenital adrenal hyperplasia (CYP21 and CYP11B1 deficiencies)
      - Virilizing adrenal neoplasm
      - Leydig cell adenoma
      - Familial testotoxicosis (sex-limited autosomal dominant pituitary gonadotropin-independent precocious Leydig cell and germ cell maturation)
      - Cortisol resistance syndrome
      - NR0B1 (DAX) mutations
  - Females
    - Ovarian cyst
    - Estrogen-secreting ovarian or adrenal neoplasm
    - Peutz-Jeghers syndrome
  - Both sexes
    - McCune-Albright syndrome
    - Hypothyroidism
    - Iatrogenic or exogenous sexual precocity (including inadvertent exposure to estrogens in food, drugs, or cosmetics)

- Variations of pubertal development
  - Premature thelarche
  - Premature isolated menarche
  - Premature adrenarche
  - Adolescent gynecomastia in boys
  - Macroorchidism
- Contrasexual precocity
  - Feminization in males
    - Adrenal neoplasm
    - Chorioepithelioma
    - CYP11B1 deficiency
    - Late-onset adrenal hyperplasia
    - Testicular neoplasm (Peutz-Jeghers syndrome)
    - Increased extraglandular conversion of circulating adrenal androgens to estrogen
    - Iatrogenic (exposure to estrogens)
  - Virilization in females
    - Congenital adrenal hyperplasia
      - CYP21 deficiency
      - CYP11B1 deficiency
      - 3β-HSD deficiency
    - Virilizing adrenal neoplasm (Cushing's syndrome)
    - Virilizing ovarian neoplasm (e.g. arrhenoblastoma)
    - Iatrogenic (exposure to androgens)
    - Cortisol resistance syndrome
    - Aromatase deficiency.

8. **Ans. (c) GnRH analogues**
   [Williams 13th ed 1181, 1182]

   Drugs used in treatment of testotoxicosis:
   - Inhibition of CYP17 (mainly 17,20-lyase activity) [suppresses gonadal and adrenal biosynthesis]: Ketoconazole
   - Antiandrogen: Spironolactone (also antimineralocorticoid), flutamide, bicalutamide, nilutamide
   - Inhibition of aromatase (blocks estrogen synthesis): testolactone, letrozole, anastrozole
   - Medroxyprogesterone acetate: Inhibition of testicular steroidogenesis.

9. **Ans. (c) Hypothyroidism**
   [Williams 13th ed 1163-72]
   See discussion of Chapter 18, Question 7.

10. **Ans. (d) Increased pigmentation**
    [Williams 13th ed pg 1185, 1186, 1190]
    See discussion of Chapter 18, Question 4.

11. **Ans. (c) Delayed puberty more common in males than females**
    [Williams 13th ed pg 1127, 1129, 1162]
    - Sexual precocity is the appearance of any sign of secondary sexual maturation before the lower limit of the normal age at onset of puberty (9 years for boys, 8 years for girls)
    - Delayed puberty is the lack of appearance of any signs of secondary sexual maturation beyond the upper limit of the normal age at onset of puberty (14 years for boys, 13 years for girls)
    - CDP is more common in boys and may be a counterpart of idiopathic CPP, a condition that is many times more common in girls.

12. **(c) GnRH antagonist**
    [Williams 13th ed pg 1174, 1182, 1184]

    Pharmacologic Therapy for Sexual Precocity

Disorder	Treatment	Action and rationale
GnRH dependent		
True or central precocious puberty	GnRH agonists (e.g. Leuprolide)	Desensitization of gonadotrophs; blocks action of endogenous GnRH
GnRH independent Incomplete sexual precocity		
Girls		
Autonomous ovarian cysts/McCune-Albright syndrome	Medroxyprogesterone acetate*	Inhibition of ovarian steroidogenesis; regression of cyst (inhibition of FSH release)
	Third-generation aromatase inhibitor (e.g. letrozole)	Inhibition of aromatase; blocks estrogen synthesis
Boys		
Familial testotoxicosis	Ketoconazole*	Inhibition of CYP17 (mainly 17,20-lyase activity)
	Antiandrogen (spironolactone, flutamide or bicalutamide) and aromatase inhibitor (testolactone, letrozole or anastrozole)	Antiandrogen Inhibition of aromatase; blocks estrogen synthesis
	Medroxyprogesterone acetate*	Inhibition of testicular steroidogenesis

    *If true precocious puberty develops, an LHRH agonist can be added.

13. **Ans. (b) Cranial tumors**
    [Williams 13th ed pg 1163-1172]
    See discussion of Chapter 18, Question 7.

14. **Ans. (a) Kallmann's syndrome**
 [Williams 13th ed pg 735, 739]
 See discussion of Chapter 12, Question 6.

15. **Ans. (c) Hypogonadism**
 [Williams 13th ed pg 271, 1168, 1170; J Neurosurg. 2004 Feb;100(2 Suppl Pediatrics):212]
 - Hypothalamic hamartomas can be associated with laughing (gelastic), petit mal, or generalized tonic-clonic seizures; mental retardation; behavioral disturbances; and dysmorphic syndromes
 - They are frequently associated with central precocious puberty
 - Hamartomas, may produce GHRH with subsequent somatotroph hyperplasia, or even a pituitary GH-cell adenoma and resultant acromegaly
 - There has been one case report of hypothalamic hamartoma secreting corticotropin-releasing hormone (CRH). The patient presented with a history of behavioral disturbances. There were no Cushing's disease-related characteristics. However, endocrinological workup revealed elevated serum CRH and adrenocorticotropic hormone levels, non-suppression with low-dose dexamethasone, and partial suppression with high-dose dexamethasone.
 - Although association of hypothalamic hamartoma and hypopituitarism have been seen in Pallister-Hall syndrome.

16. **Ans. (c) Growth velocity increased**
 [Williams 13th ed pg 1199; De Groot 7th ed pg 2131]
 See discussion of Chapter 18, Question 2.

17. **Ans. (e) More common in female than male**
 [Williams 13th ed pg 1185, 1186, 1190]
 See discussion of Chapter 18, Question 4.

18. **Ans. (b) Discordance between thelarche and menarche**
 [Williams 13th ed pg 1162-72]
 See discussions of Chapter 18, Questions 1, 7 and 11.

19. **Ans. (c) GPR52**
 [Williams 13th ed pg 702, 1138]
 Mutations in following genes are associated with hypogonadotropic hypogonadism
 - Kallmann syndrome or Normosmic IHH (with the same mutant gene)
   – KAL1
   – FGFR1 (formerly KAL2)
   – FGF8 (ligand for FGFR1)
   – NELF
   – PROK2
   – PROKR2
   – CHD7

- Normosmic isolated hypogonadotropic hypogonadism
  - *GNRH1*
  - *GNRHR*
  - *KISS1R* (formerly GPR54)
  - *KISS1*
  - *SNRPN*
  - *LEP*
  - *LEPR*
  - *NR0B1* (DAX1)
  - *TAC3*
  - *TACR3*
- Multiple pituitary hormone deficiencies
  - *PROP1* (POU1F1)
  - *HESX1* (RPX)
  - *LHX3*
  - *PHF6*.

20. **Ans. (b) Transcranial surgery is the treatment of choice**
    [Williams 13th ed pg 1168-1170]

21. **Ans. (b) Age > 13 in girls and > 14 in boys**
    [Williams 13th ed pg 1127, 1162]

    See discussion of Chapter 18, Question 11.

22. **Ans. (a) Bone age accelerated relative to height**
    [Williams 13th ed pg 1022]

    See discussion of Chapter 17, Question 1.

23. **Ans. (c) hCG secreting tumors in liver**
    [Williams 13th ed 1163-72]

    See discussion of Chapter 18, Question 7.

24. **Ans. (c) Gynecomastia absent in all**
    [Williams 13th ed pg 1134-1138]

    Features of Kallmann Syndrome
    - Anosmia or hyposmia resulting from agenesis or hypoplasia of the olfactory lobes or sulci is associated with GnRH deficiency in Kallmann syndrome
    - Most common form of IHH
    - Anatomy
      - Developmental field defect
      - Aplasia or hypoplasia of olfactory bulb and sulcus
      - Arrested migration of GnRH neurosecretory neurons from olfactory placode to medial basal hypothalamus
    - *Clinical features:*
      - Anosmia or hyposmia
      - GnRH deficiency: absent or arrested puberty

- Magnitude of the GnRH deficiency correlates with the size of the testes
- *In infancy:* Microphallus and cryptorchidism are common
- Normal stature and growth in childhood
- Normal adrenarche
- Eunuchoid proportions
- Associated defects (inconstantly present) include: cleft lip, cleft palate, imperfect facial fusion, midline cranial anomalies, seizure disorders, short metacarpals, pes cavus, neurosensory hearing loss (rarely found in the X-linked form), cerebellar ataxia and nystagmus, optic atrophy, color blindness, ocular motor abnormalities, unilateral or rarely bilateral renal aplasia or dysplasia, and mirror movements of the upper extremities (i.e. bimanual synkinesia) limited to the X-linked form.

- *MRI:* Aplasia or hypoplasia of olfactory bulbs and/or sulci
- Inheritance
  - Sporadic and familial cases; genetic heterogeneity
  - Can be
    - X linked (X-linked recessive or X chromosome deletion: Xp22.3)
    - Autosomal (Dominant: sex limitation or Recessive)
  - Genes implicated: *KAL1, FGFR1* (previously called *KAL2*), *FGF8,* PROKR2 (formerly called *KAL3*), *PROK2* (formerly called *KAL4*), *NELF, SEMA3A, SOX10, HS6ST1, HESX1, FEZF1, CHD7,* others postulated (genes for adhesion molecules e.g. NCAM, and related proteins e.g. tenascin, laminin, phosphacan)

Secondary hypogonadism, if severe enough, results in low serum testosterone and an unopposed estrogen effect from the normal conversion of adrenal precursors to estrogens. Thus, patients with Kallmann's syndrome also develop gynecomastia.

25. **Ans. (b) Short stature**
    [Williams 13th ed pg 210, 1134-1138]
    See discussion of Chapter 18, Question 24.

26. **Ans. (a) Hyperthyroidism**
    [Williams 13th ed pg 731]

    Conditions Associated with Alterations in SHBG Concentrations

Decreased SHBG concentrations	Increased SHBG concentrations
Moderate obesity, type 2 diabetes mellitus	Aging
Nephrotic syndrome	Hepatic cirrhosis and hepatitis
Glucocorticoids, progestins, and androgens	Estrogens
Hypothyroidism	Hyperthyroidism
Acromegaly	Anticonvulsants
Familial SHBG deficiency	HIV disease

CHAPTER 19

Mineral Metabolism

QUESTIONS

1. Serum phosphate is best measured in:
   a. Fasting
   b. After carbohydrate diet
   c. Without relation to food
   d. Any time of day

2. Myopathy is seen in all except:
   a. TIO
   b. XLHR
   c. Hypoparathyroidism
   d. Cushing's syndrome

3. Sarcoidosis is associated with all except:
   a. Hypocalcemia
   b. Macrophage
   c. Decreased PTH
   d. Increased 1,25(OH)D_3

4. Acute treatment of hypercalcemia- all except:
   a. Thiazide
   b. Glucocorticoid
   c. Phosphate
   d. Hydration

5. A 60-year-old lady with osteoporosis with history of wrist fracture with GERD with suspected breast lump, best treatment would be:
   a. Raloxifene
   b. Estrogen
   c. Biphosphonate
   d. Calcium

6. Asymptomatic hyperparathyroidism follow up—all except:
   a. Annual serum calcium
   b. Annual 24-hour urine calcium
   c. Annual BMD
   d. Annual creatinine

7. Vitamin D status is assessed by:
   a. 25(OH)D
   b. 1,25(OH)D
   c. 24,25(OH)$_2$D
   d. All of the above

8. Mechanisms by which glucocorticoids contribute to osteoporosis include all except:
   a. Decrease intestinal calcium absorption
   b. Decrease urinary excretion of calcium
   c. Decrease gonadal estrogen
   d. Decrease osteoblast differentiation

9. Nonhealing fractures with callus formation seen in:
   a. Cushing's syndrome
   b. Hypoparathyroidism
   c. Osteogenesis imperfect
   d. Marfan syndrome

10. Biochemical markers used mostly for:
    a. Monitoring response to treatment
    b. Defining secondary causes of osteoporosis
    c. Assessing potency of drugs
    d. Predicting fracture risk

11. Rickets in new born (infant) is characterized by all except:
    a. Craniotabes
    b. Wide open fontanelle
    c. Bow legs
    d. Rachitic rosary

12. Parathyroid carcinoma:
    a. More common in females than in males
    b. Severe hypercalcemia
    c. Presents as a lump in the neck
    d. Hypercalcemia is seen in 60%

13. Calcium response to PTH secretion curve is:
    a. Sigmoid
    b. Linear
    c. Parabola
    d. Bell-shaped

14. A 65-year-old male Ca. Prostate on GnRH analogue, smoker, hypothyroid. Least likely cause of osteoporosis in this case is:
    a. Age
    b. Smoking
    c. Hypothyroidism
    d. GnRH analogue

15. All are true about denosumab except:
    a. Antibody to RANK ligand
    b. Hypercalciuria
    c. Antiresorptive effect
    d. FDA approved for osteoporosis

16. A 17-year-old male with primary hyperparathyroidism associated with acute hypercalcemia (symptoms); serum calcium is 16 mg%. Treatment are all except:
    a. IV zolindronate
    b. IV dexamethasone
    c. SC calcitonin
    d. IVFs with diuretics

17. Osteopetrosis due to carbonic anhydride II deficiency is characterized by all except:
    a. Recurrent fractures
    b. Metabolic Acidosis
    c. Tall stature
    d. Cerebral calcification

18. **Paget's disease all except:**
    a. Increased ALP
    b. Most commonly involves long bones, hand, feet
    c. Osteoclastic activity is predominant
    d. Height loss

19. **All are true regarding osteopetrosis except:**
    a. Metabolic acidosis
    b. Tall stature
    c. Basal ganglia calcification
    d. Increased risk of fracture

20. **Paget's disease is characterized by all except:**
    a. Multinucleate giant cell osteoclasts
    b. Most common in hand and leg bones
    c. Increased ALP is common
    d. Hearing loss

21. **Hypocalcemia in all except:**
    a. Acidosis
    b. Hypomagnesemia
    c. Hypoparathyroidism
    d. Tumor lysis syndrome

22. **A 3-month-old baby with hypocalcemia with basal ganglia calcification with low PTH, next line of investigation is:**
    a. Echo   b. EEG
    c. ALP   d. PO4

23. **Risk of osteoporosis all except:**
    a. Current smoker   b. Early menopause
    c. Early menarche   d. Alcohol

24. **Osteopetrosis due to carbonic anhydrase II deficiency, all are true except:**
    a. Tall stature   b. Metabolic acidosis
    c. Basal ganglia calcification d. Increased risk of fractures

25. **In thyrotoxicosis all are true except:**
    a. Increased Ca levels   b. Increased phosphate levels
    c. Decreased PTH   d. Increased PTH

26. **Hypoparathyroidism true all except:**
    a. PTH replacement is the standard treatment
    b. Most common after surgery
    c. Basal ganglia calcification
    d. Papilledema

27. **True about cinacalcet is:**
    a. Given intravenously   b. Stimulates CaSR
    c. Inhibits CaSR   d. Currently used for osteoporosis

28. True about rickets all except:
    a. VDD type-1 less severe than VDD type-2
    b. Physiologic dose of calcitriol is useful in treatment of VDD type-1
    c. VDD type-1 is associated with alopecia
    d. Apoptosis of chondrocytes in the epiphyseal growth plates
29. Osteogenesis imperfecta true all except:
    a. Blue sclera in type I and II
    b. Dentinogenesis imperfecta may be seen
    c. Progressive hearing loss
    d. Defect in type 2 collagen
30. Richest source of vitamin D:
    a. Fish
    b. Milk
    c. Egg
    d. Greens
31. All of the steroids can be used in osteoporosis except:
    a. Nadrolone
    b. Oxandrolone
    c. Tibolone
    d. Stanozolol
32. Vitamin D has:
    a. Pro-proliferative action
    b. Antiproliferative action
    c. Both (a) and (b)
    d. None of the above
33. A 76-year-old female with T score of –2.0 with 6 month old femoral fracture.... Without h/o estrogen use, next step should be:
    a. Serum electrophoresis
    b. Vitamin D level
    c. Parathyroid scan
    d. FBS
34. Hypercalcemia is seen in all except:
    a. Lithium
    b. Thyrotoxicosis
    c. Cushing's
    d. Addison's disease
35. Osteoblast are derived from:
    a. Mesenchymal stem cell
    b. Hematopoietic stem cell
    c. Neural crest cells
    d. None of the above
36. Following are markers of osteoblastic activity except:
    a. ALP
    b. Osteocalcin
    c. Procollagen
    d. Hydroxyproline
37. Achondroplasia is due to mutation of:
    a. FGFR3
    b. FGF23
    c. IGF1
    d. FGF
38. Hypocalcemia/hyperphosphatemia/increased iPTH is most consistent with:
    a. CRF
    b. Hyperparathyroidism
    c. PHP
    d. PPHP

39. Vitamin D receptor (VDR), chromosome number:
    a. 6　　　　　　　　　　　　b. 8
    c. 12　　　　　　　　　　　　d. 20

40. Which of the following is not true about PPHP:
    a. AHO phenotype
    b. Ca^{++} decreased
    c. PTH is normal
    d. cAMP response to PTH is normal

41. Transcriptional peptide involve in the synthesis of:
    a. PTH　　　　　　　　　　　b. T4
    c. Vit-D　　　　　　　　　　d. Glucocorticoids

42. Hypo Mg^{2+} causes:
    a. Low iPTH　　　　　　　　b. High iPTH
    c. Hyper K^+　　　　　　　d. Hyper Na^+

43. $1,25(OH)_2D$ has antiproliferative action on:
    a. Prostate　　　　　　　　b. Keratinocyte
    c. Renal tubular cell　　　d. Intestine epithelium

44. Pathological fracture:
    a. Fibrous dysplasia　　　b. Fibrogenesis imperfecta ossium
    c. Paget's disease　　　　d. Acromegaly
    e. All of the above

45. Osteomalacia is characterized by:
    a. Normal osteoid volume and normal mineral/matrix ratio
    b. Increased osteoid volume and normal mineral/matrix ratio
    c. Normal osteoid volume and decreased mineral/matrix ratio
    d. Increased osteoid volume and decreased mineral/matrix ratio

46. U calcium excretion is:
    a. 1-4 mg/kg　　　　　　　b. 10-20 mg/kg
    c. 20-40 mg/kg

47. Osteomalacia may be expected in:
    a. Sarcoidosis　　　　　　b. Autoimmune adrenalitis
    c. Pseudohypoparathyroidism　　d. Pernicious anemia
    e. Mercury poisoning

48. In the treatment of osteoporosis, which of the following best describe the drug Raloxifene?
    a. Bisphosphonate
    b. Calcium receptor modulator
    c. Estrogen
    d. PTH receptor agonist
    e. Selective estrogen receptor modulator

Mineral Metabolism | 231

ANSWERS

1. **Ans. (a) Fasting**
   [Manual of Endocrinology and Metabolism- Lavin 4th ed pg 362]

2. **Ans. (c) Hypoparathyroidism**
   [Williams 13th ed pg 1305, 1306]

3. **Ans. (a) Hypocalcemia**
   [Williams 13th ed pg 1288]
   - Sarcoidosis may be associated with hypercalcemia and hypercalciuria.
   - Hypercalcemia is caused by
     - ↑ $1,25(OH)_2D_3$
     - Overproduction of bone-resorbing cytokines and PTHrP (may contribute in some patients)
   - PTH levels are suppressed.
   - Unregulated synthesis of $1,25(OH)_2D_3$ by activated macrophages occurs in sarcoid granulomas.
   - The hypercalcemia and high levels of $1,25(OH)_2D_3$ fall upon treatment with glucocorticoids.
   - Removal of a large amount of granulomatous tissue can reverse hypercalcemia.

4. **Ans. (a) Thiazide**
   [Williams 13th ed pg 1289, 1293, 1294]
   Management of Severe Hypercalcemia
   - Volume repletion (by infusing isotonic saline)
   - Bisphosphonates (intravenous)
     - e.g. Pamidronate, zoledronate, ibandronate, clodronate
     - Agents of first choice in managing severe hypercalcemia that is driven mainly by osteoclastic bone resorption
     - Serum calcium usually declines within 24 hours and reaches a nadir within a week following a single infusion
     - Contraindicated in patients with GFR ≤30 mL/minute
   - Denosumab
     - Monoclonal antibody directed against RANKL
     - Effective in managing malignancy-associated hypercalcemia
     - Effective in patients refractory to bisphosphonates
     - Alternative to intravenous bisphosphonates in patients with renal failure
   - Calcitonin
     - Directly inhibits osteoclast function
     - May be used with other antiresorptive agents
     - *Advantage:* Rapid onset of action (hours), potential to augment renal calcium excretion directly

- *Disadvantage:* Its efficacy typically is limited to a few days at most, possibly because of receptor downregulation in target cells of bone and kidney.
- Other treatments
  - Phosphate repletion (oral/enteral)
    - Appropriate for patients with significant hypophosphatemia (<2.5 mg/dL)
- Glucocorticoids (Intravenous/oral)
  - In patients with vitamin D-dependent hypercalcemia, e.g. lymphoma or granulomatous disease.
  - Response may be more delayed
- Dialytic therapy (against a low- or zero-calcium dialysate)
  - In patients with severe renal insufficiency
- Parathyroidectomy (following initial medical stabilization)
  - In patients with known primary hyperparathyroidism
- Novel approaches
  - Infliximab
    - Successful treatment of hypercalcemia in Crohn disease has been reported
  - Cinacalcet
    - Calcimimetic
    - For parathyroid carcinoma
  - Monoclonal antibodies directed against PTHrP
    - In PTHrP-dependent hypercalcemia
- Loop diuretics
  - e.g. Furosemide
  - Best avoided, except in circumstances in which vigorous rehydration fails to improve severe hypercalcemia or might precipitate congestive heart failure
- Other antiresorptives that have largely been abandoned
  - Gallium nitrate
  - Plicamycin (mithramycin)
  - Intravenous phosphate

Treatment most often entails rehydration and administration of a bisphosphonate intravenously. Calcitonin can be useful as a temporary measure early in therapy, and glucocorticoids or dialysis may be indicated in some patients.

Thiazide diuretics can exacerbate hypercalcemia and should be discontinued.

5. **Ans. (a) Raloxifene**
   [Williams 13th ed pg 1355-1358]

6. **Ans. (b) Annual 24-hour urine calcium**
   [De Groot 7th ed pg 1121]

Recommendations for follow up of patients with asymptomatic primary hyperparathyroidism who do not undergo parathyroid surgery
- *Serum calcium:* Annually
- *Serum creatinine:* Annually
- *Bone density:* Annually or biannually

Monitoring of the following are not recommended
- 24-h urinary calcium
- Creatinine clearance
- Abdominal X-ray

7. **Ans. (a) 25(OH)D**
   [Williams 13th ed pg 1277]

8. **Ans. (b) Decrease urinary excretion of calcium**
   [Williams 13th ed pg 1340, 1351]

   Mechanisms by which glucocorticoids contribute to osteoporosis:
   - Suppress bone remodeling through depletion of the osteoblastic cell population
     - Inhibit replication of osteoblast precursors and their differentiation into mature osteoblasts
     - Inhibit differentiated function of osteoblast and bone formation
     - Induce apoptosis of osteoblasts and osteocytes
   - Induce osteoclastogenesis and bone resorption
   - Decrease intestinal absorption of calcium due to impaired $1,25(OH)_2D$ production
   - Induce hypercalciuria
   - Induce hyperparathyroidism
   - Induce secondary hypogonadism
   - Induce muscle atrophy.

9. **Ans. (a) Cushing's syndrome**
   [Williams 13th ed pg 508]

10. **Ans. (a) Monitoring response to treatment**
    [De Groot 7th ed pg 1205; Williams 13th ed pg 1344, 1345; OARL Osteoporosis pg 85]

    Clinical use of Bone Markers
    - Assessment of bone loss
    - Assessment of fracture risk
    - Monitoring treatment of osteoporosis
    - Defining secondary causes of osteoporosis
    - Development of new medications (assessment of potency of drugs, their effects over time and determining optimal doses)

    Monitoring response to therapy is the best validated clinical application of bone turnover markers.

11. **Ans. (c) Bow legs**
    [Williams 13th ed pg 1233]

12. **Ans. (b) Severe hypercalcemia**
    [Groot 7th ed pg 1123; The Journal of Clinical Endocrinology & Metabolism, Volume 86, Issue 2, Feb 2001 pg 488]

    Clinical presentation of parathyroid cancer: Manifestations of hypercalcemia are the primary effects of parathyroid cancer. Hypercalcemia is present in most patients and may be severe. The disease tends not to have a bulk tumor effect, spreading slowly in the neck. Metastatic disease is a late finding—most commonly to with lung (40%), liver (10%), and lymph node (30%).

    Difference in clinical profile of parathyroid cancer and benign PHPT

	Parathyroid carcinoma	Primary hyperparathyroidism
Female:male ratio	1:1	3.5:1
Average age (yr)	48	55
Asymptomatic (%)	<5	>80
Serum calcium (mg/dL)	>14	≤1, above upper limit of normal
PTH	Markedly elevated	Mildly elevated
Palpable neck mass	Common (30–76%)	Rare
Renal involvement (%)[1]	32–80	4–18
Skeletal involvement (%)[2]	34–91	<5
Concomitant renal and skeletal disease	Common	Rare

    [1]Includes nephrolithiasis, nephrocalcinosis, and impaired renal function.
    [2]Includes osteitis fibrosa, subperiosteal resorption, "salt and pepper" skull, and diffuse osteopenia on plain radiographs.

13. **Ans. (a) Sigmoid**
    [Williams 13th ed pg 1257]

14. **Ans. (c) Hypothyroidism**
    [Williams 13th ed pg 1350; Harrison's Endocrinology 3rd ed pg 444]
    See discussion of Chapter 19, Question 23.

15. **Ans. (b) Hypercalciuria**
    [Williams 13th ed pg 1357]

16. **Ans. (b) IV dexamethasone**
    [Williams 13th ed pg 1289, 1293, 1294]
    See discussion of Chapter 19, Question 4.

17. **Ans. (c) Tall stature**
    [De Groot 7th ed pg 1173-75]

Osteopetrosis (OPT, or "Marble Bone Disease")
- Result from failure of osteoclasts to resorb skeletal tissue.
- *Forms:*
  - Autosomal recessive, infantile (malignant) type
  - Autosomal dominant, adult (benign) type
  - Autosomal recessive, childhood ("intermediate") OPT
- *Clinical features:*
  - Infantile OPT manifests in babies. Nasal stuffiness may occur due to underdeveloped sinuses. Cranial foramina do not widen, often compressing auditory, oculomotor, facial, and optic nerves. Blindness can occur. Some patients develop hydrocephalus or sleep apnea. Eruption of the dentition is delayed. There is failure to thrive. Recurrent infections, spontaneous bruising, and bleeding are common and explained by myelophthisis from excessive bone tissue, osteoclasts, and fibrosis crowding marrow spaces. This leads to severe anemia which is exacerbated by extramedullary hematopoiesis with hypersplenism and hemolysis. The skeleton is fragile. There is a large head, frontal bossing, "adenoid" appearance, nystagmus, hepatosplenomegaly, short stature, and genu valgum. Untreated patients succumb, usually during the first decade of life.
  - Intermediate OPT causes macrocephaly and short stature, sometimes with cranial nerve palsies, ankylosed teeth leading to osteomyelitis of the jaw, fractures, and anemia.
  - Adult OPT (Albers-Schönberg disease) can cause fractures within the axial as well as the appendicular skeleton, and sometimes compromised vision or hearing, facial nerve palsy, mandibular osteomyelitis, psychomotor delay, carpal tunnel syndrome, slipped capital femoral epiphysis, or osteoarthritis. Some individuals are asymptomatic.
  - Carbonic anhydrase II (CA II) deficiency, features proximal or distal renal tubular acidosis (RTA) and cerebral calcification. In infancy or early childhood, fractures, failure to thrive, developmental delay, and short stature can manifest. Mental subnormality is common. Compression of the optic nerves and dental malocclusion are further complications. Periodic hypokalemic paralysis can occur.
- *Radiographic findings:*
  - Generalized, symmetrical increase in bone mass.
  - Cortical and trabecular bone are thickened.
  - Rachitic changes in growth plates may occur if there is hypocalcemia.
  - The skull is thickened and dense, especially at its base, and the paranasal and mastoid sinuses are underpneumatized.
  - Vertebrae may show a "bone-inbone" (endobone) configuration.
  - In CA II deficiency, cerebral calcification appears on computed tomography (CT) affecting gray matter of the cortex and basal ganglia.

- In Albers-Schönberg disease, abnormalities include a dense skull base, "rugger-jersey" spine, and alternating sclerotic and lucent horizontal bands in the metaphyses of major long bones. Metaphyses are wide and may have a club shape or "Erlenmeyer flask" appearance. Rarely, distal phalanges in the hands appear eroded. Pathologic "chalk-stick" fractures occur in major long bones.
- *Laboratory findings:*
  - In infantile OPT, hypocalcemia can occur (because bone resorption is impaired), and may cause rickets. Secondary hyperparathyroidism with elevated serum levels of calcitriol is common.
  - In adult OPT, biochemical indices of mineral homeostasis are usually unremarkable. Serum PTH level can be increased. Osteoclast-derived tartrate-resistant acid phosphatase (TRAP) and the brain isoenzyme of creatine kinase are often elevated in serum.

18. **Ans. (b) Most commonly involves long bones, hand, feet**
    [De Groot 7th ed pg 1181; Harrison's Endocrinology 3rd ed pg 460-463; A.C.E.S. for P.A.C.E.S pg 548]

    Paget's Disease of Bone (PDB)
    - The principal feature is focally increased skeletal remodelling within the axial or appendicular skeleton.
    - Initially, a "wave" of osteoclast-mediated osteolysis moves slowly but relentlessly through a bone, and is then followed by disorganized skeletal repair leading to bony expansion as well as to hyperostosis and osteosclerosis.
    - The principal abnormality in Paget's disease is increased number and activity of osteoclasts. Pagetic osteoclasts are large, and have a greater number of nuclei.
    - *Clinical features:*
      - Pagetic bone is unsound and can cause pain, fracture, and deformity.
      - The skeletal sites most commonly involved are the pelvis, vertebral bodies, skull, femur, and tibia.
      - Deafness dental problems (include loosening and migration of Teeth) is common,
      - Rarely, there is malignant transformation of pagetic lesions to osteosarcoma or chondrosarcoma.
      - *Cardiovascular complications:* High-output state and cardiac enlargement; high-output heart failure is rare; calcific aortic stenosis; diffuse vascular calcifications.
    - *Radiographic findings:*
      - Typical findings include enlargement or expansion of a bone or area of a long bone, cortical thickening, coarsening of trabecular markings, and typical lytic and sclerotic changes.
      - Skull radiographs reveal regions of "cotton wool," or osteoporosis circumscripta; thickening of diploic areas; and enlargement and sclerosis of a portion or all of one or more skull bones.

- Vertebral cortical thickening of the superior and inferior end plates creates a "picture frame" vertebra. Diffuse radiodense enlargement of a vertebra is referred to as "ivory vertebra."
- Pelvic radiographs may demonstrate disruption or fusion of the sacroiliac joints; porotic and radiodense lesions of the ilium with whorls of coarse trabeculation; a thickened and sclerotic ileopectinal line (Brim sign); and protrusio acetabuli.
- Radiographs of long bones reveal bowing deformity and typical pagetic changes.
- Radionuclide 99mTc bone scans are less specific but are more sensitive than standard radiographs for identifying sites of active skeletal lesions.
- *Laboratory findings:*
  - *Markers of bone formation and resorption:* Parallel rise in markers of bone formation (ALP) and resorption (Urinary and serum deoxypyridinoline, N-telopeptide, and C-telopeptide levels, urinary hydroxyproline) respectively, confirm the coupling of bone formation and resorption in Paget's disease. The degree of bone marker elevation reflects the extent and severity of the disease.
  - Serum calcium and phosphate levels are normal in Paget's disease.
- *Agents approved for the treatment of Paget's disease:* Bisphosphonates, calcitonin.

19. **Ans. (b) Tall stature**
    [De Groot 7th ed pg 1173-75]
    See discussion of Chapter 19, Question 17.

20. **Ans. (b) Most common in hand and leg bones**
    [De Groot 7th ed pg 1181; Harrison's Endocrinology 3rd ed pg 460-463; A.C.E.S for P.A.C.E.S pg 548]
    See discussion of Chapter 19, Question 18.

21. **Ans. (a) Acidosis**
    [Williams 13th ed pg 1295; Harrison's Endocrinology 2nd ed pg 434]

    Causes of Hypocalcemia
    Parathyroid-related Disorders
    - Absence of the parathyroid glands or of PTH
      - Congenital
        - DiGeorge syndrome
        - X-linked or autosomally inherited hypoparathyroidism
        - Autoimmune polyglandular syndrome type I
        - PTH gene mutations
      - Postsurgical hypoparathyroidism
      - Infiltrative disorders
        - Hemochromatosis
        - Wilson disease
        - Metastases
      - Hypoparathyroidism following radioactive iodine thyroid ablation

- Impaired secretion of PTH
  - Hypomagnesemia
  - Respiratory alkalosis
  - Activating mutations of the calcium sensor
- Target organ resistance
  - Hypomagnesemia
  - Pseudohypoparathyroidism
    - Type I
    - Type II

Vitamin D–related Disorders
- Vitamin D deficiency
  - Dietary absence
  - Malabsorption
- Accelerated loss
  - Impaired enterohepatic recirculation
  - Anticonvulsant medications
- Impaired 25-hydroxylation
  - Liver disease
  - Isoniazid
  - CYP2R1 mutation
- Impaired 1α-hydroxylation
  - Renal failure
- Vitamin D-dependent rickets, type I
- Oncogenic osteomalacia
- Target organ resistance
  - Vitamin D-dependent rickets, type II
  - Phenytoin

Other Causes
- Excessive deposition into the skeleton
  - Osteoblastic malignancies
  - Hungry bone syndrome
- Impaired bone resorption
  - Vitamin D deficiency
  - Bisphosphonates
  - RANKL inhibition
- Severe, acute hyperphosphatemia (PTH overwhelmed)
  - Tumor lysis
  - Acute renal failure
  - Rhabdomyolysis
- Chelation
  - Foscarnet
  - Phosphate infusion
  - Infusion of citrated blood products
  - Infusion of EDTA-containing contrast reagents
  - Fluoride

- Neonatal hypocalcemia
  - Prematurity
  - Asphyxia
  - Diabetic mother
  - Hyperparathyroid mother
- HIV infection
  - Drug therapy
  - Vitamin D deficiency
  - Hypomagnesemia
  - Impaired PTH responsiveness
- Critical illness
  - Pancreatitis
  - Toxic shock syndrome
  - Intensive care unit patients.

22. **Ans. (a) Echo**
[Williams 13th ed pg 1296]

23. **Ans. (b) Early menopause**
[Harrison's Endocrinology 3rd ed pg 440; Williams 13th ed pg 1350]

Risk factors for Osteoporosis
- Nonmodifiable
  - Female sex
  - Advanced age
  - Caucasian race
- Potentially modifiable
  - Current cigarette smoking
  - Low body weight
  - Estrogen deficiency
  - Early menopause (<45 years) or bilateral ovariectomy
  - Prolonged premenstrual amenorrhea (>1 year)
  - Low calcium intake
  - Alcoholism

Causes of Secondary Osteoporosis
- Endocrine disorders
  - Diabetes mellitus
  - Hyperparathyroidism
  - Hyperthyroidism
  - Cushing's syndrome
  - Hypogonadism
  - Menstrual irregularity (even athletes)
  - Premature menopause
  - Low testosterone and estradiol levels in men
  - Hyperprolactinemia
  - Pregnancy and lactation

- Autoimmune disorders
  - Rheumatoid arthritis
  - Inflammatory bowel disease
  - Lupus erythematosus
  - Multiple sclerosis
  - Ankylosing spondylitis
- Digestive and gastrointestinal disorders
  - Celiac disease
  - Inflammatory bowel disease
  - Weight loss surgery
  - Gastrectomy
- Hematologic/blood disorders
  - Leukemia and lymphoma
  - Multiple myeloma
  - Sickle cell disease
  - Blood and bone marrow disorders
    - *Plasma cell dyscrasias:* Multiple myeloma and macroglobulinemia
    - *Myeloproliferative disorders:* Polycythemia
  - Thalassemia
- Neurologic/nervous system disorders
  - Stroke, Parkinson disease, and multiple sclerosis
  - Spinal cord injuries
- Mental illness
  - Depression
  - Eating disorders
- Cancer
  - Breast
  - Prostate
- Connective tissue disorders
  - Osteogenesis imperfecta
  - Ehlers-Danlos syndrome
  - Marfan syndorme
  - Menkes syndrome
- Drug-induced disorders
  - Glucocorticoids
  - Heparin
  - Anticonvulsants
  - Methotrexate, cyclosporine
  - Luteinizing hormone-releasing hormone (LHRH) agonist or antagonist therapy
  - Proton pump inhibitors
  - Aluminum-containing antacids
- Other diseases and conditions
  - AIDS/HIV
  - Chronic obstructive pulmonary disease

- Female athlete triad
- Kidney disease
- Liver disease
- Organ transplant
- Poliomyelitis and post-polio syndrome
- Poor diet, including malnutrition
- Weight loss
- *Lipidoses:* Gaucher disease
- Scurvy.

24. **Ans. (a) Tall stature**
    [De Groot 7th ed pg 1173-75]
    See discussion of Chapter 19, Question 17.

25. **Ans. (d) Increased PTH**
    [Werner & Ingbar's, The Thyroid 10th ed pg 469]

26. **Ans. (a) PTH replacement is the standard treatment**
    [Williams 13th ed pg 1295, 1296, 1303; Walsh and Hoyt's Clinical Neuro-ophthalmology 6th ed pg 273]

27. **Ans. (b) Stimulates CaSR**
    [Williams 13th ed pg 1259, 1283; Goodman & Gilman's, The Pharmacological Basis of Therapeutics 12th ed]

    Cinacalcet
    - Calcimimetic
    - Activator of the CaSR
    - Administered orally
    - Lowers PTH secretion and thereby lowers calcium levels
    - Approved for control of secondary hyperparathyroidism in renal disease. Also shown to lower serum calcium and PTH in primary hyperparathyroidism (and in some patients with parathyroid carcinoma).

28. **Ans. (c) VDD type-1 is associated with alopecia**
    [De Groot 7th ed pg 1161, 1163, 1230, 1240]

    Rickets is characterized by a delay in maturation and apoptosis of chondrocytes in the epiphyseal growth plates, resulting in disorganization of these chondrocytes and expansion of the growth plate.

    Pseudovitamin D–deficiency rickets (PDDR) (also referred to as vitamin D dependency type I or VDD-I)
    - Autosomal recessive disorder
    - Caused by impaired renal production of $1,25(OH)_2D$
    - Caused by mutations of the gene that encodes the $25(OH)D$ 1α-hydroxylase, the enzyme that is responsible for conversion of $25(OH)D$ to $1,25(OH)_2D$.

- Affected individuals develop the clinical and biochemical changes of rickets during the first year of life
- Characterized by hypocalcemia, hypophosphatemia, elevated serum immunoreactive PTH, and alkaline phosphatase, normal serum 25(OH)D and low or undetectable serum $1,25(OH)_2D$
- Patient responds to physiologic doses of $1,25(OH)_2D_3$.

Hereditary vitamin D-resistant rickets (HVDRR; also termed vitamin D-dependent rickets type II)
- Autosomal recessive
- Characterized by resistance of target organs to $1,25(OH)_2D$.
- Caused by mutations of the vitamin D receptor (VDR) gene
- Onset of symptoms can occur at any age from infancy to adolescence
- Patients exhibit hypocalcemia, hypophosphatemia, elevation of serum alkaline phosphatase and immunoreactive PTH, normal or increased serum 25(OH)D, and marked elevation of serum $1,25(OH)_2D$
- Patients may develop alopecia
- No treatment has been uniformly successful; treatment with parenteral calcium infusions, circumventing the intestinal resistance to 1,25-dihydroxyvitamin D, can normalize the biochemical abnormalities and lead to clinical and radiologic remission of the osteomalacic lesions.

29. **Ans. (d) Defect in type 2 collagen**
[De Groot 7th ed pg 1180, 1181; Harrison's Principles of Internal Medicine pg 2508]

Osteogenesis Imperfecta (OI)
- Often called "brittle bone disease".
- Caused by mutations in the genes that encode the pro-α1 and pro-α2 chains that combine to form the type 1 collagen heterotrimer. Additional rare types of OI involve enzymatic defects in collagen crosslinking.
- *Clinical presentation:*
  - Fractures and skeletal deformity.
  - Scleral discoloration may be present.
  - Affected individuals can manifest ligamentous laxity with joint hypermobility, diaphoresis, bruising, fragile and discoloured teeth, and hearing loss (~50% of those <30 years, and in nearly all who are older).
  - In severe OI, there is also a high-pitched voice, short stature, scoliosis, herniae, disproportionately large head compared with body size, triangular face, and chest deformity.
  - Patients generally have normal intelligence.
  - Type 1 OI features sclerae with bluish discoloration, relatively mild osteopenia with infrequent fractures (deformity is uncommon or slight), and deafness that manifests during early adult life. Type 1 OI has been subclassified into 1-A and 1-B disease depending on the absence or (more rarely) the presence, respectively, of dentinogenesis imperfecta.

- Type 2 OI is often fatal within the first weeks of life from respiratory complications. Affected newborns are often born prematurely, small for gestational age, and have short, bowed limbs, numerous fractures, markedly soft skulls, and small thoraces. Blue sclera may be present.
- Type 3 OI features recurrent fractures, including of long bone growth plates, leading to progressive skeletal deformity and short stature during childhood. Dentinogenesis imperfecta is common. Thoracic distortion predisposes to pneumonia.
- Type 4 OI frequently explains multigeneration disease. The sclerae appear normal, but skeletal deformity, dental disease, and hearing loss are typical.

- *Radiographic features:*
  - Characteristic radiographic findings include generalized osteopenia, modelling defects featuring gracile long bones, and deformities from recurrent fractures.
  - In some severely affected infants, micromelia occurs where major long bones appear wide.
  - Wormian bones in the skull is a common feature of OI.
  - Excessive pneumatization of the frontal and mastoid sinuses and platybasia that can progress to basilar impression are common with severe disease.
  - "Popcorn calcification" within metaphyses is characteristic and appears in childhood, likely from traumatic fragmentation of growth-plate cartilage. Popcorn calcification resolve when endochondral cartilage becomes fully mineralized at skeletal maturity and is replaced by bone.
  - Fractures often heal at normal rates. Occasionally, hypertrophic callus formation occurs (hallmark of type 5 OI)
  - Osteoarthritis is frequent.

- *Laboratory findings:*
  - Routine biochemical parameters of mineral metabolism are unremarkable, except hypercalciuria is common in severely affected children.
  - Elevations in serum and urinary markers of bone turnover occur in severely affected patients.

30. **Ans. (a) Fish**
    [De Groot 7th ed pg 1019]

31. **Ans. (b) Oxandrolone**
    [De Groot 7th ed 1211; Greenspan's 9th ed; Osteoporos Int (1997) 7:390-406]

32. **Ans. (b) Antiproliferative action**
    [Greenspan's 9th ed]

33. **Ans. (b) Vitamin D level**
[Menopause: The Journal of The North American Menopause Society. Vol. 17, No. 1, pp. 33]

Routine Tests for Patients with Low Bone Mass Include
- Complete blood cell count,
- Serum calcium,
- Phosphate,
- Creatinine,
- Thyroid-stimulating hormone,
- Alkaline phosphatase,
- Albumin.

Other Tests that may be Useful
- Serum 25-hydroxyvitamin D [25(OH)D]
- 24-hour urinary calcium excretion

Special Tests that may be Appropriate in Some Clinical Circumstances
- 24-hour urine free cortisol,
- Serum protein electrophoresis,
- Tissue transglutaminase antibody,
- Intact parathyroid hormone (PTH).

34. **Ans. (c) Cushing's**
[Harrison's Endocrinology 2nd ed pg 407]

Causes of Hypercalcemia
- Excessive PTH production
  - Primary hyperparathyroidism (adenoma, hyperplasia, rarely carcinoma)
  - Tertiary hyperparathyroidism (long-term stimulation of PTH secretion in renal insufficiency)
  - Ectopic PTH secretion (very rare)
  - Inactivating mutations in the CaSR (FHH)
  - Alterations in CaSR function (lithium therapy)
- Hypercalcemia of malignancy
  - Overproduction of PTHrP (many solid tumors)
  - Lytic skeletal metastases (breast, myeloma)
- Excessive $1,25(OH)_2D$ production
  - Granulomatous diseases (sarcoidosis, tuberculosis, silicosis)
  - Lymphomas
  - Vitamin D intoxication
- Primary increase in bone resorption
  - Hyperthyroidism
  - Immobilization
- Excessive calcium intake
  - Milk-alkali syndrome
  - Total parenteral nutrition

Mineral Metabolism | 245

- Other causes
  - Endocrine disorders (adrenal insufficiency, pheochromocytoma, VIPoma)
  - Medications (thiazides, vitamin A, antiestrogens).

35. **Ans. (a) Mesenchymal stem cell**
    [Williams 13th ed pg 1327]

36. **Ans. (d) Hydroxyproline**
    [Williams 13th ed pg 1344]

    Markers of Bone Turnover

Marker	Specimen
• **Markers of bone formation**	
Bone-specific alkaline phosphatase (BAP)	Serum
Osteocalcin (OC)	Serum
C-terminal propeptide of type I procollagen (PICP)	Serum
N-terminal propeptide of type I procollagen (PINP)	Serum
• **Markers of bone resorption**	
a. *Collagen-related markers*	
Hydroxyproline, total and dialyzable (HYP)	Urine
Hydroxylysine-glycosides	Urine, serum
Pyridinoline (PYD)	Urine, serum
Deoxypyridinoline (DPD)	Urine, serum
C-terminal cross-linked telopeptide of type I collagen (ICTP, CTX-MMP)	Serum
C-terminal cross-linked telopeptide of type I collagen (CTX-I)	Urine (α/β), serum (β only)
N-terminal cross-linked telopeptide of type I collagen (NTX-I)	Urine, serum
Collagen I alpha 1 helicoidal peptide (HELP)	Urine
b. *Noncollagenous proteins*	
Bone sialoprotein (BSP)	Serum
Osteocalcin fragments (uf OC, U-Mid-OC, U-Long-OC)	Urine
c. *Osteoclast enzymes*	
Tartrate-resistant acid phosphatase (TRAP)	Plasma
Cathepsins (e.g. K, L)	Plasma, serum

37. **Ans. (a) FGFR3**
    [Williams 13th ed pg 1006]

38. **Ans. (c) PHP**
    [Williams 13th ed pg 1300, 1301, Harrison's Endocrinology 3rd ed pg 434-6; De Groot 7th ed pg 1217]

Although both options (a) and (c) are correct, option (c) is more appropriate than option (a) as in CKD serum calcium and phosphate levels are maintained within the normal range until late in the course of CKD.

Type	Hypocalcemia, Hyperphosphatemia	Response of Urinary cAMP to PTH	Serum PTH	$G_s\alpha$ subunit deficiency	AHO	Resistance to hormones in addition to PTH
PHP-Ia	Yes	↓	↑	Yes	Yes	Yes
PHP-Ib	Yes	↓	↑	No	No	No
PHP-II	Yes	Normal	↑	No	No	No
PPHP	No	Normal	Normal	Yes	Yes	±

39. **Ans. (c) 12**
    [De Groot 7th ed pg 1204]

40. **Ans. (b) Ca^{++} decreased**
    [Harrison's Endocrinology 3rd ed pg 434-436]
    See discussion of Chapter 19, Question 38.

41. **Ans. (a) PTH**
    [Williams 13th ed pg 18, 19, 20, 123, 129, 137, 145, 152, 183, 188, 199, 207, 301, 492, 494, 595, 606, 704, 1256, 1267, 1269, 1270, 1703-14; Clinical Chemistry, Immunology and Laboratory Quality Control: A Comprehensive Review for Board Preparation, Certification and Clinical Practice, pg 149]
    See discussion of Chapter 1, Question 1.

42. **Ans. (a) Low iPTH**
    [Williams 13th ed pg 1310]

43. **Ans. (b) Keratinocyte**
    [Greenspan's 9th ed; Williams 13th ed pg 1272]
    $1,25(OH)_2D$ reduces the rate of proliferation of many cell lines, including normal parathyroid cells, keratinocytes, fibroblasts, lymphocytes, and thymocytes as well as abnormal cells of mammary, skeletal, intestinal, lymphatic, and myeloid origin.

44. **Ans. (e) All of the above**
    [Williams 13th ed pg 274, 275, 1186, 1278, 1350; Harrison's Endocrinology 3rd ed pg 461, 467]
    See discussion of Chapter 19, Question 23

45. **Ans. (d) Increased osteoid volume and decreased mineral/matrix ratio**
    [De Groot 7th ed pg 1230-1232]

46. **Ans. (a) 1–4 mg/kg**
    [Dynamics of Bone and Cartilage Metabolism: Principles and Clinical Applications 2nd ed pg 493]

47. **Ans. (c) Pseudohypoparathyroidism**
    [De Groot 7th ed pg 1240]

48. **Ans. (e) Selective estrogen receptor modulator**
    [Williams 13th ed pg 1355]

CHAPTER 20

Kidney Stones

QUESTIONS

1. Oxalate is produced by endogenous metabolism of:
   a. Ascorbic acid
   b. Cholesterol
   c. Protein
   d. Thiamine

2. All of the following are true about Cysteine stones except:
   a. More soluble in acidic pH
   b. D-penicillamine is drug of choice
   c. Bucillamine is alternative to D-penicillamine
   d. AR and increased excretion of dibasic AA

3. Oxalate stones, avoid all except:
   a. Milk and milk products
   b. Meat and Beef
   c. Black and green pepper
   d. Black tea, chocolate & Coke

4. Following medications are associated with renal lithiasis except:
   a. Allopurinol
   b. Sulfonamides
   c. Vitamin K
   d. Nelfinavir

5. Which vegetable has low oxalate content?
   a. Spinach
   b. Watercress
   c. Mushrooms
   d. Sorrel

ANSWERS

1. **Ans. (a) Ascorbic acid**
   [Williams 13th ed pg 1377]
   - Oxalate is produced predominantly by endogenous metabolism of glyoxylate and, to a lesser extent, by ascorbic acid.
   - Thiamine is involved in the metabolism of glyoxylate which helps in the removal of glyoxylate from being converted to oxalate. Thus, deficiency of thiamine may be associated with increased oxalate synthesis.

2. **Ans. (a) More soluble in acidic pH**
   [Williams 13th ed pg 1381]
   Cystine Stones
   - Cystinuria is AR (may be AD with incomplete penetrance).
   - Decreased renal tubular reabsorption and excessive urinary excretion of the dibasic amino acids cystine, ornithine, lysine, and arginine.
   - Cystine has low solubility of approximately 300 mg/L.
   - People with no tubular defect in cystine transport excrete approximately 30–50 mg of cystine per day. Patients heterozygous for this condition excrete about 400 mg/day, whereas homozygotes often excrete more than 600 mg/day.
   - This leads to cystine crystals precipitating and aggregating as cystine stones.
   - Stones usually develop within the second or third decade of life.
   - The stones are radiopaque.
   - *Diagnosis:*
     - Presence of the classic hexagonal cystine crystals in urine.
     - Qualitative screening with sodium nitroprusside test better confirms the presence of cystinuria.
     - Quantitative cystine measures with a 24-hour urine sample should follow to determine the risk of stone formation and to guide therapy.
   - *Therapy:*
     - Patients are advised to drink large quantities of fluids.
     - The solubility of cystine increases significantly when urine pH is greater than 6.5. Juices are encouraged because they tend to alkalinize the urine. Potassium citrate is also prescribed to maintain the urinary pH between 6.5 and 7.0.
     - Avoid: Large quantities of milk/dairy products and foods high in protein; dietary sodium restriction.
     - Chelating agents called cystine-binding thiol drugs (CBTDs) may be added: D-penicillamine, tiopronin, α-mercaptopropionylglycine, and bucillamine.

3. **Ans. (a) Milk and milk products**
   [Williams 13th ed pg 1377, 1378]
   Foods High in Oxalate
   - Beans (green and dried)
   - Beer (draft, stout, lager, pilsner)

- Beets
- Berries (blackberries, blueberries, raspberries, strawberries)
- Black tea
- Black pepper
- Celery
- Chocolate and cocoa
- Eggplant
- Figs and dried
- Greens (collard greens, dandelion greens, endive, escarole, kale, leeks, mustard greens, parsley, sorrel, spinach, Swiss chard, watercress)
- Green peppers
- Lemon, lime, and orange peel
- Nuts
- Pecans, peanuts, and peanut butter
- Okra
- Rhubarb
- Sweet potato
- Tofu

Patients should be instructed to ingest calcium containing foods, such as a glass of milk, when eating foods high in oxalate. The calcium in milk binds the dietary oxalate and may prevent its absorption.

4. **Ans. (c) Vitamin K**
   [Williams 13th ed pg 1372]

   Medications Associated with Renal Lithiasis and Nephrocalcinosis
   - Medications that promote calcium stone formation
     - Acetazolamide
     - Amphotericin B
     - Antacids (calcium and non-calcium antacids)
     - Calcium supplements
     - Glucocorticoids
     - Loop diuretics
     - Theophylline
     - Vitamin C
     - Vitamin D
   - Medications that promote uric acid lithiasis
     - Allopurinol (associated with xanthene stones)
     - Probenecid
     - Salicylates
   - Medications that can precipitate into stones or crystals
     - Acyclovir (when infused rapidly intravenously)
     - Indinavir
     - Nelfinavir
     - Sulfonamides
     - Triamterene

5. **Ans. (c) Mushrooms**
   [Williams 13th ed pg 1378]
   See discussion of Chapter 20, Question 3.

CHAPTER
21

Diabetes

QUESTIONS

1. Diabetes mellitus (DM) is associated with all except:
   a. Down syndrome
   b. Turner syndrome
   c. Kallmann syndrome
   d. Friedreich's ataxia

2. Mucormycosis treatment includes all except:
   a. Fluconazole
   b. Posaconazole
   c. Insulin
   d. Surgical debridement

3. Mucormycosis—cumulative dose of amphotericin is:
   a. 0.5 gm
   b. 2 gm
   c. 6 gm
   d. 10 gm

4. Mucormycosis is associated with DM in:
   a. 90%
   b. 75%
   c. 40%
   d. 30%

5. Diabetic ketoacidosis (DKA) 1st line of treatment is:
   a. Insulin
   b. Fluid and electrolytes
   c. Sodium bicarbonate
   d. Phosphate

6. HCO_3 is indicated in DKA if pH is:
   a. <6.9
   b. <7.0
   c. <7.1
   d. <7.2

7. All indicate a diagnosis of DKA except:
   a. RBS >250 mg/dL
   b. pH <7.3
   c. Mild ketonuria
   d. HCO_3 <13 mEq/L

8. Common cause of death due to DM in children:
   a. DKA
   b. Cardiomyopathy
   c. ESRD
   d. Infection

9. Emphysematous pyelonephritis is most commonly caused by:
   a. *E. coli*
   b. *Pseudomonas*
   c. *Klebsiella*
   d. *Proteus*

10. Post prandial hypoglycemia OHA used is:
    a. Miglitol
    b. Metformin
    c. TZD
    d. Gliclazide

11. All of the following are true about diabetic nephropathy except:
    a. Smoking accelerates decline renal function
    b. Develops in the first year
    c. Mesangial cell proliferation lead to decline in GFR after 5 years
    d. Once overt nephropathy once detected leads to ESRD in 50% cases

12. Acidosis in DKA presenting first time to the emergency has:
    a. Anion gap acidosis
    b. Hyperchloremic metabolic acidosis
    c. Mixed acidosis
    d. All of the above

13. DKA insulin infusion is started at:
    a. 0.1 u/kg/hr
    b. 0.2 u/kg/hr
    c. 0.3 u/kg/hr
    d. 0.4 u/kg/hr

14. In DKA, bicarbonate treatment may lead to adverse effects—all except:
    a. Increase tissue (intracellular) acidosis due to generation of CO_2
    b. Development of hyperkalemia
    c. Cerebral edema
    d. Cause paradoxical CNS acidosis

15. All of the following are true about HHS except:
    a. Osmolality > 300
    b. pH < 7.3
    c. Sr. Na^+ >145
    d. Glucose > 600 mg/dL

16. All are microvascular complications of DM except:
    a. CAD
    b. Nephropathy
    c. Autonomic nephropathy
    d. Retinopathy

17. Atkins diet is:
    a. Very low carbohydrate
    b. Very low protein
    c. Very high cholesterol
    d. Very low cholesterol

18. Degludec in solution:
    a. Dihexamer
    b. Dioctamer
    c. Pentamer
    d. Monomer

19. All of the following are true about insulin except:
    a. 51 amino cells
    b. Produced by β cells
    c. C-terminal cleavage
    d. Affect enzyme activity

20. Most effective diabetes prevention clinical trial:
    a. US Diabetes Prevention Program
    b. Finnish Diabetes Prevention Study
    c. Da Qing Study
    d. STOP-NIDDM

21. True about fetal pancreatic development are all except:
    a. In early pregnancy β cells > α cells
    b. At birth the ratio of β cells:α cells is 1
    c. Action starts at 14–24 weeks of pregnancy
    d. Progressive increase in β cell mass during pregnancy

22. True about CBGM:
    a. Commonly done in DM2
    b. Only used in hospitalized patients
    c. Used for diagnosis of hypoglycemia awareness and dose adjustment
    d. Severe retinopathy is C/I

23. A 25-year-old male DM1, p/w mild intermittent diarrhea and weight loss, nontender abdomen, normal USG, normal thyroid profile, HbA1c 8.1. Ix:
    a. Intestinal biopsy
    b. Anti TTG/Anti endomysial antibody
    c. Gastric emptying study
    d. Endoscopy

24. Which of the following are not included in ADA criteria for diagnosis of DM?
    a. Symptom + random plasma glucose >200 mg%
    b. Fasting plasma glucose > 126 mg%
    c. Plasma glucose >200 mg% during OGTT
    d. HbA_{1c} >8

25. Side effects of Glinides is:
    a. ↑ hematocrit
    b. CCF
    c. Edema
    d. Weight gain

26. Side effects of metformin are all except:
    a. Hepatic dysfunction
    b. Megaloblastic anemia
    c. Diarrhea
    d. Iron deficiency anemia

27. All of the following are associated with vision loss in DM except:
    a. Vitreous hemorrhage
    b. Macular edema
    c. Optic neuritis
    d. Proliferative diabetic retinopathy

28. All of the following are true about nutrition in T2DM except:
    a. Cholesterol <300 mg/d
    b. Saturated fat< 10%
    c. 60–70% is divided between MUFA and carbohydrate
    d. 40–50% protein

29. DM is associated with all except:
    a. Kallmann/McCune-Albright
    b. Down/Klinfelter
    c. Wolfram's/Turner
    d. Porphyria/FA

30. Glucokinase—all are true except:
    a. Maximum concentration in β cells
    b. Rate limiting step for entry into glycolytic pathway
    c. Mutation is associated with MODY
    d. Microvascular and macrovascular complications are common in patients with heterozygous glucokinase mutation

31. Treatment of gustatory sweating:
    a. Glycopyrrolate   b. Topical clonidine
    c. Capsaicin   d. Octreotide
    e. IVIG

32. Insulin resistance is a feature of all except:
    a. Leprechaunism   b. Rabson-Mendenhall
    c. Type 2 DM   d. MODY

33. Malnutrition related DM:
    a. Type 1 DM   b. Young type 2
    c. MODY   d. FCPD

34. Side effect of insulin therapy include all except:
    a. Weight gain   b. Hypoglycemia
    c. Retinopathy   d. Nephropathy

35. Type 2 DM concordance rate in identical twin is:
    a. 10%   b. 30%
    c. 50%   d. 70%

36. Which of the following autoantibodies found in type 1 DM?
    a. GAD-65   b. GAD-67
    c. TPO   d. All of the above

37. Synthesized earliest in fetal pancreas:
    a. Glucagon   b. Insulin
    c. PP   d. Somatostatin

38. Designer insulin include all except:
    a. Degludec   b. Glulisine
    c. Lispro   d. NPH
    e. Inhalational

39. Biochemical paradox in DKA:
    a. Hypercalcemia   b. Absent ketone bodies
    c. Hypernatremia   d. Hyperkalemia
    e. Low BUN

40. **Maturity-onset diabetes of the young (MODY):**
    a. Insulin resistance may be present
    b. Mild diabetes
    c. Chronic complications never occur
    d. Common in Gujarati people

41. **DM retinopathy is associated with all except:**
    a. VEGF
    b. GH
    c. IGF-1
    d. PKC
    e. Triamcinolone

42. **Hyperglycemic memory:**
    a. Glucometer memory
    b. Complications developing after donation of kidney from diabetic to nondiabetic
    c. Diabetic kidney rejected by nondiabetic recipient
    d. Persistence or progression of hyperglycemia-induced microvascular alterations during subsequent periods of normal glucose homeostasis

43. **Mouse models for T2DM are all except:**
    a. Ob/ob mouse
    b. Nod mouse
    c. KK mouse
    d. Agouti mouse

44. **Serum osmolality in patient of DKA is usually:**
    a. 250
    b. 270–300
    c. 350
    d. 370

45. **Hepatocyte nuclear factor (HNF) in MODY is:**
    a. Transcription factor
    b. Receptor
    c. Second messenger
    d. None of the above

46. **Glycemic load of food is obtained by:**
    a. Glycemic index multiplied by no. of grams of food
    b. Glycemic index multiplied by carbohydrate content of food
    c. Glycemic index divided by carbohydrate content of food
    d. Carbohydrate content of food divided by glycemic index

47. **Most potent entero-insulin feedback is seen with:**
    a. GLP
    b. GIP
    c. Secretin
    d. CCK

48. **Which of the following about IGF-1 is not true?**
    a. It is made up of A and B peptides linked by C-peptide
    b. It is closely homologous to proinsulin
    c. Its synthesis is dependent on GH
    d. IGF1 gene is located on chromosome 12

49. **Indirect IF used in:**
    a. IAA
    b. Islet cell antibodies
    c. GAD
    d. ICA1

50. **Legacy effect is seen in:**
    a. HTN
    b. Glucotoxicity
    c. Glycemic control
    d. Dyslipidemia

51. **All of the following statements are correct about Lispro insulin except:**
    a. 5–15 min onset
    b. Peak at 1 hr
    c. Duration is 4 hrs
    d. Preferably used in gastroparesis

52. **Lipoatrophic DM is characterized by all except:**
    a. Decreased insulin levels
    b. Decreased fat store
    c. Hypertriglyceridemia
    d. Fatty liver

53. **Thiazolidinediones—all except:**
    a. PPAR gamma agonist
    b. Action on hyperglycemia in 4–5 days
    c. Weight gain, peripheral edema
    d. ALT monitoring required

54. **A 3-year-old with diabetes, AV block, retinopathy, hypercalcemia, pigmentation, ophthalmoplegia:**
    a. Kearns-Sayre syndrome
    b. PGA1
    c. PGA2
    d. DiGeorge syndrome
    e. Sanjad-Sakati syndrome

55. **OHA to be used in hepatic failure:**
    a. Repaglinide
    b. Nateglinide
    c. Tolbutamide
    d. All of the above

56. **Dietary goals in DM:**
    a. Protein 15–20 g
    b. Saturated fat < 7% if LDL > 100 mg/dL
    c. Cholesterol < 500 mg
    d. Fiber 15–20 g

57. **Long h/o DM type 1, 40 yrs, post-menopausal with autonomic dysfunction with recurrent UTI, what can be the cause?**
    a. Cystopathy
    b. Estrogen
    c. High blood glucose
    d. All of the above

58. **Pt on 1 g Metformin TDS and 8 mg Glimepiride, with cardiomyopathy, LVEF 26%, but uncontrolled blood sugars, not ready for insulin, what can you add?**
    a. Sitagliptin
    b. Exenatide
    c. Metformin
    d. Voglibose

59. Hyperchloremic metabolic acidosis is seen in all except:
    a. Uremia
    b. RTA
    c. DKA
    d. Chronic renal failure

60. Intensive insulin therapy is used in all except:
    a. Autonomic neuropathy
    b. To prevent microvascular complications
    c. Post renal transplant in diabetic nephropathy
    d. Pregnancy

61. Not true about GDM is:
    a. Diagnosis can be made by HbA_{1c}
    b. Indian Asians are at high risk
    c. High risk patients should be evaluated at first contact
    d. Routine evaluation should be performed between 24–28 weeks

62. DKA not precipitated by:
    a. Infection
    b. Hypothyroidism
    c. Inadequate insulin
    d. Cerebral infarct

63. DKA management; not true is:
    a. I/V fluids
    b. I/V insulin
    c. Bicarbonates are routinely used
    d. Leukocytosis can be seen in the absence of infection

64. Which is not true for DKA?
    a. Bradycardia
    b. Tachypnea
    c. Dehydration
    d. Abdominal pain and tenderness

65. Which of the following is not to be mixed?
    a. Insulin lispro
    b. Insulin aspart
    c. Regular insulin
    d. Insulin glargine

66. Long acting insulin is:
    a. Insulin lispro
    b. Insulin aspart
    c. Insulin glulisine
    d. Insulin glargine

67. All are side effects of TZDs except:
    a. CCF
    b. Weight gain
    c. Increased Hematocrit
    d. Edema

68. PPAR-gamma/PPAR-alpha agonist combination is:
    a. Gemfibrozil/Pioglitazone
    b. Pioglitazone/Gemfibrozil
    c. Troglitazone/Pioglitazone

69. A 30-year-old female, ht. 5'7", wt. 75 kg, FBS 150 mg% twice; which of the following is best Rx?
    a. Life style modification
    b. Insulin
    c. OHA
    d. Statin

70. **Which of the following drugs is useful for glucotoxicity?**
    a. Metformin
    b. TZDs
    c. AGIs
    d. Sulfonylureas

71. **All are true about GLP-1 agonist except:**
    a. Glucose dependent insulin release
    b. Increases gastric emptying
    c. Inhibits glucagon release

72. **Metformin is indicated in which one of the following situations:**
    a. 60-year-old male with cardiac failure
    b. 70-year-old male with stable creatinine level of 1.5 mg%
    c. 60-year-old male with normal creatinine clearance
    d. 70-year-old female with creatinine level 1.4 mg%

ANSWERS

1. **Ans. (c) Kallmann syndrome**
   [Textbook of Diabetes 4th ed pg 27]

   Genetic Syndromes Associated with Diabetes
   - Down syndrome
   - Klinefelter syndrome
   - Turner syndrome
   - Wolfram syndrome
   - Friedreich's ataxia
   - Huntington's chorea
   - Laurence-Moon-Biedl syndrome
   - Myotonic dystrophy
   - Prader-Willi syndrome
   - Porphyria

2. **Ans. (a) Fluconazole**
   [A Practical Guide to Diabetes Mellitus, 6th ed pg 253; Therapy for Diabetes Mellitus and Related Disorders, ADA, 6th ed pg 948]
   - Rhinocerebral mucormycosis is caused by members of the order Mucorales (Mucor, Absidia, Rhizopus, Cunninghamella, and others)
   - *Treatment:*
     - Surgical debridement
     - Control of predisposing condition (hyperglycemia and metabolic acidosis)
     - Systemic antifungal therapy (Amphotericin B, Posaconazole)
   - Voriconazole, fluconazole and echinocandins are not effective.

3. **Ans. (b) 2 gm**
   [Joslin's Diabetes Mellitus 14th ed pg 1021]

4. **Ans. (d) 30%**
   [Diabetes & Metabolism 38(2012) pg 194]

5. **Ans. (b) Fluid and electrolytes**
   [Textbook of Diabetes 4th ed pg 550; Therapy for Diabetes Mellitus and Related Disorders, ADA, 6th ed pg 629]

   Four Pillars of Management of DKA
   - *Fluid and electrolyte therapy:* First priority
   - *IV insulin therapy:* Cornerstone of DKA management after initial hydration
   - Treatment of comorbidities
   - Careful monitoring of the clinical course

6. **Ans. (a) < 6.9**
   [Therapy for Diabetes Mellitus and Related Disorders, ADA, 6th ed pg 630; Williams 13th ed pg 1476]

7. **Ans. (c) Mild ketonuria**
   [Therapy for Diabetes Mellitus and Related Disorders, ADA, 6th ed pg 626; Textbook of Diabetes 4th ed pg 547]

   Diagnostic criteria for diabetic ketoacidosis (DKA) and hyperglycaemic hyperosmolar state (HHS)

	Mild DKA	Moderate DKA	Severe DKA	HHS
Glucose (mg/dL)	>250	>250	>250	>600
Arterial pH	7.25–7.30	7.00–7.24	<7.00	>7.30
Serum bicarbonate (mEq/L)	15–18	10–14	<10	>18
Urine ketone	Positive	Positive	Positive	Small
Serum ketone	Positive	Positive	Positive	Small
Effective serum osmolality (mOsm/kg)	Variable	Variable	Variable	>320
Anion gap	>10	>12	>12	Variable
Alteration in sensorial	Alert	Alert/drowsy	Stupor/coma	Stupor/coma

8. **Ans. (a) DKA**
   [Acta Endocrinol Suppl (Copenh). 1986;279:326-33]

9. **Ans. (a) *E. coli***
   [Textbook of Diabetes 4th ed pg 846]

10. **Ans. (a) Miglitol**
    [Williams 13th ed pg 1600]
    Diet, including frequent feedings, α-glucosidase inhibitor, diazoxide, or octreotide, can be tried in patients with NIPHS or post-gastric bypass hypoglycemia, but partial pancreatectomy may be required if medical therapy fails.

11. **Ans. (b) Develops in the first year**
    [Textbook of Diabetes 4th ed pg 602; Williams 13th ed pg 1517, Handbook of Nutrition and Food 2nd ed pg 793, 794; Seldin and Giebisch's The Kidney 4th ed pg 2218]

12. **Ans. (d) All of the above**
    [International Textbook of Diabetes Mellitus 4th ed pg 804]

13. **Ans. (a) 0.1 u/kg/hr**
    [Therapy for Diabetes Mellitus and Related Disorders, ADA, 6th ed pg 629]

14. **Ans. (b) Development of hyperkalemia**
    [International Textbook of Diabetes Mellitus 4th ed pg 811; Therapy for Diabetes Mellitus and Related Disorders, ADA, 6th ed pg 630]

15. **Ans. (b) pH <7.3**
    [Therapy for Diabetes Mellitus and Related Disorders, ADA, 6th ed pg 626; Textbook of Diabetes 4th ed pg 547]
    See discussion of Chapter 21, Question 7.

16. **Ans. (a) CAD**
    [Williams 13th ed pg 1484]

17. **Ans. (a) Very low carbohydrate**
    [World J Diabetes. Oct 15, 2017;8(10):441-442]

18. **Ans. (a) Dihexamer**
    [Drug Des Devel Ther. 2017 Apr 13;11:1210]
    Detemir differs from human insulin in that the amino acid threonine in B30 position (ThrB30) has been removed, and a C14 fatty acid chain has been attached to amino acid B29

    In the pharmaceutical formulation which contains zinc, phenol, and m-cresol, degludec forms finite dihexamers. After injection, with dispersal of phenol, degludec self-associates to form arrays of hundreds of hexamers that precipitate in the subcutaneous tissue environment. Slow diffusion of zinc ions from this depot results in a continuous and highly predictable slow dissociation of insulin monomers.

19. **Ans. (c) C-terminal cleavage**
    [Harrison's Endocrinology 3rd ed pg 265]
    Insulin is produced in the beta cells of the pancreatic islets. It is initially synthesized as a single-chain 86-amino-acid precursor polypeptide, preproinsulin. Subsequent proteolytic processing removes the amino terminal signal peptide, giving rise to proinsulin. Cleavage of an internal 31-residue fragment from proinsulin generates the C peptide and the A (21 amino acids) and B (30 amino acids) chains of insulin, which are connected by disulfide bonds.

20. **Ans. (a) US Diabetes Prevention Program**
    [International Textbook of Diabetes Mellitus 4th ed pg 838]
    - Numerous clinical trials have shown that in high-risk subjects, the incidence of T2DM can be prevented or delayed by lifestyle interventions or by various classes of medications.
    - The Da Qing Study (China) randomly allocated 557 persons with IGT to control, diet, exercise, or diet plus exercise. Compared with the control group, the incidence of diabetes was reduced in the three intervention groups by 31%, 46%, and 42%, respectively.
    - The Finnish Diabetes Prevention Study evaluated 522 obese persons with IGT randomly allocated to a control group or a lifestyle intervention group. The incidence of diabetes was reduced by 58% in the lifestyle group compared with the control group.

- The US Diabetes Prevention Program- 3234 overweight and obese participants with IGT were randomly allocated: control, metformin, or intensive lifestyle intervention. Nearly 20% of study participants were age 60 years and older at enrollment. Overall, the incidence of diabetes was reduced by 31% in the metformin group and 58% in the lifestyle group. Older adults had a greater benefit (71% reduction) with lifestyle intervention but did not appear to benefit from metformin.
- In the STOP-NIDDM Trial 1429 subjects with IGT were randomized to either placebo or acarbose. The incidence of diabetes was reduced by 58% in the lifestyle group compared with the control group. 221 (32%) patients randomized to acarbose and 285 (42%) randomized to placebo developed diabetes (relative hazard 0.75).

21. **Ans. (a) In early pregnancy β cells > α cells**
    [Williams 13th ed pg 874]
    - Fetal pancreas is identifiable by 4 weeks of gestation.
    - Alpha and beta cells can be recognized by 8-9 weeks.
    - Insulin, glucagon, somatostatin, and pancreatic polypeptide are measurable by 8-10 weeks of gestation.
    - Alpha cells are more numerous than beta cells in the early fetal pancreas and reach a relative peak at midgestation; beta cells continue to increase throughout the second half of gestation so that, by term, the ratio of alpha to beta cells is approximately 1 : 1.
    - Endocrine cells are dispersed throughout the exocrine tissues by 20 weeks, and the islets of Langerhans are clearly differentiated by 31 weeks.
    - Fetal beta cell is functional by 14-24 weeks of gestation.

22. **Ans. (c) Used for diagnosis of hypoglycemia awareness and dose adjustment**
    [Textbook of Diabetes 4th ed pg 407]

23. **Ans. (b) Anti TTG/Anti endomysial antibody**
    [Textbook of Diabetes 4th ed pg 873]

24. **Ans. (d) HbA$_{1c}$ >8**
    [Diabetes Care Volume 41, Supplement 1, January 2018 pg S15]

    Criteria for the Diagnosis of Diabetes (ADA)
    - FPG ≥126 mg/dL (7.0 mmol/L).
      OR
    - 2-h PG≥200 mg/dL (11.1 mmol/L) during OGTT (using a glucose load containing the equivalent of 75 g anhydrous glucose dissolved in water).
      OR
    - A1C ≥6.5% (48 mmol/mol).
      OR
    - In a patient with classic symptoms of hyperglycemia or hyperglycemic crisis, a random plasma glucose ≥200 mg/dL (11.1 mmol/L).
      NB: In the absence of unequivocal hyperglycemia, results should be confirmed by repeat testing.

25. **Ans. (d) Weight gain**
    [Williams 13th ed pg 1426]

26. **Ans. (d) Iron deficiency anemia**
    [Williams 13th ed pg 1427; International Textbook of Diabetes Mellitus 4th ed pg 651]

    ### Adverse Effects of Metformin
    - *Gastrointestinal side effects:* Nausea, diarrhea, crampy abdominal pain, dysgeusia (most common adverse events).
    - Vitamin B_{12} deficiency
    - Lactic acidosis (rare)

    Metformin is contraindicated in hepatic impairment because of risk of lactate accumulation.

27. **Ans. (c) Optic neuritis**
    [Williams 13th ed pg 1503, 1505]

    ### Causes of Vision Loss from Complications of Diabetes Mellitus Include
    - Retinal ischemia involving the fovea,
    - Macular edema at or near the fovea,
    - *Proliferative diabetic retinopathy leading to:*
        - Preretinal or vitreous hemorrhages
        - Retinal detachment and retinal tear
    - Neovascular glaucoma,
    - Retinal vessel occlusion,
    - Accelerated atherosclerotic disease,
    - Embolic phenomena.

28. **Ans. (d) 40–50% protein**
    [International Textbook of Diabetes Mellitus 4th ed pg 578; Textbook of Diabetes 4th ed pg 347; Cardiovascular Prevention and Rehabilitation pg 195, 196]

    ### Key Recommendations for Diabetic Diet and Lifestyle
    - *Dietary energy and body weight:* Achieve and/or maintain BMI of 18.5–25 kg/m^2.
    - *Dietary fat:* Total fat: <35% total energy (if overweight <30%); Saturated plus *trans* unsaturated fatty acids: <10% total energy; Polyunsaturated fatty acids: 6–10% total energy; Monounsaturated fatty acids: 10–20% total energy; Oily fish, soybean and rapeseed oil, nuts and green leafy vegetables to provide *n*-3 fatty acids; Cholesterol: <300 mg/d.
    - *Carbohydrate:* Total carbohydrate: 45–60% total energy, influenced by metabolic characteristics; Vegetables, fruits, legumes, and cereal-derived foods preferred.
    - *Sucrose and other free sugars:* If desired and blood glucose levels are satisfactory, free sugars (e.g. sucrose) up to 50 g/d may be incorporated into the diet; total free sugars should not exceed 10% total energy (less for those who are overweight).

Diabetes | **263**

- *Dietary fiber and glycemic index:* Ideally dietary fiber intake should be > 40 g/d (or 20 g/1000 kcal/d), half-soluble (lesser amounts also beneficial); Naturally occurring foods rich in dietary fiber are encouraged; Five servings per day of fiber-rich vegetables and fruit and four or more servings of legumes per week help to provide minimum requirements; Cereal-based foods should be wholegrain and high in fiber; Carbohydrate-rich low-glycemic-index foods are suitable choices.
- *Protein:* Total protein intake at lower end of normal range (0.8 g/kg/d) for type 1 patients with established nephropathy. For all others, protein should provide 10–20% total energy.
- *Vitamins, antioxidant nutrients, minerals, and trace elements:* Increase foods rich in tocopherols, carotenoids, vitamin C and flavonoids, trace elements and other vitamins; Fruits, vegetables, wholegrains rather than supplements recommended; Restrict salt to less than 6 g/d (less than 2.3 g sodium).
- *Alcohol:* Up to 10 g for women and 20 g for men per day is acceptable; Special precautions apply to those on insulin or sulfonylureas, those who are overweight and those with hypertriglyceridemia.
- *Special "diabetic" foods, or functional foods and supplements:* Non-alcoholic beverages sweetened with non-nutritive sweeteners are useful; Other special foods not encouraged; No particular merit of fructose and other "special" nutritive sweeteners over sucrose.

Also,
- In persons with plasma LDL cholesterol ≥ 100 mg/dL, the saturated fat intake should be reduced to <7%.
- Carbohydrate and monounsaturated fat together should provide 60–70% of energy intake.

29. **Ans. (a) Kallmann/McCune-Albright**
    [Textbook of Diabetes 4th ed pg 27]
    See discussion of Chapter 21, Question 1.

30. **Ans. (d) Microvascular and macrovascular complications are common in patients with heterozygous glucokinase mutation**
    [Williams 13th ed pg 1391; Textbook of Diabetes 4th ed pg 248]
    - Glucokinase is expressed at its highest levels in the pancreatic beta cell and the liver.
    - It catalyzes the transfer of phosphate from ATP to glucose to generate glucose 6-phosphate. This reaction is the first rate-limiting step in glucose metabolism.
    - Glucokinase functions as the glucose sensor in the beta cell by controlling the rate of entry of glucose into the glycolytic pathway and its subsequent metabolism.
    - Heterozygous mutations leading to partial deficiency of glucokinase are associated with MODY, and homozygous mutations resulting in complete deficiency of this enzyme lead to permanent neonatal diabetes mellitus.

31. **Ans. (a) Glycopyrrolate**
    [Williams 13th ed pg 1547]

32. **Ans. (d) MODY**
    [Williams 13th ed pg 1386; Textbook of Diabetes 4th ed pg 245, 256-259]

    Monogenic Causes of Diabetes Resulting from Insulin Resistance
    - Insulin receptor gene mutations
        - Type A insulin resistance syndrome
        - Rabson–Mendenhall syndrome
        - Leprechaunism (Donohue syndrome)
    - Inherited lipodystrophies
        - Familial partial lipodystrophy
        - Congenital generalized lipodystrophy (Berardinelli–Seip syndrome)
        - Other rare subtypes of lipodystrophy associated with dysmorphic features:
            - Mandibuloacral dysplasia
            - SHORT syndrome (short stature, hyperextensibility of joints, ocular depression, Reiger anomaly, teething delay)
            - Neonatal progeroid syndrome.
    - Other monogenic conditions associated with insulin resistance
        - Alström syndrome
        - Bardet-Biedl syndrome
        - Myotonic dystrophy
        - Friedreich ataxia
        - Werner syndrome

    T2DM Demonstrates three Cardinal Abnormalities
    - Resistance to the action of insulin in peripheral tissues, particularly muscle and fat but also liver
    - Defective insulin secretion, particularly in response to a glucose stimulus
    - Increased glucose production by the liver

    Maturity-onset diabetes of the young (MODY) results from β-cell dysfunction rather than insulin resistance.

33. **Ans. (d) FCPD**
    [Textbook of Diabetes 4th ed pg 27]

34. **Ans. (d) Nephropathy**
    [Textbook of Diabetes 4th ed pg 433, 434, 575, 578]

    Adverse Events Associated with Insulin
    - Weight gain
    - Hypoglycemia
    - Lipodystrophy/lipohypertrophy
    - *Insulin allergies (rare):* Most commonly local acute urticarial reactions.

    In the DCCT, early worsening of DR was reported at the 6- and/or 12-month visit in 13.1% of patients assigned to intensive treatment, however, the long-term benefits of intensive insulin treatment greatly outweighed the risks of early worsening.

35. **Ans. (d) 70%**
    [Harrison's Endocrinology 3rd ed pg 269]
    The concordance of type 2 DM in identical twins is between 70 and 90%.

36. **Ans. (a) GAD-65**
    [Textbook of Diabetes 4th ed pg 146-148]

    ### Islet Autoantigens and Autoantibodies
    - *GAD65Ab:* Autoantibody against glutamic acid decarboxylase- GAD65 isoform.
    - *IA-2Ab and IA-2 β Ab:* Autoantibodies against Islet antigen—2 composed of two isoforms: IA-2 (formerly known as ICA512) and IA-2 β (phogrin).
    - *IAA (Insulin autoantibodies):* Autoantibody against insulin.
    - *ZnT8Ab:* Antibody against zinc transporter ZnT8 isoform-8.

37. **Ans. (a) Glucagon**
    [Curr Opin Endocrinol Diabetes Obes. 2015 Aug;22(4):257]
    During early stages of pancreatic bud outgrowth, the vast majority of endocrine cells are α cells, followed by increased production of β, δ and ε cells during the secondary transition, and finally the pancreatic polypeptide (PP) cell population during late embryogenesis.

38. **Ans. (d) NPH**
    [Textbook of Diabetes 4th ed pg 17]
    Examples of "designer" insulins: Fast-acting insulin analogs lispro and aspart; "peakless" basal insulins such as glargine and detemir.

39. **Ans. (b) Absent ketone bodies**
    [Textbook of Diabetes 4th ed pg 550]
    - During treatment of DKA, measurements of ketone levels in urine is in general unreliable.
    - These methods measure acetoacetate (which is quantitatively of minor importance compared to 3-OH-butyrate) and acetoacetate in urine may exhibit a paradoxical initial increase because of increasing blood concentrations (and low urine production), despite successful treatment.
    - Acetone measured by standard urine dipstick methods may continue to be excreted for up to 48 hours after the onset of treatment as it is fat soluble and leaches out slowly during treatment.

40. **Ans. (b) Mild diabetes**
    [Williams 13th ed pg 1391; Textbook of Diabetes 4th ed pg 245, 247]

    ### Maturity-onset Diabetes of the Young (MODY)
    - Autosomal dominant mode of inheritance
    - Young age of onset (usually <25 years)

- Noninsulin-dependent, nonketotic
- Results from β-cell dysfunction rather than insulin resistance.
- Linked to mutations in the gene encoding the glucose sensing enzyme glucokinase (*GCK*) and mutations in several transcription factors that affect β-cell development and function.
- Clinical presentation varies greatly depending on the underlying genetic mutation–familial mild fasting hyperglycemia in glucokinase gene mutations (*GCK* MODY), familial young-onset progressive diabetes in *HNF1A* and *HNF4A* mutations (transcription factor MODY) and renal cysts and diabetes syndrome (RCAD) in *HNF1B* mutations
- Microvascular complications are rare in glucokinase MODY, but frequent in transcription factor MODY.

41. **Ans. (e) Triamcinolone**
    [International Textbook of Diabetes Mellitus 4th ed pg 893; Diabetic Retinopathy pg 270; Diabetes Mellitus: A Fundamental and Clinical Text 3rd ed pg 1471, 1472; Textbook of Diabetes 4th ed pg 589, 590]

    Intravitreal triamcinolone has shown promising results in the short term by reducing macular thickness, inducing reabsorption of hard exudates and improving the vision in eyes with chronic diabetic macular edema unresponsive to conventional laser treatment.

42. **Ans. (d) Persistence or progression of hyperglycemia-induced microvascular alterations during subsequent periods of normal glucose homeostasis**
    [Williams 13th ed pg 1486]

43. **Ans. (b) Nod mouse**
    [Williams 13th ed pg 1416-1418; 1452-1454]

    ### Rodent Models of Type 2 Diabetes Mellitus
    #### Mouse Models of Type 2 Diabetes Mellitus
    - Leptin (Lep^{ob}) and Leptin Receptor (db) Mutations (ob mouse and db mouse)
    - Agouti mouse
    - KK mouse
    - New Zealand Obese (NZO) Mouse
    - Gold thioglucose–induced diabetes
    - Diabetes induced by fat ablation
    - C57BL/6J (also known as B6) mouse fed a high-fat diet

    #### Rat Models of Type 2 Diabetes Mellitus
    - Zucker diabetic fatty rat (fa/fa)
    - Goto-Kakizaki (GK) rat
    - BHE/Cdb Rat
    - Psammomys obesus (Sand Rat)
    - Otsuka long-evans tokushima fatty (OLETF) rat
    - Neonatal streptozotocin

Animal Models of Type 1 Diabetes Mellitus
- Nonobese diabetic (NOD) mice
- Biobreeding (BB rat) rat
- *Induced Models of Type 1 Diabetes Mellitus:* Agents used—streptozotocin, copolymer of polyinosinic and polycytidylic acids (poly-IC), alloxan.

44. **Ans. (b) 270–300**

45. **Ans. (a) Transcription factor**
    [Williams 13th ed pg 1391; Textbook of Diabetes 4th ed pg 245, 247]
    See discussion of Chapter 21, Question 40.

46. **Ans. (b) Glycemic index multiplied by carbohydrate content of food**
    [Textbook of Diabetes 4th ed pg 350]
    The glycemic load considers the amount as well as the quality of carbohydrate and is defined as gram of carbohydrate within the food multiplied with the glycemic index of the food divided by 100.

47. **Ans. (a) GLP**
    [Williams 13th ed pg 1410]

48. **Ans. (b) It is closely homologous to proinsulin**
    [Williams 13th ed pg 977]
    - The IGFs (somatomedins) are a family of peptides that are, in part, GH dependent and mediate many of the anabolic and mitogenic actions of GH.
    - There are two IGFs circulating in humans, IGF-1 and IGF-2.
    - The two peptides have 50% amino acid homology to insulin. Like insulin, both IGFs have A and B chains connected by disulfide bonds.
    - The connecting C-peptide region bear no homology for the C-peptide region of proinsulin.
    - The structural similarity explains the ability of both IGFs to bind to the insulin receptor and the ability of insulin to bind to the type I IGF receptor.
    - The human IGF-1 gene (*IGF1*) is located on the long arm of chromosome 12.

49. **Ans. (b) Islet cell antibodies**
    [International Textbook of Diabetes Mellitus 4th ed pg 20]
    The first large-scale studies of the prediction of T1DM relied upon the detection of cytoplasmic islet cell autoantibodies (ICA) assays based on indirect immunofluorescence.

50. **Ans. (c) Glycemic control**
    [Textbook of Diabetes 4th ed pg 454]
    "Legacy" effect-early intensive glycemic control confers an extended reduction in complications, even when control deteriorates at later stages in the disease process.

51. Ans. (d) Preferably used in gastroparesis
[Textbook of Diabetes 4th ed pg 1431; Levin and O'Neal's The Diabetic Foot 7th ed pg 393]

Patients with gastroparesis have markedly delayed absorption of food; therefore the rapid-acting insulin analogues may cause hypoglycemia before food is absorbed.

52. Ans. (a) Decrease insulin level
[Williams 13th ed pg 1389; Textbook of Diabetes 4th ed pg 257]

Lipoatrophic Diabetes
- Monogenic form of diabetes
- Lipoatrophy and lipodystrophy—characterized by a paucity of fat
- Severe insulin resistance
- Hypertriglyceridemia
- Hepatic steatosis
- *Genetic forms:*
  - Face-sparing partial lipoatrophy (the Dunnigan or Koberling-Dunnigan syndrome)
    - Autosomal dominant form
    - Caused by mutations in the lamin A/C gene
  - Congenital generalized lipoatrophy (the Seip-Berardinelli syndrome)
    - Autosomal recessive form
    - Appears to be due to mutations in either 1-acylsn-glycerol-3-phosphate acyltransferase-2 (*AGPAT2*) or in the seipin gene product.

53. Ans. (b) Action on hyperglycemia in 4–5 days
[Textbook of Diabetes 4th ed pg 465-468]

Thiazolidinediones produce a slowly generated antihyperglycemic effect which usually requires 2–3 months to reach maximum effect.

54. Ans. (a) Kearns-Sayre syndrome
[Williams 13th ed pg 1772]

Kearns-Sayre Syndrome
- Characterized by
  - Myopathic abnormalities leading to ophthalmoplegia and progressive weakness
  - *Endocrine abnormalities:*
    - Hypoparathyroidism,
    - Primary gonadal failure,
    - Diabetes mellitus,
    - Hypopituitarism.
  - Retinitis pigmentosa
  - Heart block.
- Associated with deletions in mitochondrial DNA—usually sporadic
- May have autoimmune components.

55. **Ans. (b) Nateglinide**
   [Indian Journal of Endocrinology and Metabolism. Volume 21, Issue 2, March-April 2017 pg 344-345]

56. **Ans. (b) Saturated fat < 7% if LDL > 100 mg/dL**
   [International Textbook of Diabetes Mellitus 4th ed pg 578; Textbook of Diabetes 4th ed pg 347; Cardiovascular Prevention and Rehabilitation pg 195, 196]
   See discussion of Chapter 21, Question 28.

57. **Ans. (d) All of the above**
   [Textbook of Diabetes 4th ed pg 844, 845; Williams 13th ed pg 648, 649]

58. **Ans. (b) Exenatide**
   [Diabetes Care Volume 41, Supplement 1, January 2018 pg S75-S77]

59. **Ans. (a) Uremia**
   [Renal and Electrolyte Disorders pg 96; Harrison's Principles of Internal Medicine 19th ed pg 320]

60. **Ans. (a) Autonomic neuropathy**
   [Williams 13th ed pg 1486; Diabetes Care 2015 Jan; 38(1): 141]

   ### Patient and Disease Factors which Influence Intensiveness of Glucose Lowering
   - *Risk of hypoglycemia and other drug adverse effects:* Low-more stringent; high-less stringent
   - *Disease duration:* Newly diagnosed—more stringent; long standing—less stringent
   - *Life expectancy:* Long—more stringent; short—less stringent
   - *Comorbidities:* Absent—more stringent; severe—less stringent
   - *Established vascular complications:* Absent—more stringent; severe—less stringent
   - *Patient attitude and expected treatment efforts:* Highly motivated, adherent, excellent self-care capacities—more stringent; less motivated, nonadherent, poor self-care capacities—less stringent
   - *Resources and support system:* Readily available—more stringent; limited—less stringent.

   Thus patients with long-standing diabetes and autonomic neuropathy, may not subjectively sense symptoms of hypoglycemia even in the presence of low glucose concentrations. Glycemic targets of therapy should be adjusted upward in these patients, because they are at particularly high risk for hypoglycemia. Similarly, patients with advanced end-stage microvascular or macrovascular diabetic complications, in whom the benefit of intensive glucose control is likely to be less, should not be exposed to the increased risk of hypoglycemia that is inherent in extremely intensive insulin-treatment regimens.

61. Ans. (a) Diagnosis can be made by HbA$_{1c}$
[Diabetes Care Volume 41, Supplement 1, January 2018 pg S21, S22; International Textbook of Diabetes Mellitus 4th ed pg 824, 825]

Screening for and diagnosis of GDM

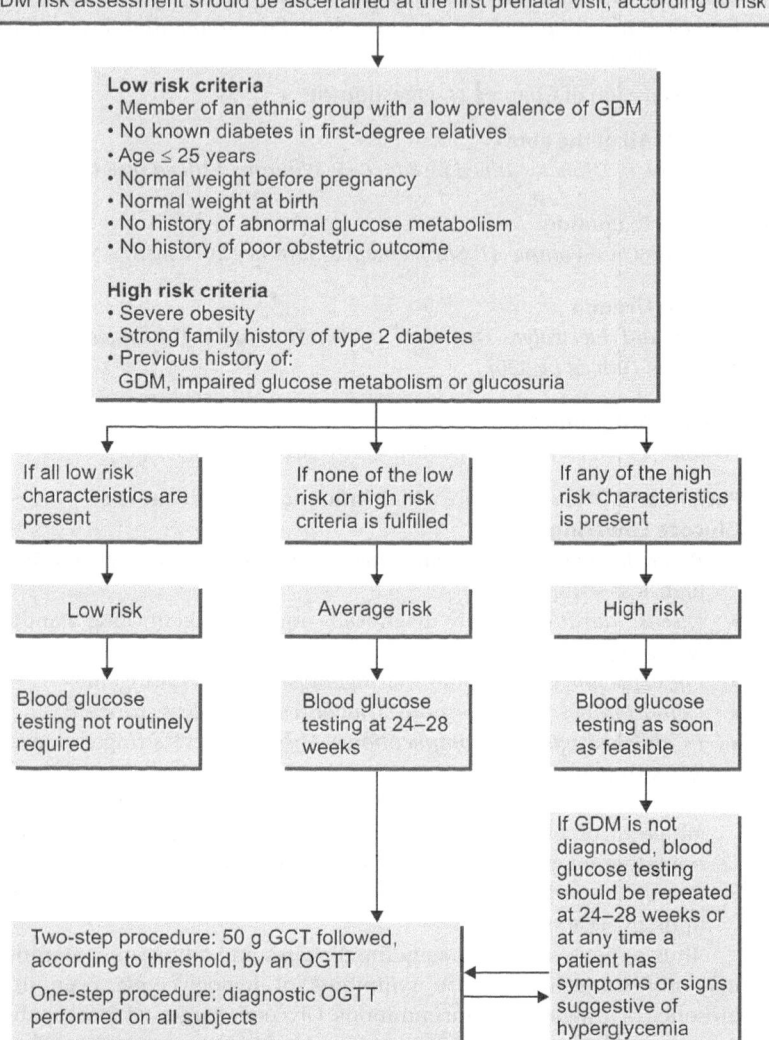

- *One-step strategy:*
  - Performa 75 g OGTT, with plasma glucose measurement when patient is fasting and at 1 and 2 hour, at 24-28 weeks of gestation in women not previously diagnosed with overt diabetes.

Diabetes | **271**

- The OGTT should be performed in the morning after an overnight fast of at least 8 hours.
- The diagnosis of GDM is made when any of the following plasma glucose values are met or exceeded:
    - *Fasting:* 92 mg/dL (5.1 mmol/L)
    - *1 hour:* 180 mg/dL (10.0 mmol/L)
    - *2 hours:* 153 mg/dL (8.5 mmol/L)
- *Two-step strategy:*
    - *Step 1:* Performa 50 g GLT (nonfasting), with plasma glucose measurement at 1 hour, at 24–28 weeks of gestation in women not previously diagnosed with overt diabetes.
        - If the plasma glucose levelmeasured 1 hour after the load is ≥130 mg/dL, 135 mg/dL, or 140 mg/dL (7.2 mmol/L, 7.5 mmol/L, or 7.8 mmol/L), proceed to a 100 g OGTT.
    - *Step 2:* The 100 g OGTT should be performed when the patient is fasting.
        - The diagnosis of GDM is made if at least two* of the following four plasma glucose levels (measured fasting and 1 h, 2 h, 3 h during OGTT) are met or exceeded:

	Carpenter-Coustan	NDDG
Fasting	95 mg/dL (5.3 mmol/L)	105 mg/dL (5.8 mmol/L)
1 h	180 mg/dL (10.0 mmol/L)	190 mg/dL (10.6 mmol/L)
2 h	155 mg/dL (8.6 mmol/L)	165 mg/dL (9.2 mmol/L)
3 h	140 mg/dL (7.8 mmol/L)	145 mg/dL (8.0 mmol/L)

NB: NDDG, National Diabetes Data Group.
- The use of A1C as a screening test for GDM does not function as well as the GLT.

62. **Ans. (b) Hypothyroidism**
[Textbook of Diabetes 4th ed pg 549]

Predisposing or Precipitating Factors for DKA
- Omission of insulin therapy (poor compliance is commonly seen in younger patients, patients with psychiatric illness)
- *Coexisting illness:*
    - Infection
    - Cardiovascular events (myocardial infarction, stroke)
    - Gastrointestinal disease
    - Inflammatory diseases
    - Pancreatitis
    - Trauma
    - Major surgery
    - Alcohol abuse
    - Drugs—especially glucocorticoids.

---

*ACOG recently noted that alternatively one elevated value can be used for diagnosis.

63. **Ans. (c) Bicarbonates are routinely used**
    [International Textbook of Diabetes Mellitus 4th ed pg 805, 808-11]

64. **Ans. (a) Bradycardia**
    [Textbook of Diabetes 4th ed pg 549]

    ### Common Clinical Features of Diabetic Ketoacidosis
    Symptoms
    - Polyuria, polydipsia
    - Rapid weight loss
    - Muscular weakness
    - Visual disturbance
    - Air hunger with Kussmaul respiration, dry lips
    - Abdominal pain, leg cramps
    - Nausea, vomiting
    - Confusion, drowsiness, coma

    Signs
    - Poor skin turgor
    - Hyperventilation (Kussmaul respirations)
    - Hypotension
    - Tachycardia
    - Impairment of mental state
    - Patients may have infections but with normothermia/hypothermia.

65. **(d) Insulin glargine**
    [Williams 13th ed pg 1469]
    - In the injection solution at pH 4, insulin glargine is completely soluble. However, it has low solubility at neutral pH.
    - After injection into the subcutaneous tissue, the acidic solution is neutralized, leading to the formation of microprecipitates from which small amounts of insulin glargine are slowly released; this results in absorption over a period of approximately 24 hours with no pronounced peak.
    - Because this insulin is provided in an acid vehicle, it cannot be mixed with other forms of insulin or intravenous fluids.

66. **Ans. (d) Insulin glargine**
    [Williams 13th ed pg 1469, 1470]

    ### Insulin Preparations
    - Rapid-acting insulins
        - Regular insulin
        - Insulin analogues
            - Insulin lispro
            - Insulin aspart
            - Insulin glulisine

Diabetes | **273**

- Intermediate- and Long-acting insulins
  - Neutral protamine hagedorn insulin
  - Insulin glargine
  - Insulin detemir insulin glargine U-300
  - Insulin degludec
  - Pegylated insulin lispro.

67. **Ans. (c) Increased Hematocrit**
    [Williams 13th ed pg 1427; [Textbook of Diabetes 4th ed pg 468]

68. **Ans. (b) Pioglitazone/Gemfibrozil**
    [Williams 13th ed pg 1694; Textbook of Diabetes 4th ed pg 465]

69. **Ans. (a) Life style modification**
    [Diabetes Care Volume 41, Supplement 1, January 2018 pg S75-S76]

70. **Ans. (a) Metformin**
    [J Diabetes Complications. 2017 Jan;31(1):21-30]

71. **Ans. (b) Increases gastric emptying**
    [Therapy for Diabetes Mellitus and Related Disorders, ADA, 6th ed pg 401]

    The Major Effects of GLP-1 include
    - Enhanced glucose-stimulated insulin biosynthesis and secretion
    - Suppression of postprandial glucagon release
    - Decreased appetite and food intake
    - Reduced hepatic glucose production
    - Delayed gastric emptying.

72. **Ans. (c) 60-year-old male with normal creatinine clearance**
    [Therapy for Diabetes Mellitus and Related Disorders, ADA, 6th ed pg 347]

CHAPTER 22

Hypoglycemia

QUESTIONS

1. Infant presented with hypoglycemia 1st investigation to be done is:
   a. Cortisol
   b. Insulin
   c. IGF-1
   d. None of the above

2. Glucagon dose in for treatment of hypoglycemia is:
   a. 1 mg
   b. 2 mg
   c. 4 mg
   d. 5 mg

3. Nonketotic hypoglycemia associated with:
   a. Glycogen storage disease
   b. FA oxidation defect
   c. Gluconeogenesis defect
   d. Hypopituitarism

4. Neonatal hypoglycemia with decreased esterified FA and ketones (BHBA):
   a. FA oxidation defect
   b. Glycogen storage disease
   c. Hyperinsulinemia
   d. Ketone synthesis defect

5. Recurrent hypoglycemia in a child seen in all except:
   a. Insulinoma
   b. Nesidioblastosis
   c. Glucagonoma
   d. Sulfonylurea administration

6. Anti-insulin antibody is detected by:
   a. Direct Immunofluorescence
   b. ELISA
   c. Indirect Immunofluorescence
   d. RIA

7. Hypoglycemia in mesenchymal tumors, due to release of:
   a. Insulin
   b. IGF-1
   c. IGF-II
   d. IGFBP3

8. **Cause of reactive hypoglycemia:**
   a. Gastrectomy
   b. Increase IGF2
   c. Galactosemia
   d. Hereditary fructose intolerance
   e. Congenital hyperinsulinism

9. **Hypoglycemic attacks do not occur in:**
   a. Glycogen storage diseases 1 and 3
   b. Pyruvate kinase deficiency
   c. Glycogen synthase deficiency
   d. Hereditary fructose intolerance

10. **Hypoglycemia in infants of diabetic mother latest in:**
    a. 1–4 hours
    b. 4–6 hours
    c. 6–12 hours
    d. 12–72 hours

11. **Insulinoma diagnostic criteria:**
    a. C-peptide >0.6
    b. Insulin >6
    c. Glucose <45
    d. All of the above
    e. Any of the above

12. **All of the following are correct about sulphonylurea induced hypoglycemia except:**
    a. Increased insulin
    b. Dilution antibodies not seen
    c. Low C-peptide
    d. Increased insulin/glucose ratio

13. **Insulinoma:**
    a. Serum insulin/glucose ratio more than 0.9 is diagnostic
    b. 32-hour fast required for diagnosis
    c. Diazoxide is Rx of choice
    d. Intraoperative pancreatic USG is helpful

14. **Which one of the following statements is true?**
    a. C-peptide levels differentiate between insulinoma and repaglinide toxicity
    b. Type 1 glycogen storage disease causes fasting hypoglycemia
    c. Cortisol plays an important role in acute hypoglycemia
    d. None of the above

15. **A 30-year-old lady presented to the casualty with coma. On admission her blood sugar level was 1.3 mmol/L; C-peptide level is low; plasma insulin levels are high. What is diagnosis?**
    a. Insulinoma
    b. Surreptitious use of sulfonylureas
    c. Exogenous use of insulin
    d. Psychogenic

16. **Physiological responses to hypoglycemia:**
    a. Decreased cognition
    b. Decreased glucagon
    c. Decreased cortisol
    d. Cholinergic activation

17. Low blood glucose level typically results in the secretion of all of the following except:
    a. Glucagon
    b. Thyroxine (T4)
    c. hGH
    d. PTH
    e. None of the above
18. The general adaptation syndrome (GAS) is activated by the:
    a. Hypothalamus
    b. Adrenal gland
    c. Pituitary gland
    d. Thyroid gland
    e. Release of glucocorticoids
19. A meal rich in proteins but low in carbohydrates does not cause hypoglycemia because:
    a. Glucagon secretion is stimulated by meals
    b. The meal causes compensatory increase in T4 secretion
    c. Cortisol in circulation prevents glucose from entering the muscles
    d. The amino acids in the meal are converted to glucose
20. Which of the following investigations is least common to order during hypoglycemia?
    a. Glucose level
    b. Insulin
    c. Cortisol
    d. Ketone
    e. Catecholamine
21. Which of the following is used in preparation prior to resection of an insulinoma?
    a. Propranolol
    b. Octreotide
    c. Phentolamine
    d. Phenoxybenzamine
22. All of the following can cause hypoglycemia except:
    a. Pentamidine
    b. Phenytoin
    c. Alcohol
    d. Quinine
23. Hepatic glycogen content is usually sufficient to maintain plasma glucose level for:
    a. 6 hours
    b. 4 hours
    c. 10 hours
    d. 8 hours

ANSWERS

1. **Ans. (d) None of the above**
   [J Pediatr. 2015 Aug;167(2):240, 242]

   Approach to Hypoglycemia in Neonates, Infants and Children
   - Whenever possible, specimens for identifying the etiology of hypoglycemia should be obtained at the time of spontaneous or induced hypoglycemia.
   - Assays for plasma glucose, bicarbonate, BOHB, and lactate are readily available and useful for distinguishing categories of hypoglycemia disorders.
   - Extra plasma can be held in reserve for specific tests based on the suspected diagnosis, additional tests can be performed, such as growth hormone (for suspected GHD), cortisol (for suspected adrenal insufficiency), total and free carnitine, acyl-carnitine profile, (for a suspected disorder of fatty acid oxidation) plasma insulin, FFA, C-peptide and proinsulin (for suspected hyperinsulinism), and drug screening.
   - For suspected hyperinsulinism, the fasting test can be terminated with administration of glucagon (1 mg IV, intramuscularly, or subcutaneously) to evaluate the glycemic response. An exaggerated glycemic response (>30 mg/dL [>1.7 mmol/L]) is nearly pathognomonic of hyperinsulinism.

   Adrenal insufficiency, congenital or acquired, may manifest with hypoglycemia. Simultaneous measurement of plasma adrenocorticotropic hormone and cortisol is recommended if primary adrenal insufficiency is suspected. An adrenocorticotropic hormone stimulation test may be needed.

Metabolic Clues of Hypoglycemia Diagnosis

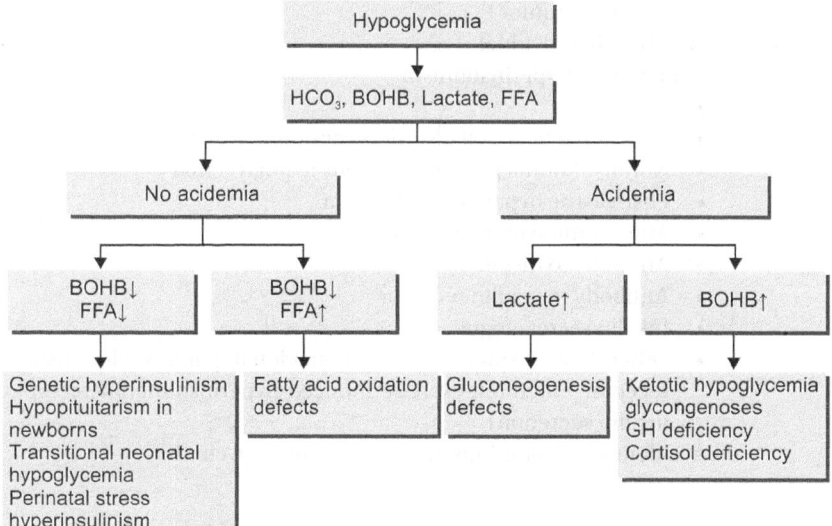

2. **Ans. (a) 1 mg**
   [Williams 13th ed pg 1595]

3. **Ans. (b) FA oxidation defect**
   [J Pediatr. 2015 Aug;167(2):240]
   See discussion of Chapter 22, Question 1.

4. **Ans. (b) Hyperinsulinemia**
   [J Pediatr. 2015 Aug;167(2):240]
   See discussion of Chapter 22, Question 1.

5. **Ans. (c) Glucagonoma**
   [Williams 13th ed pg 1587, 1600-02, 1730]
   Glucagonoma is characterized by hyperglycemia.

   Causes of Hypoglycemia in Adults
   - Ill or Medicated individual
     - Drugs
       - Insulin or insulin secretagogue
       - Alcohol
       - Others
     - Critical illnesses
       - Hepatic, renal, or cardiac failure
       - Sepsis
       - Inanition
     - Hormonal deficiency
       - Cortisol
       - Glucagon and epinephrine (in insulin-deficient diabetes mellitus)
     - Non-islet cell tumor
   - Seemingly well individual
     - Endogenous hyperinsulinism
       - Insulinoma
       - Functional beta-cell disorders (nesidioblastosis)
       - Noninsulinoma pancreatogenous hypoglycemia
       - Post-gastric bypass hypoglycemia
       - Autoimmune hypoglycemia
       - Antibody to insulin
       - Antibody to insulin receptor
       - Insulin secretagogue
       - Other (e.g. insulin binding monoclonal paraprotein, insulin receptor mutation, exercise induced hyperinsulinemia, ectopic insulin secretion)
     - Accidental, surreptitious, or malicious hypoglycemia.

Hypoglycemia in children can be caused by the same mechanisms as in adults. In addition, several hypoglycemic disorders are unique to, or have their onset in, infancy and childhood.

Causes of Hypoglycemia Unique to, or Typically with Onset in, Infancy and Childhood

- Intolerance of fasting
  - Preterm or small-for-gestational-age infants
  - Hypopituitarism, adrenal hypoplasia, congenital adrenal hyperplasia
  - Ketotic hypoglycemia of childhood
- Hyperinsulinism
  - Infant of a diabetic mother
  - Maternal drugs (sulfonylurea, β2-adrenergic agonist)
  - *Congenital hyperinsulinism:* Mutations in sulfonylurea receptor-1 (SUR1), the potassium inward rectifying channel (Kir6.2), glucokinase (GK), glutamate dehydrogenase (GDH), short-chain 3-hydroxyacyl-CoA dehydrogenase (SCHAD), monocarboxylate transporter 1 (MCT1), HNF4A and HNF1A; Insulinoma
  - *Others:* Rh incompatibility, Beckwith-Wiedemann syndrome, exchange transfusions, perinatal stress
- Activating mutations in the postreceptor insulin signalling pathway (e.g. *AKT2* gene)
- Enzyme defects
  - *Carbohydrate metabolism:* Glycogen storage disease types Ia (von Gierke disease, glucose-6-phosphatase deficiency), Ib (glucose-6-phosphate transporter defect), III (amylo-1,6-glucosidase deficiency), VI (glycogen phosphorylase deficiency) and IX (phosphorylase kinase deficiency); glycogen synthase deficiency (GSD type 0); fructose-1,6-bisphosphatase deficiency, phosphoenolpyruvate carboxykinase deficiency, and pyruvate carboxylase deficiency; hereditary fructose intolerance (Fructose-1-phosphate aldolase deficiency); galactosemia (Galactose-1-phosphat-Uridyltransferase deficiency, GALT), GLUT2 deficiency (in Fanconi-Bickel syndrome)
  - *Protein metabolism:* Branched-chain α-keto acid dehydrogenase complex deficiency
  - *Fat metabolism:* Fatty acid oxidation defects including deficiencies in the carnitine cycle [primary carnitine deficiency due to autosomal recessive mutations in the carnitine transporter (OCTN2), carnitine palmitoyltransferase 1, CPT1 deficiency, carnitine acylcarnitine translocase (CACT) deficiency, and carnitine palmitoyltransferase 2, CPT2 deficiency], the β-oxidation spiral [e.g. very long-, long-, medium- and short-chain acyl-CoA dehydrogenase deficiency], the electron transport system [glutaric acidemia type 2], and the ketogenesis sequence [3-hydroxy-3-methylglutaryl coenzyme A (HMG-CoA) synthase deficiency, and HMG-CoA lyase deficiency].

6. **Ans. (d) RIA**
   [https://www.mayomedicallaboratories.com/test-catalog/Overview/8666]

7. **Ans. (c) IGF-II**
   [Williams 13th ed pg 1597]

   Non-islet cell tumor hypoglycemia (NICTH) is caused by mesenchymal tumors. The tumors are usually large. NICTH is often the result of overproduction of incompletely processed pro-insulin-like growth factor 2 (pro-IGF-2), but overproduction of insulin-like growth factor 1 (IGF-1) has also been reported. Concentrations of plasma free IGF-2 (or IGF-1) are elevated. Because of suppression of growth hormone secretion and the resulting low IGF-1 levels, the ratio of plasma IGF-2 to IGF-1 is elevated.

8. **Ans. (a) Gastrectomy**
   [De Groot 7th ed pg 826]

   Reactive hypoglycemia refers to hypoglycemia that occurs after meals. Conditions associated with hypoglycemia only after meal ingestion include:
   - *Alimentary:* gastrectomy, vagotomy and pyloroplasty, esophageal resection, altered gastric motility, peptic ulcer disease, renal glycosuria.
   - Prediabetes (usually seen during OGTT).
   - *Idiopathic:* Some of these patients have noninsulinoma pancreatogenous hypoglycemia syndrome (NIPHS).

9. **Ans. (b) Pyruvate kinase deficiency**
   [Williams 13th ed pg 1587, 1600-1602]

   See discussion of Chapter 22, Question 5.

10. **Ans. (d) 12-72 hours**
    [https://www.uptodate.com/contents/infant-of-a-diabetic-mother]

11. **Ans. (d) All of the above**
    [Greenspan's 9th ed]

Diagnostic criteria for insulinoma after a 72-hour fast	
Plasma glucose	<45 mg/dL
Plasma insulin (RIA)	≥6 µU/mL
Plasma insulin (ICMA)	≥3 µU/mL
Plasma C-peptide	≥200 pmol/L
Plasma proinsulin	≥5 pmol/L
β-hydroxybutyrate	≥2.7 nmol/L
Sulfonylurea screen (including repaglinide and nateglinide)	Negative

12. **Ans. (c) Low C-peptide**
    [Williams 13th ed pg 1598, 1599]

    ### Approach to Hypoglycemia
    - Document Whipple's triad (symptoms, signs, or both consistent with hypoglycemia; a low plasma glucose concentration; and resolution of those symptoms or signs after the plasma glucose concentration is raised).
    - Seek clues to specific disorders such as drugs, critical illnesses, hormone deficiencies, or non-islet cell tumors.
    - If the cause of a hypoglycemic disorder is not evident (i.e. in a seemingly healthy individual) assess the following during an episode of hypoglycemia:
        - Plasma glucose
        - Insulin
        - C-peptide
        - Proinsulin
        - β-hydroxybutyrate
        - Screen for oral hypoglycemic agents
        - Plasma glucose response to IV glucagon 1.0 mg
        - Insulin antibodies.2
    - If Whipple's triad has not been documented an attempt should be made to recreate the circumstances in which symptomatic hypoglycemia is likely to occur. This can be accomplished by a prolonged supervised fast in a patient with a history suggestive of fasting hypoglycemia or by providing a mixed meal in a patient with a history suggestive of postprandial hypoglycemia.

Interpretation of Results

Patterns of findings during fasting or after a mixed meal in normal individuals and in individuals with hyperinsulinemic (or IGF-mediated) hypoglycemia or hypoglycemia caused by other mechanisms

Symptoms, signs or both	Glucose (mg/dL)	Insulin (μU/mL)	C-Peptide (nmol/L)	Proinsulin (pmol/L)	β-hydro-xybutyrate (mmol/L)	Glucose increase after glucagon (mg/dL)	Circulating oral hypoglycemic agent	Antibody to insulin	Diagnostic interpretation
No	<55	<3	<0.2	<5	<2.7	<25	No	No	Normal
Yes	<55	>>3	<0.2	<5	≤2.7	>25	No	Neg (Pos)	Exogenous insulin
Yes	<55	≥3	≥0.2	≥5	≤2.7	>25	No	Neg	Insulinoma, NIPHS, PGBH
Yes	<55	≥3	≥0.2	≥5	≤2.7	>25	Yes	Neg	Oral hypoglycemic agent
Yes	<55	>>3	>>0.2	>>5	≤2.7	>25	No	Pos	Insulin autoimmune
Yes	<55	<3	<0.2	<5	≤2.7	>25	No	Neg	IGF
Yes	<55	<3	<0.2	<5	>2.7	<25	No	Neg	Not insulin- or IGF-mediated

13. **Ans. (d) Intraoperative pancreatic USG is helpful**
    [Williams 13th ed pg 1598-1600; De Groot 7th ed pg 835, 836, 2611; The Journal of Clinical Endocrinology & Metabolism, Volume 94, Issue 3, 1 March 2009, Pages 715]
    - Insulinomas are insulin-secreting pancreatic β-cell tumors.
    - Typically presents in the postabsorptive (fasting) state. However, some report symptoms exclusively in the postprandial state.
    - Mostly benign (<10% are malignant insulinomas, multiple insulinomas, or the multiple endocrine neoplasia type 1 (MEN1) syndrome].
    - 99% of insulinomas occur within the pancreas. Others are mostly found in the wall of the duodenum or gastrosplenic omentum.
    - Pancreatic insulinomas average about 2 cm in diameter and appear with equal frequency in the head, body, and tail.
    - Diagnostic approach
      Documentation of hypoglycemia associated with inappropriate hyperinsulinemia:
      – A patient with documented whipple triad, inappropriately high levels of insulin, C-peptide, and proinsulin and no detectable circulating oral hypoglycemic agent; suppressed β-hydroxybutyrate levels; a brisk glycemic response to IV glucagon during hypoglycemia; and no circulating insulin antibody may have an insulinoma. (See discussion of Chapter 22, Question 12)
      – If Whipple triad has not been documented a patient with a history suggestive of fasting hypoglycemia should undergo a prolonged supervised fast (72-hour fast).
      Localization:
      – Available modalities
        ♦ Computed tomography (CT)
        ♦ Magnetic resonance imaging (MRI)
        ♦ Transabdominal ultrasonography
        ♦ *Endoscopic pancreatic ultrasonography (EUS):* Sensitivity >90%
        ♦ Somatostatin receptor scintigraphy
        ♦ Positron emission tomography with radiotracers such as fluorine-18-labeled dihydroxyphenylalanine
        ♦ Selective pancreatic arterial calcium injections (end point: at least a twofold increase in hepatic venous insulin levels over baseline)
        ♦ *Intraoperative pancreatic ultrasonography:* Most sensitive
      – Currently, preoperative transabdominal ultrasonography followed by intraoperative ultrasonography is considered the most sensitive and specific approach and has been recommended for routine use; this approach along with palpation can be used to detect >95% of tumors.
    - *Treatment:*
      – Surgery is the treatment of choice for insulinoma

- In unresectable disease empirical treatments (diet, diazoxide, octreotide, everolimus) can be tried; there has been progress with chemotherapy (streptozocin ± fluorouracil, mithramycin, doxorubicin have been tried).
- Ratios employing insulin and glucose have no diagnostic utility.

14. **Ans. (b) Type 1 glycogen storage causes fasting hypoglycemia**
    [Williams 13th ed pg 1584,1601]
    See discussion of Chapter 22, Questions 5, 12 and 16.

15. **Ans. (c) Exogenous use of insulin**
    [Williams 13th ed pg 1599]
    See discussion of Chapter 22, Question 12.

16. **Ans. (d) Cholinergic activation**
    [Williams 13th ed pg 1584]

Physiologic responses to decreasing plasma glucose concentrations			
Response	*Glycemic threshold [mmol/L (mg/dL)]*	*Physiologic effects*	*Role in prevention or correction of hypoglycemia (Glucose counter-regulation)*
↓ Insulin	4.4–4.7 (80–85)	↑ Ra (↓ Rd)	Primary glucose regulatory factor, first defense against hypoglycemia
↑ Glucagon	3.6–3.9 (65–70)	↑ Ra	Primary glucose counter-regulatory factor, second defense against hypoglycemia
↑ Epinephrine	3.6–3.9 (65–70)	↑ Ra, ↓ Rc	Involved, critical when glucagon is deficient, third defense against hypoglycemia
↑ Cortisol and growth hormone	3.6–3.9 (65–70)	↑ Ra, ↓ Rc	Involved, not critical
Symptoms	2.8–3.1 (50–55)	↑ Exogenous glucose	Prompt behavioral defense (food ingestion)
↓ Cognition	<2.8 (50)	—	(Compromises behavioral defense)

Symptoms of Hypoglycemia Include
- Neurogenic (or autonomic) symptoms
  - Caused by sympathoadrenal (particularly the sympathetic neural) discharge
  - Include:
    - *Adrenergic (catecholamine-mediated) symptoms:* Palpitations, tremor, anxiety/arousal
    - *Cholinergic (acetylcholine-mediated) symptoms:* Sweating, hunger, paresthesias.

- Neuroglycopenic symptoms
  - Direct result of brain glucose deprivation.
  - *Include:* Cognitive impairments, behavioral changes, psychomotor abnormalities, seizure and coma.

17. **Ans. (b) Thyroxine (T4)**
    [Williams 13th ed pg 1584; Metabolism Clinical and Experimental, 2002 Oct, Volume 51, Issue 10, pg 1370-1374; PLoS One. 2013;8(1):e54209]

18. **Ans. (a) Hypothalamus**
    [British Medical Journal, June 1950, pg 1383-1392]

19. **Ans. (a) Glucagon secretion is stimulated by meals**
    [Diabetes Mellitus: A Fundamental and Clinical Text 3rd ed pg 662]

20. **Ans. (e) Catecholamine**
    [Williams 13th ed pg 1598]
    See discussion of Chapter 22, Question 12.

21. **Ans. (b) Octreotide**
    [Indian Journal of Anaesthesia. 2012 Mar-Apr; 56(2): 117-122]

    Perioperative management prior to resection of an insulinoma: Intravenous infusion of 10% dextrose should be started for the fasting period. Frequent glucose monitoring is important to prevent plasma glucose level to fall below 40-50 mg/dL at any time. Diazoxide and somatostatin analogues are continued in the morning of surgery to reduce insulin secretion intraoperatively while handling of the tumor.

22. **Ans. (b) Phenytoin**
    [Williams 13th ed pg 1597]

    ### Drugs (Other Than Antihyperglycemic Agents and Alcohol) causing Hypoglycemia
    - Moderate quality of evidence
      - Cibenzoline
      - Gatifloxacin
      - Pentamidine
      - Quinine
      - Indomethacin
      - Glucagon (during endoscopy)
    - Low quality of evidence
      - Chloroquinoxaline sulfonamide
      - Artesunate/artemisinin/artemether
      - Insulin-like growth factor type 1
      - Lithium
      - Propoxyphene/dextropropoxyphene
    - Very low quality of evidence
      - Angiotensin-converting enzyme inhibitors

- Angiotensin receptor antagonists
- β-adrenergic receptor antagonists
- Levofloxacin
- Mifepristone
- Disopyramide
- Trimethoprim-sulfamethoxazole
- Heparin
- 6-Mercaptopurine

23. **Ans. (d) 8 hours**
    [Williams 13th ed pg 1584]
    - The glucose pool (free glucose in the extracellular fluids and in the cells of certain tissues, primarily liver) is 15–20 g. Glycogen contains approximately 70 g glucose (*range:* 25–130 g).
      Therefore, in an adult of average size, preformed glucose can provide < 8-hour supply.
    - If fasting is prolonged 24–48 hours, hepatic glycogen content falls to less than 55 mmol (10 g), and gluconeogenesis becomes the sole source of glucose production.

CHAPTER 23

Obesity

QUESTIONS

1. Prader-Willi syndrome is characterized by all except:
   a. Hypertonia
   b. Obesity
   c. Short stature
   d. Hypogonadism

2. In android obesity waist hip ratio is:
   a. > 0.65
   b. > 0.85
   c. > 0.25
   d. > 0.75

3. Increased in obesity are all except:
   a. IGF-1
   b. IGF-BP3
   c. Insulin
   d. Impaired GTT

4. Fatty liver defined as increase in weight of liver due to:
   a. > 5% TG
   b. > 10% TG
   c. > 5% cholesterol
   d. > 10% cholesterol

5. Prader-Willi syndrome is characterized by all except:
   a. Obesity
   b. Hyperphagia
   c. IGT
   d. Short height
   e. Retinitis pigmentosa

6. Anorexigenic agents:
   a. Ghrelin
   b. NPY
   c. Leptin
   d. CRH

7. True about leptin is:
   a. Decreases in obesity
   b. Suppresses appetite
   c. Stimulates appetite
   d. Secreted by hypothalamus

8. All is true about metabolic syndrome in Indians except:
   a. Waist circumference > 90 cm in males and > 80 cm in females
   b. TG levels > 150 mg%
   c. BP > 130/85 mm Hg
   d. FBS < 100 mg%

9. Clinical features of Bardet–Biedl syndrome include all except:
   a. Mental retardation
   b. Obesity
   c. GnRH deficiency
   d. Central DI
   e. Short stature

10. True about leptin—all except:
    a. 167 amino acids
    b. Level increased in night
    c. Released from adipocytes
    d. Increase body fat

11. A 38-year-old male presents with gross obesity. What is the average daily energy used by a male of this age?
    a. 1500 kcal
    b. 2000 kcal
    c. 2500 kcal
    d. 3000 kcal
    e. 3500 kcal

Obesity | **289**

ANSWERS

1. **Ans. (a) Hypertonia**
   [Williams 13th ed pg 1143]

   Prader-Willi Syndrome
   - Autosomal dominant disorder
   - Lack of a functional paternal 15q11-q13 region, caused by any of a variety of genetic mechanisms, can result in the syndrome.
     - 70% of Prader-Willi cases are caused by a paternal deletion of 15q11-q13;
     - 20-25% of cases involve maternal uniparental disomy in which both chromosomes 15 are derived from the mother (genomic imprinting);
     - In 2-5% of cases, an imprinting center defect has been detected.
   - *Characterized by:*
     - Intrauterine growth retardation, delayed onset and poor fetal activity
     - Infantile central hypotonia, and lethargy
     - Early-onset childhood hyperphagia, pathologic obesity
     - Carbohydrate intolerance (leading to type 2 diabetes)
     - Short stature,
     - Small hands and feet
     - Mild to moderate mental retardation
     - Emotional instability, including perseveration, obsessions, and compulsions
     - Almond-shaped eyes, a triangular mouth, and narrow bifrontal diameter
     - Delayed puberty and hypogonadotropic hypogonadism caused by combined hypothalamic and gonadal dysfunction
     - *Male subjects:* Micropenis, cryptorchidism, underdeveloped scrotum
     - *Female subjects:* Underdevelopment of the labia majora, labia minora, or clitoris; amenorrhea/irregular menses/spotting
     - Risk for sudden death due to gastrointestinal, respiratory, or cardiac complications.

2. **Ans. (b) > 0.85**
   [Clinical Gynecologic Endocrinology and Infertility 7th ed pg 479]

3. **Ans. (a) IGF-1**
   [Curr Opin Endocrinol Diabetes Obes. 2013 Feb;20(1):45, 47; Obesity: Mechanisms and Clinical Management pg 159; Greenspan's 9th ed]

   Obesity is associated with decreased baseline GH levels and responses to stimuli while IGF-1 is concentration may be normal, high or slightly reduced. Changes in the production of IGF binding proteins (decreased IGFBP-1 and IGFBP-2 and increased IGFBP-3) may result in increased free IGF-1 fractions.

4. **Ans. (a) >5% TG**
   [Zakim and Boyer's Hepatology 7th ed pg 391]

5. **Ans. (e) Retinitis pigmentosa**
   [Williams 13th ed pg 1143]
   See discussion of Chapter 23, Question 1.

6. **Ans. (c) Leptin**
   [Greenspan's 9th ed; De Groot 7th ed pg 459, 461; Harrison's Endocrinology 3rd ed pg 236]

   Factors that Regulate Appetite

Increase appetite	Decrease appetite
Adipose tissue derived peptide	
	Leptin
GI and pancreatic peptides	
Ghrelin	Cholecystokinin (CCK)
	Peptide YY3-36 (PYY)
	Glucagon-like peptide 1 (GLP-1)
	Pancreatic polypeptide (PP)
Hypothalamic neuropeptides	
Neuropeptide-Y (NPY)	α-melanocyte-stimulating hormone (α-MSH)
Melanin-concentrating hormone (MCH)	Cocaine-amphetamine-regulated transcript (CART)
Agouti-related peptide (AgRP)	GLP-1
Orexin	Serotonin
Endocannabinoid	Corticotropin-releasing hormone
Galanin	Urocortin
β-endorphin	Neurotensin
Dynorphin	Neuromedin
Enkephalin	

7. **Ans. (b) Suppresses appetite**
   [Williams 13th ed pg 1616; De Groot 7th ed pg 461]

8. **Ans. (d) FBS < 100 mg%**
   [Harrison's Endocrinology 3rd ed pg 253]

   NCEP-ATPIII 2001 Criteria for Metabolic Syndrome
   Three or more of the following:
   - *Central obesity:* Waist circumference >102 cm (M), >88 cm (F)
   - *Hypertriglyceridemia:* Triglycerides 150 mg/dL or specific medication
   - *Low HDL cholesterol:* <40 mg/dL and <50 mg/dL, respectively, or specific medication

- *Hypertension:* Blood pressure ≥130 mm Hg systolic or ≥85 mm Hg diastolic or specific medication
- Fasting plasma glucose ≥100 mg/dL or specific medication or previously diagnosed type 2 diabetes.

IDF Criteria for Metabolic Syndrome
- *Waist circumference:*
  - Men: ≥94 cm / Women: ≥80 cm (Europid, Sub-Saharan African, Eastern and Middle Eastern)
  - Men: ≥90 cm / Women: ≥80 cm (South Asian, Chinese, and ethnic South and Central American)
  - Men: ≥85 cm / Women: ≥90 cm (Japanese)
- *Two or more of the following:*
  - Fasting triglycerides >150 mg/dL or specific medication
  - HDL cholesterol <40 mg/dL and <50 mg/dL for men and women, respectively, or specific medication
  - Blood pressure >130 mm Hg systolic or >85 mm Hg diastolic or previous diagnosis or specific medication
  - Fasting plasma glucose ≥100 mg/dL or previously diagnosed type 2 diabetes.

9. **Ans. (d) Central DI**
   [De Groot 7th ed pg 182]

Bardet-Biedl Syndrome
- Autosomal recessive
- *Clinical features:*
  - Obesity and poor growth,
  - Retinitis pigmentosa,
  - Renal and urogenital abnormalities,
  - Hypogonadotropic hypogonadism,
  - Polydactyly.
- *Neurobehavioral Profile:* Spastic paraplegia, developmental delay, decreased IQ, altered fine-motor function, and reduced olfactive function.
- *Other abnormalities:*
  - Hearing loss,
  - Hepatic fibrosis,
  - Diabetes mellitus,
  - Hypertension,
  - Congenital heart disease.
- Ciliary defects are likely the predominant cause of BBS phenotypes.
- Hyperleptinemia consequent to hypothalamic leptin resistance is the main abnormality in the neuroendocrine control of food intake in BBS resulting in increased appetite, and obesity.

10. **Ans. (d) Increase body fat**
    [Williams 13th ed pg 1616; De Groot 7th ed pg 169]
    Leptin is synthesized within the adipocyte and plasma concentrations are directly related to adipocyte (fat) mass. It acts on centres within the hypothalamus to produce satiety.

11. **Ans. (c) 2500 kcal**
    [Park's Textbook of Preventive and Social Medicine 23rd ed pg 636]

CHAPTER
24

Disorders of Lipid Metabolism

QUESTIONS

1. True about triglycerides are all except:
   a. Fibrate and niacin are used in Rx of hypertriglyceridemia
   b. Does not specifically increase risk of CAD
   c. Chylomicronemia syndrome is associated with severe hypertriglyceridemia
   d. Omega-6 FA are used in Rx

2. All of the following have LDL receptor mediated effect except:
   a. Simvastatin
   b. Ezetimibe
   c. Cholestyramine
   d. Niacin

3. Increased HDL is associated with all except:
   a. Alcohol
   b. Exercise
   c. Fibrates
   d. Progesterone

4. True about estrogen are all except:
   a. ↓ TBG
   b. ↑ HDL
   c. ↓ LDL
   d. ↑ LDL receptor in liver

5. Hypertriglyceridemia is a feature of all except:
   a. Lipodystrophy
   b. Alcohol
   c. AIP
   d. DM/obesity

6. Hyper cholesterolemia is seen in all except:
   a. Cigarette smoking
   b. Nephrotic syndrome
   c. Chronic obstructive lung disease
   d. Hypothyroidism

7. Side effects of niacin are all except:
   a. Myopathy
   b. Hepatic dysfunction
   c. Flushing
   d. Hyperglycemia

8. Most prominent Apo lipoprotein in HDL:
   a. Apo A1
   b. Apo B100
   c. Apo AIII
   d. Apo B 250

9. ↑mortality seen in:
   a. Gemfibrozil
   b. CETP inhibitors
   c. Rosuvastatin

10. Action of HDL include all except:
    a. Apoptotic
    b. Anti-inflammatory
    c. Antioxidant
    d. Endothelial repair

11. Niacin induced flushing treatment of choice:
    a. Aspirin
    b. Paracetamol
    c. Steroids
    d. Cetirizine

12. Apo A1 present in:
    a. HDL
    b. Lp(a)
    c. LDL
    d. VLDL

13. An HIV patient is on protease inhibitor therapy, his lipid profile shows TG of 1500 mg/dL and LDL-C of 400 mg%. Best drug for him is:
    a. Gemfibrozil
    b. Statins
    c. Cholesterol absorption inhibitors
    d. Omega-3 fatty acids

14. Which of the following statements is true?
    a. Familial hypertriglyceridemia is associated with isolated increase in TG level and normal LDL
    b. ApoB-100 is the structural protein of HDL
    c. Familial dysbetalipoproteinemia is caused by defect in gene for hepatic lipase
    d. ApoB-48 is the structural protein of LDL

15. All of the following drugs reduce LDL cholesterol by increasing LDL receptor activity except:
    a. Ezetimibe
    b. Simvastatin
    c. Bile acid binding drugs
    d. Niacin

ANSWERS

1. **Ans. (d) Omega-6 FA are used in Rx**
   [Williams 13th ed pg 1686, 1687, 1695]
   Omega-3 fatty acids (EPA and DHA) decrease triglyceride secretion from the liver, and lower triglycerides by 20-50%.

2. **Ans. (d) Niacin**
   [Williams 13th ed pg 1690, 1691]
   Drugs that interfere with bile acid absorption from the gut (Bile acid sequestrants, e.g. Cholestyramine, Colestipol, Colesevelam), inhibit cholesterol synthesis in cells (HMG-CoA reductase inhibitors, e.g. Lovastatin, Pravastatin, Simvastatin, Fluvastatin, Atorvastatin, Rosuvastatin, Pitavastatin), or block cholesterol absorption from the gut (Intestinal cholesterol absorption inhibitor, e.g. ezetimibe) work mainly by inducing LDL-receptor expression in hepatocytes.

3. **Ans. (d) Progesterone**
   [Harrison's Endocrinology 3rd ed pg 327, 339]

   Causes of Altered LDL- and HDL-C

LDL	Elevated	Hypothyroidism, nephrotic syndrome, cholestasis, acute intermittent porphyria, anorexia nervosa, hepatoma, drugs (e.g. thiazides, cyclosporine, carbamazepine)
	Reduced	Severe liver disease, malabsorption, malnutrition, Gaucher's disease, chronic infectious disease, hyperthyroidism, drug (e.g. niacin toxicity)
HDL	Elevated	Alcohol, exercise, exposure to chlorinated hydrocarbons, drug (e.g. estrogen)
	Reduced	Smoking, type 2 DM, obesity, malnutrition, Gaucher's disease, drugs (e.g. anabolic steroids, beta blockers)

   - Progestins generally have androgen like effects on lipid and lipoproteins and therefore progestin administration decreases HDL cholesterol and triglyceride levels but has little or no effect on LDL cholesterol levels. There is a considerable variation among progestins in influencing lipid and lipoprotein metabolism depending on their androgenic potency.
   - *Measures useful in patients with low HDL-C:*
     - Removal of secondary cause
     - Discontinuation of smoking
     - Weight loss (in obese persons)
     - Exercise
     - Optimal control of diabetes

- Niacin is the most effective HDL-C–raising therapeutic agent (up to ~30%)
- Fibrates have only a modest effect on plasma HDL-C levels (~5–15%), except in patients with coexisting hypertriglyceridemia, where the effect on HDL levels can be greater.
- Statins increase plasma levels of HDL-C only modestly (~5–10%).

4. Ans. (a) ↓ TBG

[De Groot LJ, Chrousos G, Dungan K, et al., editors. South Dartmouth (MA): MDText.com, Inc.; 2000-.; Greenspan's 9th ed; Endocrine Secrets 6th ed pg 337]

Effect of Oral Estrogen Treatment on Lipid and Lipoproteins

Lipids/lipoproteins	Estrogen treatment
LDL-C	Decrease
HDL-C	Increase
Triglycerides	Increase
Lp(a)	Decrease

Mechanisms of Estrogen Induced Lipid and Lipoprotein Changes

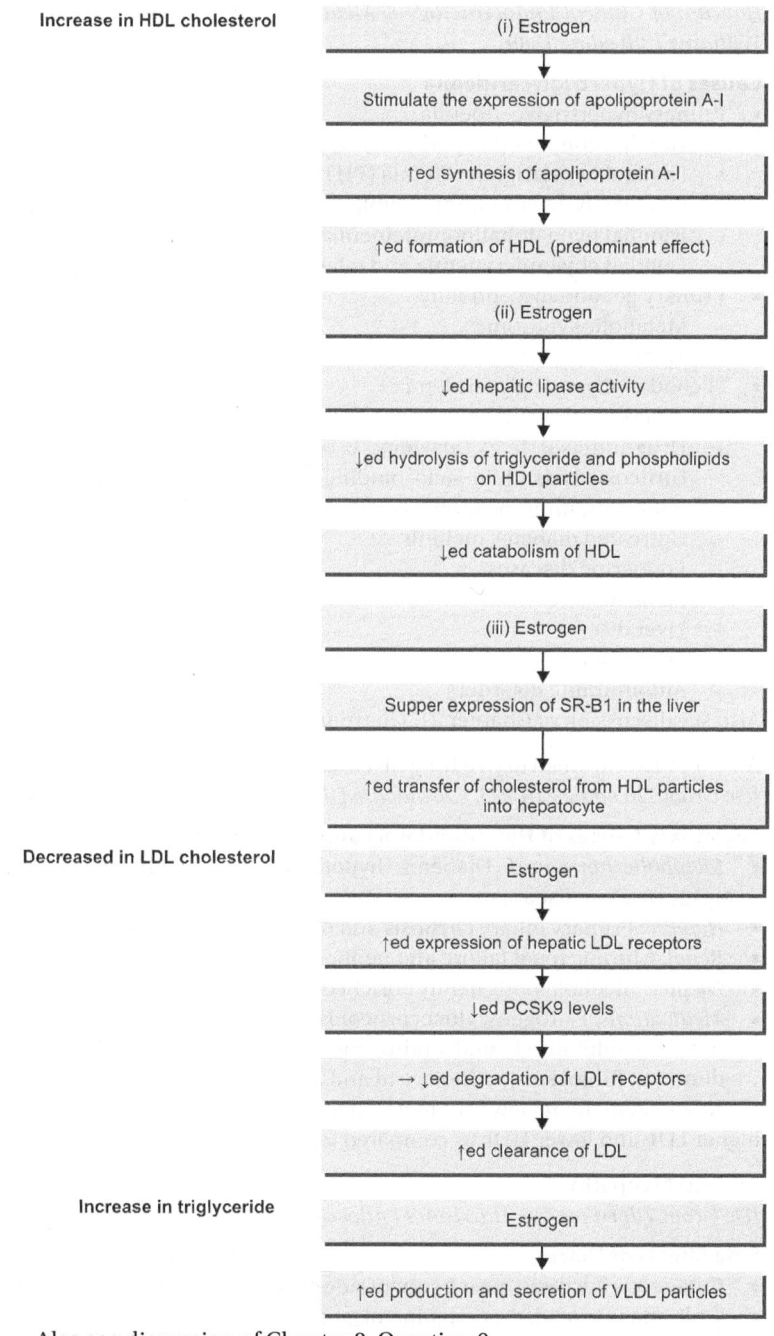

Also see discussion of Chapter 8, Question 9.

5. **Ans. (c) AIP**
   [Journal of Clinical Endocrinology & Metabolism, September 2012;97:2972; Williams 13th ed pg 1389]

   Causes of Hypertriglyceridemia
   - Primary hypertriglyceridemia
     - Familial combined hyperlipidemia (FCHL)
     - Familial hypertriglyceridemia (FHTG)
     - Familial dysbetalipoproteinemia
     - Familial hypoalphalipoproteinemia (FHA)
     - Familial chylomicronemia and related disorders
   - Primary genetic susceptibility
     - Metabolic syndrome
     - Treated type 2 diabetes
   - Secondary hypertriglyceridemia
     - Excess alcohol intake
     - Drug-induced (e.g. thiazides, b-blockers, estrogens, isotretinoin, corticosteroids, bile acid-binding resins, antiretroviral protease inhibitors, immunosuppressants, antipsychotics)
     - Untreated diabetes mellitus
     - Endocrine diseases
     - Renal disease
     - Liver disease
     - Pregnancy
     - Autoimmune disorders

   Also see discussion of Chapter 21, Question 52.

6. **Ans. (c) Chronic obstructive lung disease**
   [De Groot 7th ed pg 719,723; Cardiovasc Diabetol. 2016 Nov 24;15(1):158]

   Secondary Causes of Hyperlipidemia and Dyslipidemias
   - *Metabolic/hormonal:* Diabetes, hypothyroidism, lipodystrophy, polycystic ovarian disease
   - *Hepatic:* Primary biliary cirrhosis and other forms of cirrhosis
   - *Renal:* Chronic renal failure and nephrotic syndrome
   - *Dietary:* Alcohol, foods highly enriched in cholesterol and saturated fat
   - *Medications:* Estrogens, glucocorticoids, anti-HIV treatments (especially protease inhibitors), oral androgens and anabolic steroids, thiazide diuretics, β-blockers, retinoic acid and antipsychotics

   In a systematic review and meta-analysis, smokers were found to have higher LDL and lower HDL as compared to non smokers.

7. **Ans. (a) Myopathy**
   [De Groot 7th ed pg 735; Harrison's Endocrinology 3rd ed pg 338]

   Side Effects of Niacin
   - Cutaneous flushing (most frequent side effect), postural lightheadedness
   - ↑ plasma uric acid, exacerbation of gout
   - Exacerbation of diabetes (impact is modest with less than 0.3 unit rise in glycated hemoglobin)

Disorders of Lipid Metabolism

- Elevation of liver enzymes (up to 15% of patients)
- Rashes
- Nausea, vomiting, exacerbation of symptoms of esophageal reflux
- Acanthosis nigricans (infrequent)
- Maculopathy (infrequent)

8. **Ans. (a) Apo A1**
   [Harrison's Endocrinology 3rd ed pg 318]

   Major Apoliprotein in Various Lipoprotein Classes
   - *Chylomicrons, chylomicron remnants:* Apo B 48
   - *VLDL, IDL, LDL, Lp(a):* Apo B 100
   - *HDL:* Apo A I

9. **Ans. (b) CETP inhibitors**
   [De Groot 7th ed pg 734, 735]

10. **Ans. (a) Apoptotic**
    [De Groot 7th ed pg 719; High Density Lipoproteins- From Biological Understanding to Clinical Exploitation pg 210, 348, 351, 373, 374]

    HDL has anti apoptotic activity

11. **Ans. (a) Aspirin**
    [Williams 13th ed pg 1693]

12. **Ans. (a) HDL**
    [Williams 13th ed pg 1668]

    Major Apolipoproteins

Apolipoprotein	Synthesis	Functions
Apo A I	Liver, intestine	Structural protein (HDL) Cofactor for LCAT Crucial role in reverse cholesterol transport Ligand for ABC-A1 and SR-BI
Apo A II	Liver	Inhibits apoE binding to receptors Activates hepatic lipase Inhibits LCAT
Apo B 48	Intestine	Structural protein (chylomicrons)
Apo B 100	Liver	Structural protein (VLDL and LDL) Ligand for LDL receptor
Apo C I	Liver	Modulates remnant binding to receptors Activates LCAT
Apo C II	Liver	Cofactor for LPL
Apo C III	Liver	Modulates remnant binding to receptors Inhibitor of LPL
Apo E	Liver, brain, skin, testes, spleen	Ligand for LDL and remnant receptors Local lipid redistribution Reverse cholesterol transport (HDL with Apo E)

13. **Ans. (b) Statins**
    [Williams 13th ed pg 1689, 1690, 1692, 1793]

14. **Ans. (a) Familial hypertriglyceridemia is associated with isolated increase in TG level and normal LDL**
    [Harrison's Endocrinology 3rd ed pg 326, 327; Williams 13th ed pg 1668]
    Also see discussion of Chapter 24, Question 12.

15. **Ans. (d) Niacin**
    [Williams 13th ed pg 1690, 1691]
    See discussion of Chapter 24, Question 2.

CHAPTER 25

Statistics

QUESTIONS

1. Coefficient of variation:
   a. (Standard deviation/mean) × 100
   b. (Mean/standard deviation) × 100
   c. Square of standard deviation
   d. Square root of standard deviation

2. Not true:
   a. In normal distribution mean, median and mode do not coincide
   b. Mode is most commonly occurring value
   c. Median has equal no. of values above and below
   d. ± 2 SD covers 95% of values

3. Nonparametric test include all except:
   a. Kaplan-Meier curve
   b. McNemar test
   c. Chi-square
   d. Independent samples t-test
   e. None of the above

4. Bayes' theorem predicts:
   a. Pre-test predictive value
   b. Post-test probability
   c. Likelihood ratio
   d. Number needed to treat (NNT)

5. Type 2 error in biostatistics means:
   a. Accepting null hypothesis when it is false
   b. Rejecting null hypothesis when it is true
   c. Also known as alpha error
   d. Enumerating error in predicting outcome of a randomized control trial

ANSWERS

1. **Ans. (a) (Standard deviation/mean) × 100**
   [Statistics at Square One 11th ed pg 21]
   The *coefficient of variation* (CV%) is the intrasubject standard deviation divided by the mean, expressed as a percentage. It is a measure of repeatability for biochemical assays, when an assay is carried out on several occasions on the same sample.

2. **Ans. (a) In normal distribution mean, median and mode do not coincide**
   [Statistics at Square One 11th ed pg 4,13,14,15,21,174; Basics of Biostatistics: A Manual for Medical Practitioners pg 165]
   - Central tendency (also known as statistical average) is given by mean, median and mode
     - Median:
       + The median (or midpoint) is the point which has the property that half the data are greater than it, and half the data are less than it.
       + It is the middle value in a set of data.
       + If n is odd, the median is the $(n+1)/2$th largest observation.
       + If n is even, to find the median average the $(n/2)$th largest and the $(n/2+1)$th largest observations.
       + The main advantage of median is that it is "robust" to outliers.
       + It is most often used when describing skewed data.
     - Mean:
       + An average value that is computed by adding together all of the values and dividing by the number of values.

       $$\bar{x} = \frac{\sum x}{n}$$

       $\bar{x}$ signifies the mean; x is each of the values; n is the number of these values; and Σ denotes "sum of".
       + A major disadvantage of the mean is that it is sensitive to outlying points.
     - Mode:
       + The most frequently occurring value.
       + It can be used for grouped continuous data, for count data and for categorical data.
   - Standard deviation
     - The standard deviation is a measure of spread or variability.
     - It is a summary measure of the differences of each observation from the mean of all the observations.

     $$SD = \sqrt{\frac{\sum(x-\bar{x})^2}{n-1}}$$

- In a normal distribution mean, median & mode coincide (mean = median = mode)
- If the observations follow a Normal distribution, a range covered by one standard deviation above the mean and one standard deviation below it ($x \pm 1$ SD) includes about 68% of the observations; a range of two standard deviations above and two below ($x \pm 2$ SD) about 95% of the observations; and of three standard deviations above and three below ($x \pm 3$ SD) about 99.7% of the observations.

3. **Ans. (d) Independent samples t-test**
   [Basics of Biostatistics: A Manual for Medical Practitioners pg 301-320; Clinical Prediction Models: A Practical Approach to Development, Validation, and Updating pg 79; Statistics in Plain English, Third Edition pg 161]

   Nonparametric tests can be applied in situations
   - When assumption of population being a normal distribution is not true or doubtful
   - When test is being done for randomness, ranks, association or independence

   The nonparametric tests assume that the variable and its probability density function are continuous and all sample observations are independent

   Examples of nonparametric tests
   - Run test- test for randomness in a series of observations
   - Signed-rank test- for testing specified mean or median of a population
   - Wilcoxon Signed Rank Test- for paired data
   - Kolmogorov-Smirnov test for one sample
   - Kolmogorov-Smirnov test- for comparing two populations
   - Mann-Whitney "U" test- for equality of two means
   - Wilcoxin-Wilcox test- for comparison of multiple treatment on a series
   - Kruskal–Wallis rank sum test (H-Test)
   - Kruskal–Wallis analysis of variance
   - Friedman test (two-way ANOVA)
   - Test of significance of Spearman's rank correlation
   - Test of significance of Kendall rank correlation
   - McNemar's test for paired samples
   - Cochran Q test
   - Kaplan-Meier Analysis test for survival outcome
   - Chi-square test

4. **Ans. (b) Post-test probability**
   [Statistics at Square One 11th ed pg 68, 106]

   If D represents data and H the null hypothesis, the P-value is P(D|H) (probability of the data given the hypothesis) and not P(H|D) (probability of the hypothesis given the data).

   To get from one to the other we need Bayes' theorem.

This states that P(H|D) is proportional to P(D|H) × P(H).

The term P(H) is the prior distribution and measures our prior beliefs about the distribution (based on earlier studies and clinical judgement).

Odds of disease after positive test is derived from Bayes' theorem as follows:

Odds of disease after positive test = odds of disease before test × likelihood ratio for a positive test [LR(+)]

Likelihood ratio for a positive test LR(+) is defined as:

$$LR(+) = \frac{\text{Probability of positive test given the disease}}{\text{Probability of postitive test without disease}}$$

$$= \frac{\text{Sensitivity}}{1-\text{specificity}}$$

5. **Ans. (a) Accepting null hypothesis when it is false**
   [Statistics at Square One 11th ed pg 179]
   - *Type I error (α):* Rejecting the null hypothesis when it is true (i.e. claiming to have found an effect that is not really there).
   - *Type II error (β):* Failing to reject the null hypothesis when it is false (i.e. not finding an effect even though it is there).